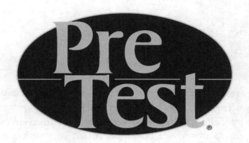

Medicine

PreTest® Self-Assessment and Review

Notice

Medicine is an ever-changing science. As new research and clinical experience broaden our knowledge, changes in treatment and drug therapy are required. The authors and the publisher of this work have checked with sources believed to be reliable in their efforts to provide information that is complete and generally in accord with the standards accepted at the time of publication. However, in view of the possibility of human error or changes in medical sciences, neither the authors nor the publisher nor any other party who has been involved in the preparation or publication of this work warrants that the information contained herein is in every respect accurate or complete, and they disclaim all responsibility for any errors or omissions or for the results obtained from use of the information contained in this work. Readers are encouraged to confirm the information contained herein with other sources. For example and in particular, readers are advised to check the product information sheet included in the package of each drug they plan to administer to be certain that the information contained in this work is accurate and that changes have not been made in the recommended dose or in the contraindications for administration. This recommendation is of particular importance in connection with new or infrequently used drugs.

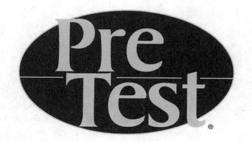

Medicine

PreTest® Self-Assessment and Review
14th Edition

Robert S. Urban, MD
Professor, Internal Medicine
Department of Internal Medicine
Texas Tech University Health Sciences Center
Amarillo, Texas

J. Rush Pierce Jr, MD, MPH
Professor, Internal Medicine
Vice-Chair for Faculty Development
Division of Hospital Medicine
University of New Mexico School of Medicine
Albuquerque, New Mexico

Roger D. Smalligan, MD, MPH
Professor and Regional Chair
Internal Medicine
Department of Internal Medicine
Texas Tech University Health Sciences Center
Amarillo, Texas

New York   Chicago   San Francisco   Athens   London   Madrid   Mexico City
Milan   New Delhi   Singapore   Sydney   Toronto

Medicine: PreTest® Self-Assessment and Review, 14th Edition

Copyright © 2016 by McGraw-Hill Education. All rights reserved. Printed in the United States of America. Except as permitted under the United States Copyright Act of 1976, no part of this publication may be reproduced or distributed in any form or by any means, or stored in a data base or retrieval system, without the prior written permission of the publisher.

Previous editions copyright © 2012, 2009, 2006, 2003, 2001, 1998, 1995, 1992, 1989, 1987, 1985, 1982, 1978 by The McGraw-Hill Companies, Inc.

PreTest® is a registered trademark of McGraw-Hill Education. All rights reserved.

2 3 4 5 6 7 8 9 10   LCR   21 20 19 18 17

ISBN 978-0-07-185005-6
MHID 0-07-185005-8

This book was set in Minion pro by Cenveo® Publisher Services.
The editors were Catherine A. Johnson and Cindy Yoo.
The production supervisor was Richard Ruzycka
Project management was provided by Sonam Arora, Cenveo Publisher Services.
RR Donnelley was printer and binder.

This book is printed on acid-free paper.

Library of Congress Cataloging-in-Publication Data

Medicine (Dwyer)
Medicine : pretest self-assessment and review / R. Steven Urban, J. Rush Pierce Jr.,
    Roger D. Smalligan.—14th edition.
        p. ; cm.
    Includes bibliographical references and index.
    ISBN 978-0-07-185005-6 (pbk. : alk. paper)—ISBN 0-07-185005-8
I. Urban, Robert S., editor.   II. Pierce, J. Rush, Jr., editor.   III. Smalligan,
Roger D., editor.
[DNLM: 1. Clinical Medicine—Examination Questions.   W 18.2]
R834.5
616.0076—dc23   2015010473

McGraw-Hill Education books are available at special quantity discounts to use as premiums and sales promotions or for use in corporate training programs. To contact a representative, please visit the Contact Us pages at www.mhprofessional.com.

Contributors

Mashrafi Ahmed, MD
Assistant Professor, Internal Medicine
Texas Tech University Health Sciences
  Center
Amarillo, Texas
Hematology/Oncology

Ravindra M. Bharadwaj, MD, MPH
Associate Professor, Internal Medicine
Geriatrics Clerkship Director
Texas Tech University Health Sciences
  Center
Amarillo, Texas
Geriatrics

ASM Islam, MD
Assistant Professor, Internal Medicine
Texas Tech University Health Sciences
  Center
Amarillo, Texas
Hospital Medicine

Faisal A. Khasawneh, MD
Associate Professor, Infectious Diseases and
  Critical Care
Department of Internal Medicine
Texas Tech University Health Sciences
  Center
Amarillo, Texas
Infectious Disease

J. Rush Pierce Jr, MD, MPH
Professor, Internal Medicine
Vice-chair for Faculty Development
Division of Hospital Medicine
University of New Mexico School of
  Medicine
Albuquerque, New Mexico
Gastroenterology
General Medicine and Prevention
Pulmonology

Roger D. Smalligan, MD, MPH
Professor and Regional Chair
Internal Medicine
Department of Internal Medicine
Texas Tech University Health Sciences
  Center
Amarillo, Texas
Endocrinology and Metabolic Disease
Nephrology
Rheumatology

Robert S. Urban, MD
Professor, Internal Medicine
Department of Internal Medicine
Texas Tech University Health Sciences
  Center
Amarillo, Texas
Allergy and Immunology
Cardiology
Dermatology
Neurology
Women's Health

Student Reviewer

Nina Hooshvar, MD
Class of 2015
Tulane University School of Medicine

Contents

Introduction

Medicine: PreTest® Self-Assessment and Review, 14th Edition, is intended to provide medical students, as well as house officers and physicians, with a convenient tool for assessing and improving their knowledge of medicine.

The 500 questions in this book are similar in format and complexity to those included in Step 2 CK of the United States Medical Licensing Examination (USMLE). They may also be a useful study tool for Step 3 and for the National Board of Medical Examiners (NBME) medical student exam for the internal medicine clerkship.

For multiple-choice questions, the **one best** response to each question should be selected. For matching sets, a group of questions will be preceded by a list of lettered options. For each question in the matching set, select **one** lettered option that is **most** closely associated with the question.

Each question in this book has a corresponding answer and a short discussion of various issues raised by the question and its answer. A listing of references for the entire book follows the last chapter.

To simulate the time constraints imposed by the qualifying examinations for which this book is intended as a practice guide, the student or physician should allot about one minute for each question. After answering all questions in a chapter, as much time as necessary should be spent in reviewing the explanations for each question at the end of the chapter.

Attention should be given to all explanations, even if the examinee answered the question correctly. Those seeking more information on a subject should refer to the reference materials listed or to other standard texts in medicine.

Acknowledgments

We would like to offer special thanks to:

Joan Urban, David Urban, Elizabeth Urban, and Catherine Urban.

Diane Goodwin, Read Pierce, Rebecca Pierce Martin, Cason Pierce, and Susanna Pierce.

Annye Smalligan, Dean Smalligan, Abby Smalligan, Tate Smalligan, and Jack Smalligan.

To the medical students, residents, faculty, and staff of Texas Tech University School of Medicine—in pursuit of excellence.

Infectious Disease

Questions

1. A 30-year-old man complains of fever and sore throat for several days. The patient presents to you today with additional complaints of hoarseness, difficulty breathing, and drooling. On examination, the patient is febrile and has inspiratory stridor. Which of the following is the best course of action?

a. Begin outpatient treatment with ampicillin.
b. Culture throat for beta-hemolytic streptococci.
c. Admit to intensive care unit and obtain otolaryngology consultation.
d. Obtain chest x-ray.
e. Obtain Epstein-Barr serology.

2. A 70-year-old patient with long-standing type 2 diabetes mellitus presents with complaints of pain in the left ear with purulent drainage. On physical examination, the patient is afebrile. The pinna of the left ear is tender, and the external auditory canal is swollen and edematous. The white blood cell count is normal. Which of the following organisms is most likely to grow from the purulent drainage?

a. *Pseudomonas aeruginosa*
b. *Streptococcus pneumoniae*
c. *Candida albicans*
d. *Haemophilus influenzae*
e. *Moraxella catarrhalis*

3. A 25-year-old male student presents with the chief complaint of rash. He denies headache, fever, or myalgia. A slightly pruritic maculopapular rash is noted over the abdomen, trunk, palms of the hands, and soles of the feet. Inguinal, occipital, and cervical lymphadenopathy is also noted. Hypertrophic, flat, wart-like lesions are noted around the anal area. Laboratory studies show the following:

Hct: 40%
Hgb: 14 g/dL
WBC: 13,000/μL
Diff: 50% segmented neutrophils, 50% lymphocytes
Which of the following is the most useful laboratory test in this patient?

a. Human papillomavirus (HPV) serology
b. Rapid Plasma Reagin (RPR) test
c. Nucleic acid amplification test for *Chlamydia*
d. Blood cultures
e. Biopsy of perianal lesions

4. A 35-year-old previously healthy man develops cough with purulent sputum over several days. On presentation to the emergency room, he is lethargic. Temperature is 39°C (102°F), pulse is 110, and blood pressure is 100/70 mm Hg. He has rales and dullness to percussion at the left base. There is no rash. Flexion of the patient's neck when supine results in spontaneous flexion of hip and knee. Neurologic examination is nonfocal. There is no papilledema. A lumbar puncture is performed in the emergency room. The cerebrospinal fluid (CSF) shows 8000 leukocytes/μL, 90% of which are polymorphonuclear cells. Glucose is 30 mg/dL with a peripheral glucose of 80 mg/dL. CSF protein is elevated to 200 mg/dL. CSF Gram stain is pending. Which of the following is the correct treatment option?

a. Begin acyclovir for herpes simplex encephalitis.
b. Obtain emergency magnetic resonance imaging (MRI) scan before beginning treatment.
c. Begin dexamethasone, followed by ceftriaxone and vancomycin, for pneumococcal meningitis.
d. Begin ceftriaxone, vancomycin, and ampicillin to cover both pneumococci and *Listeria*.
e. Begin high-dose penicillin for meningococcal meningitis.

5. A 56-year-old woman presents with a 3-day history of fever, headache, fatigue, and myalgia, along with nausea and vomiting. She reports cough with minimal hemoptysis but denies abdominal pain and dysuria. About a week ago, she came back from a month-long missionary trip to a small village in Liberia. She had received appropriate pre-travel vaccines including the yellow fever vaccine. She was also compliant with her malaria prophylaxis as prescribed. On examination, she is tachypneic, tachycardic, and in mild respiratory distress. She has generalized petechiae but no other rashes or lymphadenopathy. What is the most likely infectious pathogen?

a. *Plasmodium malariae*
b. *Salmonella typhi*
c. Influenza virus
d. Ebola virus
e. *Mycobacterium tuberculosis*

6. A 79-year-old nursing home patient presents with fever, confusion, productive cough, and shortness of breath. He has diabetes, hypertension, and dementia. He takes insulin, metoprolol, and aspirin. He is allergic to eggs, sulfa, and angiotensin-converting enzyme inhibitors. He is diagnosed with a left lower lobe health care–associated pneumonia. On admission, he is given linezolid, meropenem, and levofloxacin. His condition improves markedly, and on the fifth hospital day he is ready to be discharged back to his nursing home. His sputum and blood cultures grow *Klebsiella pneumoniae*. It is resistant to ampicillin and cefazolin but susceptible to ceftriaxone, piperacillin/tazobactam, meropenem, ciprofloxacin, and trimethoprim/sulfamethoxazole. Which of the following statements regarding discharge antibiotics is correct?

a. Discharge the patient on the same intravenous antibiotics since his condition improved on them.
b. Discharge the patient on oral trimethoprim/sulfamethoxazole.
c. Discharge the patient on oral amoxicillin.
d. Discharge the patient on oral ciprofloxacin.
e. Discharge the patient on intravenous piperacillin/tazobactam.

7. A 19-year-old male patient presents with a 1-week history of malaise and anorexia followed by fever and sore throat. On physical examination, the throat is inflamed without exudate. There are a few palatal petechiae. Cervical adenopathy is present. The liver span is 12 cm and the spleen is palpable.

> Throat culture: negative for group A streptococci
> Hgb: 12.5 g/dL, Hct: 38%
> Reticulocytes: 4%
> WBC: 14,000/μL
> Segmented neutrophils: 30%
> Lymphocytes: 60%
> Monocytes: 10%
> Total bilirubin: 2.0 mg/dL (normal 0.2-1.2)
> Lactate dehydrogenase (LDH) serum: 260 IU/L (normal 20-220)
> Aspartate aminotransferase (AST): 60 U/L (normal 8-40 U/L)
> Alanine aminotransferase (ALT): 55 U/L (normal 8-40 U/L)
> Alkaline phosphatase: 40 IU/L (normal 35-125)

Which of the following is the most important initial test combination to order?

a. Liver biopsy and hepatitis antibody
b. Streptococcal screen and antistreptolysin O (ASO) titer
c. Peripheral blood smear and heterophile antibody
d. Toxoplasma IgG and stool sample
e. Lymph node biopsy and cytomegalovirus serology

8. A 30-year-old man presents with right upper quadrant (RUQ) pain. He has been well except for an episode of diarrhea that occurred 4 months ago, just after he returned from a missionary trip to Mexico. He has lost 7 lb. He is not having diarrhea. His blood pressure is 140/70, pulse 80, and temperature 37.5°C (99.5°F). On physical examination there is RUQ tenderness without rebound. There is some radiation of the pain to the shoulder. The liver is percussed at 14 cm. There is no lower quadrant tenderness. Bowel sounds are normal and active. Which of the following is the most appropriate next step in evaluation of the patient?

a. Serology and RUQ ultrasound
b. Stool for ova and parasite
c. Blood cultures
d. Diagnostic aspirate
e. Empiric broad-spectrum antibiotic therapy

9. An 80-year-old female patient complains of a 3-day history of a painful rash extending over the right half of her forehead and down to her right eyelid. There are weeping vesicular lesions on physical examination. Which of the following is the most likely diagnosis?

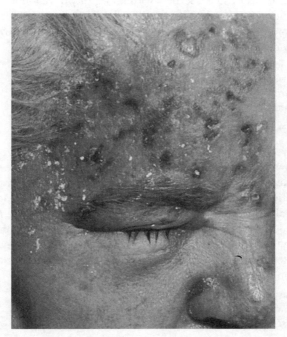

Reproduced, with permission, from Wolff K, et al. *Fitzpatrick's Color Atlas & Synopsis of Clinical Dermatology*. 6th ed. New York, NY: McGraw-Hill Education, 2009.

a. Impetigo
b. Adult chickenpox
c. Herpes zoster
d. Coxsackie A virus
e. Herpes simplex virus

10. A 58-year-old woman presents to her internist with a 2-day history of low-grade fever and RUQ abdominal pain. She reports nausea but denies vomiting or diarrhea. On physical examination, she is pale and jaundiced. Her temperature is 38.3°C (100.9°F). She has reduced air entry at the right lung base and has RUQ tenderness without rigidity or rebound tenderness. Bowel sounds are normal. Her white blood cell count is 16,000/μL and urinalysis shows no red or white blood cells. Which of the following is the most likely diagnosis?

a. Right-sided pyelonephritis
b. Right lower lobe pneumonia
c. High retrocecal appendicitis
d. Cholangitis
e. Gastritis

11. A 35-year-old man complains of inability to close his right eye. Examination shows facial nerve weakness of the right side of the face; both forehead and lower face are involved. There are no other cranial nerve abnormalities, and the rest of the neurological examination is normal. The patient is afebrile. Examinations of the heart, chest, abdomen, and skin show no additional abnormalities. There is no lymphadenopathy. About 1 month ago the patient was seen by a dermatologist for a bull's-eye skin rash 2 weeks after returning from a camping trip in upstate New York. Which of the following is the most likely diagnosis?

a. Sarcoidosis
b. Idiopathic Bell palsy
c. Lyme disease
d. Syphilis
e. Lacunar infarct

12. A 67-year-old man presents to the emergency department in mid-August with fever, headache, and right arm and leg weakness. His symptoms progressed over the preceding 2 days. He has diabetes mellitus controlled with oral hypoglycemic agents. He is retired, denies recent travel, and spends most of his afternoons gardening. On physical examination he appears healthy but confused. He has neck rigidity and 4 out of 5 strength in his right arm and leg. Cranial nerve examination is within normal limits. CT head is negative. Lumbar puncture reveals a white blood cell count of 158 with predominance of lymphocytes and 21 red blood cells. Cerebrospinal fluid (CSF) glucose level is normal, while CSF protein level is mildly elevated. Which of the following is the most likely diagnosis?

a. Embolic stroke
b. West Nile virus (WNV) encephalitis
c. Subarachnoid hemorrhage
d. Bacterial meningitis
e. Tuberculous meningitis

13. A 59-year-old man undergoes coronary bypass surgery. He receives vancomycin prophylactically for 24 hours. On the ninth postoperative day, he develops a fever of 39.8°C (103°F) with a heart rate of 115 beats/min and a blood pressure of 105/65 mm Hg. The surgical site is healing well with no redness or discharge. His white blood cell count is 14,000/mm³ and urinalysis reveals many white blood cells per high-power field. Blood and urine cultures grow a non–lactose-fermenting oxidase-positive gram-negative rod. Which of the following antibiotics is most appropriate to treat this infection?

a. Moxifloxacin
b. Ceftriaxone
c. Imipenem
d. Trimethoprim-sulfamethoxazole
e. Tigecycline

14. You are a physician in charge of patients who reside in a nursing home. Several of the patients have developed influenza-like symptoms, and the community is in the midst of an influenza A outbreak. None of the nursing home residents have received the influenza vaccine. Which course of action is most appropriate?

a. Give the influenza vaccine to all residents who do not have a contraindication to the vaccine (ie, allergy to eggs).
b. Give the influenza vaccine to all residents who do not have a contraindication to the vaccine; also give oseltamivir for 2 weeks to all residents.
c. Give amantadine alone to all residents.
d. Give azithromycin to all residents to prevent influenza-associated pneumonia.
e. Do not give any prophylactic regimen, but treat with oseltamivir if a clinical outbreak should occur.

15. A 60-year-old male patient complains of low back pain, which has intensified over the past 3 weeks. He had experienced some fever at the onset of the pain. He was treated for acute pyelonephritis about 4 months ago. Physical examination shows tenderness over the L2-3 vertebra and paraspinal muscle spasm. Laboratory data show an erythrocyte sedimentation rate of 80 mm/h and elevated C-reactive protein. Which of the following statements is correct?

a. Hematogenous osteomyelitis rarely involves the vertebra in adults.
b. The most likely initial focus of infection was soft tissue.
c. Blood cultures will be positive in most patients with this process.
d. An MRI scan is both sensitive and specific in defining the process.
e. Surgery will be necessary if the patient has osteomyelitis.

16. A 39-year-old man with sickle cell anemia is admitted with cough, rusty-colored sputum, and shaking chills. Physical examination reveals rales and bronchial breath sounds in the left posterior chest. The patient's sputum grows penicillin-resistant *S pneumoniae*. Which of the following best describes the mechanism of penicillin resistance in this *S pneumoniae*?

a. Penicillinase production
b. Reduced cell wall permeability to penicillin
c. Altered penicillin binding protein
d. Penicillin efflux pump
e. Down regulation of cell wall porins

17. A family of four presents to the emergency room with sudden-onset abdominal cramps, nausea, and vomiting. None of them has fever or diarrhea. Four hours earlier, they had lunch at a roadside restaurant. They ate a variety of grilled meats, fried rice, and seasoned vegetables. What is the most likely mechanism of their symptoms?

a. Ingestion of preformed toxins.
b. Bacterial invasion of stomach and small intestine wall.
c. Proliferation of ingested bacteria with subsequent production of toxin active against small bowel mucosal cells.
d. Bacterial invasion of large intestine wall.
e. Secondary malabsorption caused by the pathogen's overgrowth in the proximal small intestine.

18. A 61-year-old woman presents to the hospital with perforated diverticulitis. She undergoes laparotomy and left-sided hemicolectomy. She is started on intravenous fluids and broad-spectrum antibiotics through a central venous catheter. Her sepsis resolves, but she continues to have ileus and subsequently is started on total parenteral nutrition. On the 10th postoperative day, she develops new fever. Physical examination does not reveal any obvious foci of infection. Blood white blood cell count is high with 6% bands but no eosinophils; her kidney and liver function tests are normal. Urine culture and blood cultures continue to be negative. Her chest x-ray is negative. CT abdomen and pelvis does not reveal any abscess or fluid collections. Despite multiple broad-spectrum antibiotics and changing her central venous catheter, she continues to be febrile with significant leukocytosis. Which of the following is the most likely cause of her fever of unknown origin?

a. Drug fever
b. Tumor fever
c. Central fever
d. Herpes simplex virus
e. Candidemia

19. An 18-year-old woman presents with a 2-day history of sore throat. Which of the following constellation of symptoms and signs is most consistent with group-A streptococcal pharyngitis?

a. Fever, anorexia, dysphagia, and hoarseness
b. Fever, runny nose, cough, myalgia, and poor appetite
c. Fever, no cough, tonsillar exudates, and tender anterior cervical lymphadenopathy
d. Fever, cough, pharyngeal erythema, and dysphagia
e. Fever, trismus, dysphagia, and neck swelling

20. A 78-year-old-woman presents to the emergency room in mid-December with 1-week history of shortness of breath and dry cough. She denies fever but reports chills. She denies chest pain or sick contacts. She is up to date on her vaccination including influenza and pneumococcal vaccines. She has diabetes and hypertension. Her medications, which she takes regularly, include insulin, lisinopril, metoprolol, hydrochlorothiazide, and aspirin. On examination, she has basal rales with no wheezing. Heart examination reveals regular heart sounds with no gallops. She has 1+ lower limb edema. Blood white blood cell count is 12,000/μL with no bands. Her kidney function tests and liver enzymes are within normal levels. Chest x-ray shows basal opacities bilaterally. Which of the following supports a diagnosis of pneumonia?

a. High B-natriuretic peptide level
b. High procalcitonin level
c. High D-dimer level
d. High troponin level
e. Low C-reactive protein

21. A 32-year-old male patient complains of fever and shortness of breath. There is no pleuritic chest pain or rigors and no sputum production. A chest x-ray shows diffuse perihilar infiltrates. The patient's condition worsens while on levofloxacin. A methenamine silver stain of bronchial washings shows cyst-like structures. Which of the following is correct?

a. Definitive diagnosis can be made by serology.
b. The organism will grow after 48 hours.
c. History will likely provide important clues to the diagnosis.
d. Cavitary disease is likely to develop.
e. The infection is unlikely to recur.

22. A 40-year-old woman cuts her finger while cooking in her kitchen. Two days later she becomes rapidly ill with fever and shaking chills. Her hand becomes painful and mildly erythematous. Later that evening her condition deteriorates as the erythema progresses and the hand becomes dusky red. Bullae and decreased sensation to touch develop over the involved hand. What is the most important next step in the management of this patient?

a. Surgical consultation and exploration of the wound
b. Treatment with clindamycin for mixed aerobic-anaerobic infection
c. Treatment with penicillin for clostridial infection
d. Vancomycin to cover community-acquired methicillin-resistant *Staphylococcus aureus* (CA-MRSA)
e. Evaluation for acute osteomyelitis

23. A 25-year-old man from East Tennessee has been ill for 5 days with fever, chills, and headache when he notes a rash that develops on his palms and soles. In addition to macular lesions, petechiae are noted on the wrists and ankles. The patient has recently returned from a summer camping trip. Which of the following is the most important aspect of the history?

a. Exposure to contaminated springwater
b. Exposure to raw pork
c. Exposure to ticks
d. Exposure to prostitutes
e. Exposure to mosquitos

24. A 49-year-old man has a history of athlete's foot but is otherwise healthy when he develops sudden onset of fever and pain in the right foot and leg. On physical examination, the foot and leg are fiery red with a well-defined indurated margin that appears to be rapidly advancing. There is tender inguinal lymphadenopathy. Which organism is the most likely cause of this infection?

a. *Staphylococcus epidermidis*
b. Tinea pedis
c. *Streptococcus pyogenes*
d. Mixed anaerobic infection
e. Alpha-hemolytic streptococci

25. An 18-year-old male patient has been seen in the clinic for urethral discharge. He is treated with IM ceftriaxone, but the discharge has not resolved and the culture has returned as no growth. Which of the following is the most likely etiologic agent to cause this infection?

a. Ceftriaxone-resistant gonococci
b. *Chlamydia psittaci*
c. *Chlamydia trachomatis*
d. Herpes simplex virus
e. *Chlamydia pneumoniae*

26. A 70-year-old nursing home resident is admitted to the hospital for pneumonia and treated for 10 days with levofloxacin. She improves but develops diarrhea 1 week after discharge, with low-grade fever, mild abdominal pain, and 2 to 3 watery, nonbloody stools per day. Polymerase chain reaction (PCR) for *Clostridium difficile* toxin in a stool sample is positive. The patient is treated with oral metronidazole, but does not improve after 10 days. Diarrhea has increased and fever and abdominal pain continue. What is the best next step in the management of this patient?

a. Obtain *C difficile* enzyme immunoassay.
b. Continue metronidazole for at least 2 more weeks.
c. Switch treatment to oral vancomycin.
d. Hospitalize patient for fulminant *C difficile*–associated disease.
e. Use fecal microbiota transplantation.

27. A college wrestler develops cellulitis after abrading his skin during a match. He is afebrile and appears well, but the lateral aspect of his arm is red and swollen with a draining pustule. Gram stain of the pus shows gram-positive cocci in clusters. Which of the following statements is correct?

a. The patient will require hospital admission and treatment with intravenous vancomycin.
b. The organism will almost always be sensitive to oxacillin.
c. The organism is likely to be sensitive to trimethoprim-sulfamethoxazole.
d. Community-acquired methicillin-resistant staphylococci have the same sensitivity pattern as hospital-acquired methicillin-resistant staphylococci.
e. The infection is likely caused by streptococci.

28. A 27-year-old man has fever, macular rash, and lymphadenopathy. He had unprotected sex with a male partner 2 weeks before the onset of these symptoms and has just learned that the partner is infected with human immunodeficiency virus (HIV). The patient's rapid HIV test is negative. What is the best test to evaluate this patient for HIV infection?

a. HIV enzyme-linked immunosorbent assay (ELISA)
b. PCR for HIV RNA
c. Western blot testing
d. Glycoprotein 120 ELISA testing
e. PCR for HIV DNA

29. A businessman traveling around the world asks about prevention of malaria. He will travel to India and the Middle East and plans to visit several small towns. What is the most appropriate advice for the traveler?

a. Common sense measures to avoid malaria such as use of insect repellants, bed nets, and suitable clothing have not really worked in preventing malaria.
b. The decision to use drugs effective against resistant-*P falciparum* malaria will depend on the knowledge of local patterns of resistance and the patient's very specific travel plans.
c. Prophylaxis should be started the day of travel.
d. Chemoprophylaxis has been proven to be entirely reliable.
e. He should stay inside at the noon as this is the mosquito's peak feeding time.

30. A 36-year-old man with history of acute myelogenous leukemia is admitted to the ICU with neutropenic fever and low blood pressure that requires norepinephrine drip. The patient finished his first cycle of chemotherapy 10 days ago. He denies respiratory, gastrointestinal, or urinary symptoms. CBC reveals mild thrombocytopenia and an absolute neutrophil count of 100/μL. Urinalysis is within normal limits and chest x-ray does not show any infiltrate. Awaiting culture results, which of the following antibiotic regimens is most appropriate?

a. Imipenem
b. Vancomycin
c. Vancomycin, piperacillin/tazobactam, and tobramycin
d. Cefepime, levofloxacin, and amphotericin B
e. Continue supportive measures awaiting culture results

31. A 62-year-old man presents to his new primary care physician for a first visit. The patient has not seen a doctor for more than 10 years. He has mild intermittent bronchial asthma. The patient is sexually active with a single long-term partner. He does not recall receiving any vaccines since childhood. Which of the following vaccines should be offered?

a. Pneumococcal, influenza, zoster, and tetanus-diphtheria-acellular pertussis (Tdap)
b. Pneumococcal, influenza, zoster, and tetanus-diphtheria (Td)
c. Pneumococcal, influenza, and HPV
d. Pneumococcal, influenza, and tetanus-diphtheria-acellular pertussis (Tdap)
e. Pneumococcal, influenza, and meningococcal

32. A 60-year-old woman is admitted to the hospital in septic shock secondary to a urinary tract infection (UTI). The patient is started on antibiotics awaiting culture results. She improves with complete resolution of her symptoms. The patient continues to have a urinary catheter in place. On the 10th hospital day, she is discharged to a rehabilitation facility. As a part of the routine admission orders, urinalysis and culture are ordered. The patient denies fever, abdominal pain, nausea, or vomiting. The urinalysis shows 5 to 10 white blood cells and a negative dipstick for nitrite and leukocyte esterase, but the culture grows more than 10^5 colonies of *Candida albicans*. Which of the following is the best course of action?

a. Start antifungal therapy with fluconazole
b. Continue broad-spectrum antibiotics
c. Remove the urinary catheter
d. Encourage water intake and continue to observe
e. Remove the urinary catheter and start liposomal amphotericin B

33. An 18-year-old high school student presents to the emergency room with a 1-day history of right knee pain, swelling, and redness. He is a quarterback on the school's football team. He remembers falling on the knee while practicing 2 days ago. The knee is tapped and 15 mL of cloudy fluid is sent for cell count, Gram stain, and culture. The Gram stain shows gram-positive cocci in clusters. Which of the following is the best course of action?

a. Start vancomycin and consult orthopedic surgery.
b. Consult orthopedic surgery.
c. Start linezolid awaiting culture results.
d. Start ceftriaxone.
e. Start telavancin and order MRI of the knee.

34. A 40-year-old man presents to the emergency room with a 1-week history of fever, rigors, and generalized weakness. The patient denies recent travel or sick contacts but admits to intravenous drug use. On examination, he has splinter and subconjunctival hemorrhages. Cardiac examination shows a holosystolic murmur over the left lower sternal boarder. There are no other localizing signs. Chest x-ray and urinalysis are negative. After obtaining blood cultures, the patient is started on intravenous antibiotics and admitted to the medical floor. Twenty-four hours later, all sets of blood cultures grow gram-positive cocci in clusters. A transthoracic echocardiogram is negative for vegetations. Which of the following is the best course of action?

a. Place a peripherally inserted central catheter (PICC) and start vancomycin.
b. Repeat blood cultures to confirm the positive cultures were not contaminants.
c. Order a transesophageal echocardiogram.
d. Continue vancomycin till the patient becomes afebrile, then discharge him on PO linezolid to finish a total of 2 weeks.
e. Order a three-phase bone scan.

35. A 20-year-old woman presents with a 2-day history of dysuria, lower abdominal pain, and low-grade fever. Her urine is cloudy with pyuria and abundant gram-positive bacteria. She is a college student who is sexually active with no previous history of sexually transmitted diseases. Which organism is most likely responsible for this woman's symptoms?

a. *Enterococcus faecalis*
b. *Escherichia coli*
c. *Neisseria gonorrhoeae*
d. *Staphylococcus saprophyticus*
e. *Candida albicans*

Questions 36 and 37

Select the fungal agent most likely responsible for the disease process described. Each lettered option may be used once, more than once, or not at all.

a. *Histoplasma capsulatum*
b. *Blastomyces dermatitidis*
c. *Coccidioides immitis*
d. *Cryptococcus neoformans*
e. *Candida albicans*
f. *Aspergillus fumigatus*
g. *Mucor* species

36. A 48-year-old painter presents with fever, cough, and shortness of breath. His symptoms develop 10 days after he remodeled a house in Indiana. Chest x-ray shows interstitial infiltrates and hilar lymphadenopathy.

37. A diabetic patient is admitted with elevated blood sugar and acidosis. The patient complains of headache and sinus tenderness and has black, necrotic material draining from the nares.

Questions 38 and 39

Match each clinical description with the appropriate infectious agent. Each lettered option may be used once, more than once, or not at all.

a. Herpes simplex virus
b. Epstein-Barr virus
c. Parvovirus B19
d. *Listeria monocytogenes*
e. *Acinetobacter baumannii*
f. *Enterococcus faecalis*

38. A 33-year-old elementary school teacher presents with fever, sore throat, and diffuse, lacy rash. She subsequently develops arthralgia of small joints of the hand.

39. A 30-year-old pregnant woman develops severe sepsis with headache and neck stiffness after eating coleslaw, soft cheese, and cantaloupes at a potluck dinner. Two other women who attended the event develop self-limiting abdominal cramps, nausea, and vomiting.

Questions 40 and 41

Match the clinical description with the most appropriate isolation precaution. Each lettered option may be used once, more than once, or not at all.

a. Standard precautions
b. Contact precautions
c. Droplet precautions
d. Airborne precautions

40. An 18-year-old college student presents with fever, headache, neck stiffness, and petechial rash on his ankles. Lumbar puncture shows abundance of white blood cells with extracellular as well as intracellular gram-negative diplococci.

41. A 60-year-old nursing home resident presents with a 3-day history of progressive shortness of breath and cough. The lung examination reveals right basilar crackles. The chest x-ray shows right lower lobe consolidation. Sputum culture grows methicillin-resistant *Staphylococcus aureus* (MRSA).

Questions 42 to 45

Match the clinical description with the most likely etiologic agent. Each lettered option may be used once, more than once, or not at all.

a. *Aspergillus flavus*
b. *Coccidioides immitis*
c. Herpes simplex virus type 1
d. Herpes simplex virus type 2
e. Hantavirus
f. Coxsackievirus B
g. Human parvovirus

42. A 50-year-old develops sudden onset of bizarre behavior. CSF shows 80 lymphocytes; MRI shows temporal lobe abnormalities.

43. A patient with a previous history of tuberculosis now complains of hemoptysis. Chest x-ray reveals an upper lobe mass with a cavity and a crescent-shaped air-fluid level.

44. A Filipino patient develops a pulmonary nodule after travel through Arizona and South California.

45. A 35-year-old male patient complains of fever, cough, and sore throat. Several days later, he develops retrosternal chest pain, with diffuse ST-segment elevations on ECG.

Infectious Disease

Answers

1. The answer is c. This patient, with the development of hoarseness, breathing difficulty, and stridor, is likely to have acute epiglottitis. Because of the possibility of impending airway obstruction, the patient should be admitted to an intensive care unit for close monitoring. The diagnosis can be confirmed by indirect laryngoscopy or soft tissue x-rays of the neck, which may show an enlarged epiglottis. Otolaryngology consult should be obtained. The most likely organism causing this infection is *H influenzae*. Many of these organisms are lactamase producing and would be resistant to ampicillin. A third-generation cephalosporin or beta-lactamase-resistant semisynthetic penicillin would be appropriate empiric choices for therapy. Streptococcal pharyngitis can cause severe pain on swallowing, but the infection does not descend to the hypopharynx and larynx. Lateral neck films would be more useful than a chest x-ray. Classic finding on lateral neck films would be the thumbprint sign. Infectious mononucleosis often causes exudative pharyngitis and cervical lymphadenopathy but not stridor.

2. The answer is a. Ear pain and drainage in an elderly diabetic patient must raise concern about malignant external otitis. The swelling and inflammation of the external auditory meatus strongly suggest this diagnosis. This infection usually occurs in older, poorly controlled diabetics and is almost always caused by *P aeruginosa*. It can invade contiguous structures including facial nerve or temporal bone and can even progress to meningitis. *Streptococcus pneumoniae, H influenzae,* and *M catarrhalis* frequently cause otitis media, but not external otitis. *Candida albicans* almost never affects the external ear.

3. The answer is b. Diffuse rash involving palms and soles should suggest the possibility of secondary syphilis. The hypertrophic, wart-like lesions around the anal area, called *condyloma lata,* are specific for secondary syphilis. The VDRL slide test will be positive in all patients with secondary syphilis. Rash and lymphadenopathy would not be found if the perianal lesions were due to HPV. *Chlamydia* infections cause urethritis with mucopurulent discharge from the penile meatus but not the rash or hypertrophic skin changes. Blood cultures might be drawn to rule out bacterial infection such as chronic meningococcemia; however, the clinical picture is not consistent with a systemic bacterial infection. Biopsy of the condyloma is not necessary in this setting, as regression of the lesion with treatment will distinguish it from genital wart (condyloma acuminatum) or squamous cell carcinoma. Penicillin continues to be the drug of choice for all stages of syphilis.

4. The answer is c. This previously healthy male has developed acute bacterial meningitis as evident by meningeal irritation with a positive Brudzinski sign, and a CSF profile typical for bacterial meningitis (elevated white blood cell count, high percentage of polymorphonuclear leukocytes, elevated protein, and low glucose). The patient likely has concomitant pneumonia. This combination suggests pneumococcal infection. Because of the potential for beta-lactam resistance, the recommendation for therapy prior to availability of susceptibility data is ceftriaxone and vancomycin. A short course of dexamethasone started before or with the first dose of antibiotics is recommended in suspected bacterial meningitis cases. Dexamethasone decreases adverse neurological sequelae of meningitis and has been associated with lower mortality. Though herpes simplex can be seen in young healthy patients, the clinical picture and CSF profile are not consistent with this infection. The CSF in herpes simplex encephalitis shows a lymphocytic predominance and normal glucose. *Listeria monocytogenes* meningitis is a concern in alcoholic, immunocompromised, or elderly patients. Gram stain would show gram-positive rods. *Neisseria meningitidis* is the second commonest cause of bacterial meningitis but rarely causes pneumonia (the portal of entry is the nasopharynx). Although penicillin G still kills the meningococcus, empiric therapy should cover all likely pathogens until Gram stain and culture results are available. Because the patient has no papilledema and no focal neurologic findings, treatment should not be delayed to obtain CT or MRI scan.

5. The answer is d. The patient has a flu-like illness with hemorrhagic tendency as manifested by hemoptysis and petechiae. A hemorrhagic fever, which is worrisome for Ebola virus in this case, is the most likely diagnosis given her signs, symptoms, and recent travel to an area of Africa known to have Ebola virus present. Other hemorrhagic fever syndromes include yellow fever, dengue fever, Lassa fever, Marburg, and hantavirus. The pathogenesis of this illness involves vascular bed infection leading to microvascular damage and changes in vascular permeability with subsequent organ dysfunction. The patient should be admitted under strict airborne and contact precautions and supportive measures provided for any ensuing organ failure. There is no known effective antiviral therapy for Ebola virus, and vaccine development is in progress at the time of this writing. Furthermore, this symptomatic patient's close contacts should be identified and observed closely for 21 days since last exposure to the index patient's body fluids.

Malaria, caused by *Plasmodium* species, could present in a similar fashion but taking her malaria prophylaxis makes the diagnosis less likely. *S typhi* and *S paratyphi,* are the most common causes of typhoid fever in the returning traveler but the petechiae, hemoptysis, and lack of abdominal pain make this diagnosis unlikely. Influenza is endemic in the tropics year round, but hemorrhagic tendencies are uncommon with this viral infection. Tuberculosis has a subacute presentation and would be unlikely to present as an acute hemorrhagic fever.

6. The answer is d. The patient has health care–associated pneumonia. He was started on broad-spectrum antibiotics to cover likely pathogens, which include MRSA and resistant gram-negative bacteria such as *P aeruginosa*. His condition improved markedly and the culprit bacterium in his case was not as resistant as feared. Furthermore, his pneumonia was not complicated by cavitation or empyema, and he did not have vomiting or diarrhea to preclude finishing his antibiotic course orally. This case represents an opportunity for antibiotic de-escalation, which involves the practice of starting with a broad-spectrum empiric antibiotic regimen (designed to avoid inadequate therapy) combined with a commitment to change from broad to narrow-spectrum therapy and from multiple agents to fewer medications. Continuing all of the empirically chosen antibiotics puts this patient at risk for drug-drug interaction and *C difficile* infection and is not justifiable given the susceptible culprit isolated. De-escalation is an example of antimicrobial stewardship, a coordinated effort that aims at optimizing clinical outcomes while minimizing antibiotic toxicity, cost, and resistant bacteria selection. Discharging the patient on meropenem or piperacillin/tazobactam would have been an appropriate choice had this been a mixed infection (aspiration pneumonia, for example). Trimethoprim/sulfamethoxazole is an inappropriate choice given the reported sulfa allergy. This patient's *Klebsiella* is resistant to ampicillin and cefazolin.

7. The answer is c. This young man presents with classic signs and symptoms of infectious mononucleosis. In a young patient with fever, pharyngitis, lymphadenopathy, and lymphocytosis, the peripheral blood smear should be evaluated for atypical lymphocytes. A heterophile antibody test should be performed. The symptoms described in association with atypical lymphocytes and a positive heterophile test are virtually always caused by Epstein-Barr virus. Neither liver biopsy nor lymph node biopsy is necessary. Workup for toxoplasmosis, cytomegalovirus infection, or HIV infection would be considered in heterophile-negative patients. Antistreptolysin O titer is used to diagnose acute rheumatic fever (ARF) but ARF causes joint and cardiac manifestations, not lymphadenopathy and hepatitis as in this case.

8. The answer is a. The history and physical examination suggest amebic liver abscess. Symptoms usually occur 2 to 5 months after travel to an endemic area. Diarrhea usually occurs first but resolves before the hepatic symptoms develop. The most common presentation for an amebic liver abscess is abdominal pain, usually in the RUQ. Amebic serology using enzyme immunoassay (EIA) is a sensitive test and is positive in more than 90% of patients. Ultrasound has 75% to 85% sensitivity and shows abscess with well-defined margins. Stool will not show the trophozoite at this stage of the disease process. Blood cultures and broad-spectrum antibiotics would be ordered in cases of pyogenic liver abscess, but this patient's travel history, the chronicity of his illness, and his lack of clinical toxicity suggest *Entamoeba histolytica* as the probable cause. Aspiration is not necessary unless rupture of abscess is imminent. Metronidazole remains the drug of choice for amebic liver abscess.

9. The answer is c. A painful vesicular rash in a dermatomal distribution strongly suggests herpes zoster, although other viral pathogens may also cause vesicles. Herpes zoster may involve the eyelid when the first or second branch of the fifth cranial nerve is affected. Prompt treatment with an antiviral such as acyclovir, valacyclovir, or famciclovir shortens symptomatic illness and decreases the chance of post-zoster neuralgia. Impetigo is a cellulitis caused by group A-hemolytic streptococci. It often involves the face and can occur after an abrasion of the skin. Its distribution is not dermatomal, and it rarely causes severe pain. Chickenpox produces vesicles in various stages of development that are diffuse and produce more pruritus than pain. Coxsackievirus can produce a morbilliform vesiculopustular rash, often with a hemorrhagic component and with lesions of the throat, palms, and soles. Herpes simplex virus (HSV) causes lesions of the lip (herpes labialis) but does not spread in a dermatomal pattern.

10. The answer is d. All of the given diagnoses can cause epigastric or RUQ abdominal pain, but jaundice makes cholangitis the most likely diagnosis. Fever, RUQ abdominal pain, and jaundice are called Charcot triad and are highly suggestive of cholangitis. The bacteria implicated in this infection include gut flora including Enterobacteriaceae and anaerobes. The negative urinalysis argues against UTI, and the presence of leukocytosis and fever would be unusual in uncomplicated gastritis. Upper abdominal pathologies are often associated with basal atelectasis and sometimes sympathetic effusion, accounting for the diminished breath sounds in this case. Right lower lobe pneumonia can cause abdominal pain, but you would expect cough with sputum production and signs of consolidation on physical examination. Alongside broad-spectrum antibiotics, this patient needs abdominal ultrasound to evaluate the biliary tree; she might need endoscopic retrograde cholangiopancreatography (ERCP) or surgery to relieve any biliary obstruction.

11. The answer is c. This patient's symptoms and time course are consistent with stage 2 Lyme disease. A few weeks after a camping trip and presumptive exposure to the *Ixodes* tick, the patient developed a rash consistent with erythema migrans (stage 1). Secondary neurologic, cardiac, or arthritic symptoms occur weeks to months after the rash. Facial nerve palsy is one of the more common signs of stage 2 Lyme disease; it may be unilateral (as in this case) or bilateral. Stage 3 Lyme disease occurs months to years later and is characterized by recurrent and sometimes destructive oligoarticular arthritis. Sarcoidosis can cause facial palsy, but there are no other signs or symptoms (such as lymphadenopathy) to suggest this disease. Idiopathic Bell palsy would not account for the previous rash or the exposure history. Syphilis always needs to be considered in the same differential with Lyme disease, but the rash described would be atypical, and the neurologic findings of secondary syphilis are usually associated with mild meningeal inflammation. The upper motor neuron involvement of lacunar infarct would spare the upper forehead.

12. The answer is b. The patient's presentation and laboratory workup strongly suggest encephalitis. Currently, WNV is the most common cause of epidemic viral encephalitis in the United States; it is transmitted via mosquito bites hence cases present during summer months. The majority of WNV infections are subclinical or cause a flu-like illness called West Nile fever. Elderly and immunocompromised patients are at high risk for encephalitis. They present with headache, fever, altered level of consciousness, and, in some cases, focal weakness and extrapyramidal features such as tremor. HSV is the most common cause of endemic viral encephalitis. The virus has a predilection to involve the temporal lobes and to cause seizures.

Patients with bacterial meningitis have higher white blood cell counts with predominance of neutrophils, low CSF glucose levels, and elevated CSF protein levels.

The negative CT head despite symptoms present for 48 hours argues against an embolic stroke or subarachnoid hemorrhage. Patients with ischemic strokes do not have CSF pleocytosis, and patients with subarachnoid hemorrhage have much higher CSF red blood cell count. Tuberculosis can cause chronic aseptic meningitis and can be associated with cranial nerve palsies. The case at hand did not have any risk factors for tuberculosis.

13. The answer is c. The patient has a health care–associated UTI complicated by gram-negative bacteremia. The complete identification of gram-negative rods might take 48 hours. Knowing the ability of the growing bacteria to ferment lactose might help in the early prediction of the likely pathogen at hand. Among lactose fermenting gram-negative rods, Enterobacteriaceae such as *E coli* are most common. Among non–lactose-fermenting oxidase-positive gram-negative bacteria, *Pseudomonas aeruginosa* is most common. Ceftriaxone, imipenem, and trimethoprim-sulfamethoxazole can be used to treat UTIs while moxifloxacin and tigecycline do not achieve high enough concentration in urine to be used for this indication. Of the listed antibiotics, imipenem, which is a carbapenem beta-lactam antibiotic, is the only one with anti-pseudomonal activity. Antibiotics with anti-pseudomonal activity include certain penicillins (piperacillin/tazobactam and ticarcillin/clavulanate), cephalosporins (ceftazidime and cefepime), carbapenems (imipenem, meropenem, and doripenem), fluoroquinolones (ciprofloxacin and levofloxacin), and aminoglycosides (gentamicin, tobramycin, and amikacin).

14. The answer is b. Influenza A is a potentially lethal disease in the elderly and chronically debilitated patient. In institutional settings such as nursing homes, outbreaks are likely to be particularly severe. Thus, prophylaxis is extremely important in this setting. All residents should receive the influenza vaccine unless they have known egg allergy (patients can choose to decline the vaccine). Since protective antibodies to the vaccine will not develop for 2 weeks, oseltamivir can be used for protection against influenza A during the interim 2-week period. Because of increasing resistance, amantadine is no longer recommended for prophylaxis. The best way to prevent influenza-associated pneumonia is to prevent the outbreak in the first place.

15. The answer is d. The presentation strongly suggests vertebral osteomyelitis. MRI is sensitive and specific for the diagnosis of vertebral osteomyelitis and is the diagnostic procedure of choice. MRI will reveal the extent of contiguous disc and soft tissue involvement and will help assess for pending neurological compromise. The vertebrae are a common site for hematogenous osteomyelitis. Prior UTI is often the primary mechanism for bacteremia and vertebral seeding. Blood cultures at the time of presentation are positive in fewer than half of all cases. Treatment requires 6 to 8 weeks of antibiotics, but surgery is rarely required for cure.

16. The answer is c. Multiple mechanisms account for bacterial antibiotic resistance. They can be classified into three major groups: enzymatic antimicrobial breakdown, reduced intracellular antibiotic concentration, and alteration of the antibiotic target. The above mechanisms can coexist. Penicillin resistance in *S pneumoniae* (and in *S aureus* and some gram-negative bacteria) is mediated through changing the antibiotic target. In the case of *S pneumonia* that target is the penicillin-binding protein. Beta-lactamases are the most common example of the first mechanism. Beta-lactamase inhibitors such as sulbactam and tazobactam can inactivate those enzymes. Downregulation of small cell membrane channels (porins) prevents antibiotics from entering bacterial cells. On the other hand, some bacteria are able to pump the antibiotics that have already entered the cell out using efflux pumps. Those pumps can coexist in the setting of downregulated porins, both of which prevent the antibiotics from achieving high enough concentration at their intracellular site of action.

17. The answer is a. The symptoms and time of onset after consumption of contaminated food determine the pathogenesis and agents likely responsible for food-borne illness. Nausea and vomiting within 1 to 6 hours of consumption of food are caused by preformed toxins of *Bacillus cereus* and *S aureus* or heavy metals such as copper or zinc. Abdominal cramps and diarrhea that develop more than 8 hours after a meal are caused by *Campylobacter jejuni, E coli, Salmonella, Shigella,* and *Vibrio parahae-molyticus.* It takes more than 8 hours for the bacteria to proliferate in the gut, invade intestinal mucosa, and initiate the infection. Invasion of colonic mucosa is expected to cause diarrhea. Watery diarrhea can also be caused by enterotoxigenic *E coli, Vibrio cholerae,* and Norovirus. Enterotoxigenic *E coli* and *V cholerae,* in particular, produce toxins that target enterocytes and cause the previously described manifestations. *Yersinia enterocolitica* can cause fever and abdominal cramps without diarrhea—a presentation closely resembling acute appendicitis. Cryptosporidiosis, cyclosporiasis, and giardiasis cause diarrhea that can persist for 1 to 3 weeks. *Giardia* proliferates in the proximal small intestine and can cause malabsorption symptoms. The onset of symptoms in these parasitic diseases is more gradual; fever and systemic toxicity are absent.

18. The answer is e. Patients may develop fever as a result of infectious or noninfectious diseases. The term *fever of unknown origin* (FUO) is applied when significant fever (usually defined as >38.3°C or >101°F) persists without known cause after an adequate evaluation. The leading causes of FUO are infections, malignancies, and collagen vascular diseases. As our ability to diagnose these entities increases, their likelihood of causing FUO lessens. Infections such as intra-abdominal abscesses, tuberculosis, hepatobiliary disease, endocarditis (especially if the patient had previously taken antibiotics), and osteomyelitis may cause FUO. The presented patient's history and workup are not consistent with any of these entities, nor has she had rash suggestive of herpes infection.

In immunocompromised patients, such as those infected with HIV, a number of opportunistic infections or lymphomas may cause fever and escape early diagnosis. Neoplastic diseases such as lymphomas and some solid tumors (eg, renal cell carcinoma and primary or metastatic disease of the liver) are associated with FUO. A number of collagen vascular diseases such as adult Still disease may cause FUO. Other causes of FUO include granulomatous diseases (ie, giant cell arteritis, regional enteritis, sarcoidosis, and granulomatous hepatitis), drug fever, deep venous thrombosis, pulmonary emboli, and central nervous processes such as intracerebral bleed. In drug fever, patients might have rash, eosinophilia, and elevated liver enzymes, but central fever and drug fever are diagnoses of exclusion.

The presence of bandemia in our patient supports an infectious etiology. The presented case has multiple risk factors for candidemia, namely, central venous catheterization, total parenteral nutrition, and broad-spectrum antibiotics. *Candida* does not grow on blood cultures in up to 40% of candidemia cases. Response to empiric treatment with antifungal agents can be the only measure to diagnose patients with occult *Candida* infection.

19. The answer is c. Viruses are the most common cause of pharyngitis in adults. Group-A beta-hemolytic streptococci (*S pyogenes*) accounts for 50% of pharyngitis cases in children but only 10% of cases in adults. Centor criteria (fever, absence of cough, tonsillar exudate, and tender anterior cervical lymphadenopathy) are widely used to identify patients at risk for group-A streptococcal pharyngitis. Patients with two or three criteria should have a positive rapid streptococcal antigen test or positive throat culture before being given antibiotics. A negative rapid streptococcal antigen test needs to be confirmed by a throat culture. Patients meeting all four Centor criteria should also have either of the previously described confirmatory tests but may be treated empirically while awaiting results. A 10-day course of oral penicillin continues to be the treatment of choice for streptococcal pharyngitis. A 5-day course of azithromycin can be used in penicillin-allergic patients.

Trismus, hoarseness, and neck swelling are concerning for more serious infections such as epiglottitis. Runny nose, cough, and myalgia suggest a viral illness such as the common cold.

20. The answer is b. This patient is at risk for multiple illnesses that can account for her presentation. She is at risk for pneumonia given her age and comorbidities. She is also at risk for heart failure and coronary artery disease. Furthermore, angiotensin-converting enzyme inhibitors frequently cause dry cough.

Respiratory complaints are a common cause for emergency room visits. Multiple biomarkers have been studied as tools to differentiate among different etiologies of shortness of breath. B-natriuretic peptide is secreted from the ventricles and is elevated in heart failure. Procalcitonin is the precursor of the hormone calcitonin and is produced by many cells in the body following inflammation, especially inflammation of bacterial origin as in bacterial pneumonia. Procalcitonin elevation can lag several hours following the onset of bacterial pneumonia. It may not increase at all in localized bacterial infections such as empyema and lung abscess. D-dimer is produced during coagulation and is expected to rise in patients with deep venous thrombosis and pulmonary embolism. Troponin I is released in the circulation once myocardial cells are damaged; it is elevated in myocardial infarction. C-reactive protein is an inflammatory marker that is very sensitive but not specific. It goes up (not down) in inflammation irrespective of its etiology.

None of the above biomarkers is a stand-alone test. Their results need to be interpreted within the clinical context and in light of other laboratory values and imaging studies. Furthermore, the indiscriminant use of those tests can be confusing and costly. They should be ordered if they are likely to change management.

21. The answer is c. Patients with *Pneumocystis jiroveci* (formerly *carinii*) frequently present with shortness of breath and no sputum production. The interstitial pattern of infiltrates on chest x-ray distinguishes the pneumonia from most bacterial infections. Diagnosis is made by review of methenamine silver stain. Serology is not sensitive or specific enough for routine use. The organism does not grow on any media. Cavitation is quite unusual. The history is likely to suggest risk factors for HIV disease. The disease commonly recurs in patients with CD4 counts below 200/L unless prophylaxis (usually with trimethoprim-sulfamethoxazole) is employed.

22. The answer is a. The striking features of this infection are its rapid onset and progression to a cellulitis characterized by dusky dark-red erythema, bullae formation, and anesthesia over the area. The patient is acutely ill with fever, tachycardia, and other evidence of systemic inflammatory response syndrome (SIRS). These are clues to necrotizing fasciitis, a rapidly spreading deep soft tissue infection. The organism, usually *Streptococcus pyogenes*, reaches the deep fascia from the site of penetrating trauma. Prompt surgical exploration down to fascia or muscle may be lifesaving. Necrotic tissue is Gram-stained and cultured—streptococci, staphylococci, mixed anaerobic infection, or clostridia are all possible pathogens. Antibiotics to cover these organisms are important but not as important as prompt surgical debridement. Acute osteomyelitis is considered when cellulitis does not respond to antibiotic therapy, but would not present with this rapidity.

23. The answer is c. The rash of Rocky Mountain spotted fever (RMSF) occurs about 5 days into an illness characterized by fever, malaise, and headache. The rash may be macular or petechial, but almost always spreads from the ankles and wrists to the trunk. The rash indicates endothelial infection, which in severe cases can lead to capillary leak and shock. North Carolina and East Tennessee have a relatively high incidence of disease. RMSF is a rickettsial disease with the tick as the vector, and the disease is more common in warm months when ticks are active. About 80% of patients will give a history of tick exposure. Doxycycline is considered the drug of choice, but chloramphenicol is preferred in pregnancy because of the effects of tetracycline on fetal bones and teeth. Overall mortality from the infection is now about 5%.

24. The answer is c. Erysipelas, the cellulitis described, is typical of infection caused by *S pyogenes* (group A-hemolytic streptococci). There is often a preceding event such as a cut in the skin, dermatitis, or superficial fungal infection that precedes this rapidly spreading cellulitis. Patients are usually febrile and may appear toxic. *Staphylococcus epidermidis* does not cause rapidly progressive cellulitis. *Staphylococcus aureus* can cause cellulitis that is difficult to distinguish from erysipelas, but it is usually more focal and likely to produce furuncles or abscesses. Tinea infections spread slowly and are confined to the epidermis; they do not cause fever, dermal edema, or tender lymphadenopathy. Anaerobic cellulitis is more often associated with underlying diabetes. Alpha-hemolytic streptococci rarely cause skin and soft tissue infections.

25. The answer is c. About half of all cases of nongonococcal urethritis are caused by *C trachomatis*. *Ureaplasma urealyticum* and *Trichomonas vaginalis* are rarer causes of urethritis. Herpes simplex would present with vesicular lesions and pain, not with a meatal discharge. *Chlamydia psittaci* is the etiologic agent in psittacosis. Almost all gonococci are susceptible to ceftriaxone at recommended doses.

26. The answer is c. The presentation is very consistent with *C difficile* disease. The patient is elderly, has been in both a nursing home and hospital setting and received more than 1 week of a fluoroquinolone antibiotic. Mild fever, abdominal pain, and watery diarrhea are all consistent with the diagnosis, and the PCR test is the most specific of diagnostic tests. Failure on metronidazole is increasingly reported, with at least a 25% failure rate. Switching to oral vancomycin is recommended. The patient does not have fulminant disease with acute abdomen, sepsis, or toxic megacolon; so hospitalization is not necessary. Fecal microbiota transplantation is a potential treatment for recurrent and refractory *C difficile* infection.

27. The answer is c. Community-onset skin infection is often caused by CA-MRSA. Over 63% of *S aureus* isolates from the community were methicillin-resistant in one study. However, these isolates are different from the MRSA seen in the hospital setting. CA-MRSA isolates are sensitive to linezolid and trimethoprim-sulfamethoxazole and to a lesser degree to clindamycin and tetracyclines. They are resistant to beta-lactams and erythromycin. In healthy individuals such as the wrestler described, hospitalization and treatment with vancomycin would not be necessary. Telavancin, ceftaroline, and daptomycin are alternatives to vancomycin in some circumstances for the management of community-acquired or hospital-acquired MRSA. Streptococci usually cause a rapidly spreading cellulitis without pustule formation.

28. The answer is b. HIV infection is usually diagnosed by the detection of HIV-specific antibodies using rapid HIV test or a conventional enzyme-linked immunosorbent assay (ELISA), which are highly sensitive tests, and confirmed by Western blot or indirect immunofluorescence assay, which are highly specific tests. Antibodies appear in few weeks after infection, sometimes after the development of acute HIV symptoms (acute retroviral syndrome). Clinicians should maintain a high level of suspicion for acute HIV infection in all patients who have a compatible clinical syndrome and who report recent high-risk behavior. When acute retroviral syndrome is a possibility, a plasma RNA PCR should be used in conjunction with an HIV antibody test to diagnose acute HIV infection. Although HIV DNA testing is available, it offers no added advantages over the more readily available and FDA-approved HIV RNA testing. The patient's HIV serology (antibody testing) is negative, so repeating the serology testing by ELISA or ordering Western blot is not indicated at this point. It is appropriate to repeat the serology testing in 4 to 6 weeks.

29. The answer is b. Whether or not to use drugs such as atovaquone-proguanil, mefloquine, or primaquine for resistant-*Plasmodium falciparum* will depend on knowledge of specific local patterns of drug sensitivity of plasmodia. Specific information can be obtained from the CDC website or malaria hotline. The common sense measures described are extremely important and part of the overall worldwide plan to contain the spread of malaria. Prophylaxis should begin 2 days to 2 weeks before departure in order to have adequate levels of drug on arrival and to identify potential side effects before leaving. Chemoprophylaxis is not entirely reliable, and malaria should always be in the differential diagnosis of a febrile illness in a traveler to endemic regions, even if the drug regimen has been faithfully followed. Mosquitoes' peak feeding periods are dawn and dusk.

30. The answer is c. Neutropenic fever is a medical emergency. Infections, most commonly gram-negative bacteria such as *P aeruginosa*, are responsible for most cases. Prompt empiric antibiotic therapy with two antibiotics from two different antibiotic classes (double coverage) that have anti-pseudomonal activity is most appropriate. Adding an antibiotic with anti–methicillin-resistant *S aureus* (anti-MRSA) activity to the initial antibiotic regimen is indicated if the patient was on antibiotic prophylaxis before the onset of the neutropenic fever or if he has any of the following conditions: skin infection, moderate to severe mucositis, central venous catheter, or shock (as in this vignette). Imipenem alone is not enough because it lacks anti-MRSA activity. Vancomycin does not provide gram-negative coverage and should never be used alone in the treatment of neutropenic fever. Awaiting culture results without initiating empirical antibiotic coverage is inappropriate because it increases the patient's mortality risk. Antifungal therapy is often added in the subsequent days if the patient fails to respond to broad-spectrum antibiotics.

31. The answer is a. Assessment for adult vaccination should be based on age, comorbidities, immunization history, and other risk factors such as travel plans and sexual behaviors. Adults should get tetanus and diphtheria vaccine (Td) every 10 years. Tetanus, diphtheria, and acellular pertussis (Tdap) vaccine should replace one of the Td vaccines if not given before or during adult life. Zoster vaccine is indicated for individuals over 60 years of age. The influenza vaccine is recommended for all persons aged 6 months and older, including all adults. Pneumococcal vaccine is indicated in patients with chronic illnesses such as heart failure, bronchial asthma, chronic obstructive pulmonary disease, chronic kidney disease, and diabetes mellitus. Otherwise, the pneumococcal vaccine is administered once at the age of 65. HPV vaccine is indicated in females and males who are 11 to 26 years of age. The meningococcal vaccination is recommended for adults with anatomic or functional asplenia or persistent complement component deficiencies, as well as adults with HIV infection. Meningococcal vaccine is also indicated for patients traveling to meningitis endemic areas.

32. The answer is c. Every positive culture requires interpretation. A positive culture could represent a pathogen, a colonizer, or a contaminant. The presence of symptoms and signs of infection in addition to supportive laboratory and radiologic data indicates that a cultivated microbe is a true pathogen. The patient has no symptoms or signs of infection, and her urinalysis shows no pyuria. In this case, *C albicans* is a colonizer, and no antifungal therapy is indicated. Predisposing risk factors need to be eliminated to reduce the chances of colonization and to prevent a colonizer from becoming a pathogen. Removing a Foley catheter, controlling hyperglycemia, and stopping broad-spectrum antibiotics, when feasible, represent some examples of risk factor elimination. Antifungal therapy (such as with fluconazole or amphotericin B) is inappropriate for fungal colonization alone.

33. The answer is a. The patient has right knee septic arthritis caused by bacteria that form gram-positive cocci in clusters. This is an orthopedic emergency requiring prompt management. *Staphylococcus aureus* is the most likely agent. Involvement in a contact sport puts the patient at risk for infections caused by CA-MRSA. Consulting orthopedic surgery and starting an antibiotic with activity against MRSA while awaiting culture results is the most appropriate course of action. Antibiotics with activity against MRSA include vancomycin, linezolid, daptomycin, and telavancin. Appropriate antibiotics alone without getting orthopedic surgery involved are not enough. Antibiotics are much less effective in undrained abscesses. Joint drainage through daily closed-needle aspiration, arthroscopy, or arthrotomy helps in removing thick purulent material and lysis of adhesions. Ceftriaxone is not active against MRSA. Further testing, such as MRI, will not add useful information at this point.

34. The answer is c. The patient is an intravenous drug user who presents with fever, gram-positive bacteremia, a murmur, and evidence of systemic embolization—a picture consistent with infective endocarditis (IE). The positive blood cultures in this case are highly unlikely to represent contaminants. Ordering transesophageal echocardiogram (TEE) despite the negative transthoracic echocardiogram (TTE) is appropriate, given TEE's higher sensitivity. Repeating blood cultures 2 to 4 days after initial positive cultures and as needed thereafter is recommended to document clearance of bacteremia. In the case of gram-positive bacteremia, the duration of treatment is counted from the first negative blood culture. Placing long-term intravenous catheters such as peripherally inserted central catheter (PICC) should be delayed, if possible, until the gram-positive bacteremia clears. It is not appropriate to treat IE with oral or bacteriostatic antibiotics. Once IE is confirmed, the patient will require 6 weeks of intravenous antibiotics. There is nothing in the patient's presentation that is suggestive of osteomyelitis to require a bone scan.

35. The answer is d. The patient's UTI is caused by gram-positive bacteria. This excludes *E coli* and *N gonorrhoeae*, both of which are gram-negative, and *C albicans*, which is a yeast. *Enterococcus faecalis* and *S saprophyticus* are gram-positive bacteria that can cause UTI, but the second agent is a more likely cause of UTI in young women. *Staphylococcus saprophyticus* colonizes the rectum or the urogenital tract of approximately 5% to 10% of women and is second only to *E coli* as the causative agent of uncomplicated UTIs in young sexually active women. Such infections are successfully treated with trimethoprim-sulfamethoxazole. Other acceptable treatment options for acute uncomplicated cystitis include nitrofurantoin and fosfomycin. Fluoroquinolones are highly efficacious in a 3-day regimen but should be reserved for treating complicated UTI or patients who are allergic or intolerant of the above options.

36 and 37. The answers are 36-a, 37-g. Many fungal infections have a geographic predilection. Coccidioidomycosis occurs in the Southwest (California, Arizona), while histoplasmosis and blastomycosis occur in the Ohio and Mississippi basins. Histoplasmosis usually affects the lungs as the primary site and can cause atypical pneumonia with hilar lymphadenopathy. It disseminates, however, to the reticuloendothelial system, causing hepatosplenomegaly and bone marrow involvement. It can also cause chronic pneumonia with pulmonary nodules and cavities. Blastomycosis presents with signs and symptoms of chronic respiratory infection. The organism has a tendency to produce skin lesions in exposed areas that become crusted, ulcerated, or verrucous. Bone pain is caused by osteolytic lesions. Mucormycosis originates in the nose and paranasal sinuses. Sinus tenderness, bloody nasal discharge, and obtundation occur usually in the setting of diabetic ketoacidosis.

Cryptococcosis, candidiasis, aspergillosis, and mucormycosis are ubiquitous diseases without geographic pattern. Invasive disease tends to occur in immunocompromised patients. Cryptococcal meningitis and esophageal candidiasis afflict patients with impaired T-cell function (ie, AIDS patients), while invasive candidiasis, aspergillosis, or mucormycosis attack patients with neutrophil dysfunction, such as those with acute leukemia or uncontrolled diabetes.

38 and 39. The answers are 38-c, 39-d. Parvovirus B19 is the agent responsible for erythema infectiosum, also known as fifth disease. This disease most commonly affects children between the ages of 5 and 14 years, but it can also occur in adults. The disease in children is characterized by low-grade fever, followed several days later by a slapped-cheek rash. Adults develop fever and a diffuse lacelike rash. Some adults progress to a symmetric polyarthropathy that can mimic rheumatoid arthritis but is self-limited after several weeks to months. Complications in adults also include aplastic crisis in patients with chronic hemolytic anemia (especially sickle cell disease), spontaneous abortion, and hydrops fetalis.

Listeriosis is caused by eating food contaminated with *L monocytogenes*. It is a gram-positive rod that has a predilection to infect older adults, pregnant women, immunocompromised patients, and newborns. It can cause sepsis, meningitis, and miscarriages. Deli meats, unwashed vegetables, raw milk, soft cheeses, and cantaloupes have been implicated in causing *Listeria* outbreaks. Ampicillin is the antibiotic of choice for treating this infection.

HSV causes vesicular rash and can cause meningitis and encephalitis. Epstein-Barr virus causes infectious mononucleosis. A significant proportion of patients with infectious mononucleosis develop macular rash if they are treated with amoxicillin. *Enterococcus faecalis* is a gram-positive coccus that can cause UTI, infective endocarditis, and line infections. *Acinetobacter baumannii* is a gram-negative coccobacillus that can cause hospital-acquired infections. The latter two bacteria are often multidrug resistant and difficult to treat. They are transmitted through contact with infected or colonized individuals.

40 and 41. The answers are 40-c, 41-b. There are four types of isolation precautions that can be implemented in health care settings. Any given patient might require more than one type of precaution. Standard precautions apply when interacting with any patient, regardless of the diagnosis. They include hand washing before and after contact with every patient and the use of gloves, gowns, masks, and eye protection when contact with open sores, blood, or body secretions is anticipated. Contact precautions reduce the risk of spreading microorganisms that are transmitted by direct or indirect contact. They include private room placement of the patient and the use of gloves and gowns when in contact with the patient or the immediate environment. Contact precautions are indicated in patients colonized or infected with MRSA, vancomycin-resistant enterococci (VRE), and *C difficile*.

Droplet precautions limit the transmission of infections that are carried in respiratory droplets (>5 μm in size) such as influenza and meningococcal meningitis. Droplet precautions include placing the patient in a private room and asking health care professionals to use surgical masks within 3 ft from the patient. Airborne precautions reduce the risk of airborne particulate (particles less than 5 μm in size) transmission of infectious agents such as tuberculosis. The patient is placed in a private negative-pressure room with high-efficiency masks, such as the N95 mask, worn by all health care professionals upon entering those rooms. The patient in question 40 has meningococcal meningitis and requires droplet precautions for 24 hours of effective antibiotic therapy. The patient in question 41 has health care–associated MRSA pneumonia and requires contact precautions.

42 to 45.   The answers are 42-c, 43-a, 44-b, 45-f. Herpes simplex encephalitis can occur in patients of any age—usually in immunocompetent patients. Most adults with HSV encephalitis have previous infection with mucocutaneous HSV-1. The bizarre behavior includes personality aberrations, hypersexuality, or sensory hallucinations. CSF shows lymphocytes with a near-normal sugar and protein. Focal abnormalities are seen in the temporal lobe by CT scan, MRI, or electroencephalogram.

The patient who has a history of tuberculosis and now complains of hemoptysis would be reevaluated for active tuberculosis. However, the chest x-ray described is characteristic of a fungus ball—almost always the result of an aspergilloma growing in a previous cavitary lesion.

The Filipino patient who has developed a pulmonary nodule after travel through the Southwest would be suspected of having developed coccidioidomycosis. Individuals from the Philippines have a higher incidence of the disease and are more likely to have complications of dissemination.

The 35-year-old with cough, sore throat, and fever went on to develop symptoms of myopericarditis with typical ECG findings. Coxsackievirus B infection is the most likely cause of upper respiratory tract infection (URI) symptoms that evolve into a picture of myopericarditis. Pericarditis may be asymptomatic or can present with chest pain, both pleuritic and ischemic-like. Enteroviruses rarely, if ever, attack the pericardium alone without involving the subepicardial myocardium.

HSV type 2 typically causes genital ulcers, although it can cause mild encephalitis with headache and cerebellar ataxia. Hantavirus often leads to a severe pulmonary infection with a diffuse acute respiratory distress syndrome (ARDS)-like picture; thrombocytopenia can provide an important diagnostic clue. Parvovirus B19 usually causes a benign undifferentiated viral syndrome, with transient skin manifestations.

Suggested Readings

1. Southwick F. *Infectious Diseases: A Clinical Short Course*, 3rd ed. New York: McGraw-Hill; 2013. Chapters: 1, 2, 3, 4, 6, 9, and 10.
2. Clinical practice guidelines at the Infectious Diseases Society of America, available at: www.idsociety.org/IDSA_Practice_Guidelines
3. Hoen B, Duval X. Infective endocarditis. *N Engl J Med*. 2013;368:1425-1433.
4. Musher DM, Thorner AR. Community-acquired pneumonia. *N Engl J Med*. 2014;371:1619-1628.
5. Zumla A, Raviglione M, Hafner R, von Reyn CF. Tuberculosis. *N Engl J Med*. 2013;368:745-755.
6. Schuetz P, Amin DN, Greenwald JL. Role of procalcitonin in managing adult patients with respiratory tract infections. *Chest*. 2012;141:1063-1073.
7. Doron S, Davidson LE. Antimicrobial stewardship. *Mayo Clin Proceedings*. 2011;86:1113-1123.

Hospital-Based Medicine

Questions

46. You are covering a busy hospital service at night when you are paged to evaluate a 78-year-old man with sudden onset of dyspnea. A review of the patient's chart reveals that he was diagnosed with small cell lung cancer 2 months earlier. He was subsequently treated with radiation therapy and chemotherapy. He was admitted to the hospital 3 days earlier with a suspected pathologic fracture of the right femur. He has no other known metastases. Thirty minutes ago he became acutely short of breath. Current vital signs include a heart rate of 115 beats/min, blood pressure of 92/69 mm Hg, and respiratory rate of 32/min. Oxygen saturation is 94% on 4 L of oxygen via nasal cannula. He is anxious and tachypneic, but lung sounds are clear and symmetric. The heart rhythm is regular and no murmurs are appreciated. What is the best next step in the management of this patient?

a. Immediately administer empiric antibiotics for coverage of hospital-acquired pneumonia.
b. Immediately administer therapeutic dose of intravenous heparin.
c. Arrange for synchronized electrical cardioversion.
d. Order a ventilation/perfusion (V/Q) scan of the chest.
e. Administer a benzodiazepine.

47. You respond to the cardiopulmonary arrest of a 72-year-old woman in the intensive care unit. She has no palpable pulse, but the cardiac monitor shows sinus tachycardia at 124/min. Breath sounds are symmetric with bag-mask positive-pressure ventilation. What is the best next step in the management of this patient?

a. Immediate electrical cardioversion
b. Immediate transthoracic cardiac pacing
c. Immediate administration of high-volume normal saline
d. Immediate large-bore pericardiocentesis
e. Immediate administration of extended-spectrum antibiotics

48. You are asked to provide preoperative risk assessment for a 72-year-old woman who was admitted with a hip fracture after a fall. She had a myocardial infarction 4 months ago. She has infrequent exertional chest pain that resolves with sublingual nitroglycerine. She has never had congestive heart failure or a stroke. She has well-controlled diabetes. Her medications include lisinopril, metoprolol, atorvastatin, metformin, nitroglycerin, and aspirin. Laboratory testing reveals hemoglobin of 10.5 g/dL and creatinine of 1.5 mg/dL. An electrocardiogram (ECG) reveals evidence of a remote inferior myocardial infarction. Chest x-ray shows normal cardiac size and no evidence of congestive heart failure. Which underlying risk factor places her at highest risk for a major perioperative cardiovascular event?

a. Diabetes mellitus
b. Elevated creatinine of 1.5 mg/dL
c. Age greater than 70 years
d. History of ischemic heart disease
e. Hemoglobin of 10.5 mg/dL

49. A 71-year-old woman is brought to the emergency room by her daughter because of sudden onset of right-sided weakness and slurred speech. The patient, a recent immigrant from Southeast Asia, has not seen a doctor in two decades. Her symptoms began 75 minutes ago while she was eating breakfast. A stat noncontrast CT scan of the head is normal. Labs are normal. Physical examination reveals an anxious appearing woman with dense hemiplegia of the R upper and lower extremities. Deep tendon reflexes are not discernible on the R side and are 2+ on the left. What is the best next step in management of this patient?

a. Immediate intravenous unfractionated heparin
b. Immediate thrombolytic therapy
c. Immediate administration of interferon-beta
d. Emergent MRI/MRA of head
e. Emergent cardiac catheterization

50. A 64-year-old man with cirrhosis and pneumonia is admitted to your service toward the end of your shift. Some important laboratory tests are still outstanding when you are scheduled to turn care over to the cross-covering team. Which of the following provides the safest way to transfer care to the cross-covering team overnight?

a. Add an addendum to your written history and physical about the outstanding laboratory tests.
b. Call the cross-covering team and provide a list of the outstanding tests.
c. Leave a written list of the outstanding laboratory test for the cross-covering team.
d. Check on the outstanding laboratory test early the next morning.
e. Prepare a written list of all your patients that includes tasks to be done overnight, and review this list with the oncoming team.

51. An 84-year-old woman develops confusion and agitation after surgery for hip fracture. Her family reports that prior to her hospitalization she functioned independently at home, but has some memory problems and needed help balancing her checkbook and paying bills. Her current medications include intravenous fentanyl for pain control, lorazepam for control of her agitation, and deep vein thrombosis (DVT) prophylaxis. She has also been started on ciprofloxacin for pyuria (culture pending). In addition to frequent reorientation of the patient, which of the following series of actions would best manage this patient's delirium?

a. Increase lorazepam to more effective dose, repeat urinalysis.
b. Discontinue lorazepam, remove Foley catheter, add haloperidol for severe agitation, and change to non-fluoroquinolone antibiotic.
c. Continue lorazepam at current dose, discontinue fentanyl, and add soft restraints.
d. Continue lorazepam at current dose, add alprazolam 0.25 mg for severe agitation, repeat urinalysis, and restrain patient to prevent self-harm.
e. Discontinue lorazepam, remove Foley catheter, add alprazolam 0.25 mg for severe agitation, and place the patient on telemetry.

52. You are caring for a 72-year-old man admitted to the hospital with an exacerbation of congestive heart failure. Before admission he was able to ambulate two blocks before stopping because of dyspnea. He has now returned to baseline and is ready for discharge. His preadmission medications include aspirin, metoprolol, and furosemide. Systolic blood pressure has ranged from 110 to 128 mm Hg over the course of his hospitalization. Heart rate was in 120 s at the time of presentation, but has been consistently around 70/min over the past 24 hours. An echocardiogram performed during this hospitalization revealed global hypokinesis with an ejection fraction of 30%. Which of the following medications, when added to his preadmission regimen, would be most likely to decrease his risk of subsequent mortality?

a. Digoxin
b. Enalapril
c. Hydrochlorothiazide
d. Propranolol
e. Spironolactone

53. A 64-year-old woman presents to the emergency room with flank pain and fever. She noted dysuria for the past 3 days. Blood and urine cultures are obtained, and she is started on intravenous ciprofloxacin. Six hours after admission, she becomes tachycardic and her blood pressure drops. Her intravenous fluid is normal saline (NS) at 100 mL/h. Her current blood pressure is 79/43 mm Hg, heart rate is 128/min, respiratory rate is 26/min, and temperature is 39.2°C (102.5°F). She seems drowsy yet uncomfortable. Extremities are warm with trace edema. What is the best next course of action?

a. Administer IV hydrocortisone at stress dose.
b. Begin norepinephrine infusion and titrate to mean arterial pressure greater than 65 mm Hg.
c. Add vancomycin to her antibiotic regimen for improved gram-positive coverage.
d. Administer a bolus of NS.
e. Place a central venous line to monitor central venous oxygen saturation.

54. An 84-year-old woman presents to the ED with shortness of breath. She has been coughing for the past 2 to 3 days. The patient has a history of mild dementia, but she has been able to maintain independent living at home with the assistance of her daughters and a home health agency. Her daughter denies any fever at home. Vital signs include a heart rate of 102/min, respiratory rate of 24/min, blood pressure 142/58 mm Hg, and temperature of 37.8°C (100°F) with a weight of 52 kg. Oxygen saturation is 93% on room air. Upon examination, she appears to be in mild respiratory distress. She is pleasant but oriented only to self. Chest auscultation reveals few crackles in the left upper lung field. WBC count is 12,500, BUN is 30 mg/dL, and creatinine is 1.3 mg/dL. A chest radiograph shows an infiltrate in the left upper lung lobe. What is the best initial course of therapy for this patient?

a. Begin a third-generation cephalosporin and admit her to the hospital.
b. Begin a renal-dosed third-generation cephalosporin and a macrolide, and admit her to the hospital.
c. Begin a respiratory fluoroquinolone and discharge her home with outpatient follow-up.
d. Begin a loop diuretic and monitor her oxygen saturation.
e. Begin bronchodilator therapy with an inhaled beta-agonist.

55. A 78-year-old man presents to the emergency department with acute onset of bright red blood per rectum. Symptoms started 2 hours earlier, and he has had three bowel movements since then with copious amounts of blood. He denies prior episodes of rectal bleeding. He notes dizziness with standing but denies abdominal pain. He has had no vomiting or nausea. A nasogastric lavage is performed and shows no coffee-ground material or blood. Lab evaluation reveals hemoglobin of 10.5 g/dL. What is the most likely source of the bleeding?

a. Internal hemorrhoids
b. Dieulafoy lesion
c. Diverticulosis
d. Mallory-Weiss tear
e. Sessile polyp

56. You are covering the general medical service one evening when contacted by the nursing staff about a "critical" laboratory test on a patient. The patient in question is a 62-year-old man who was admitted to the hospital with community-acquired pneumonia. His comorbidities include diabetes mellitus and chronic kidney disease. The patient had a scheduled chemistry panel, which showed potassium of 6.5 mEq/L. You immediately order an ECG (see the following figure). What is the next best step in management of this patient's hyperkalemia?

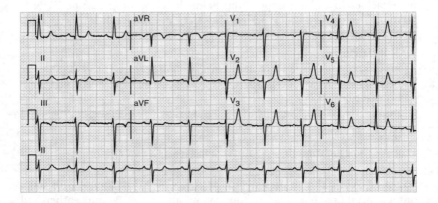

a. Administer IV calcium gluconate.
b. Administer oral sodium polystyrene sulfonate (Kayexalate).
c. Administer subcutaneous insulin.
d. Administer IV sodium bicarbonate.
e. Repeat the serum potassium.

57. A 48-year-old man is admitted to your service after an inhalational chemical exposure. He develops respiratory distress and requires endotracheal intubation and mechanical ventilation. Which of the following is the best way to decrease his risk of developing ventilator-acquired pneumonia?

a. Daily interruption of sedation to assess respiratory status
b. Nasopharyngeal rather than oropharyngeal endotracheal intubation
c. Institution of protocol to keep bed flat during ventilation
d. Intermittent nasopharyngeal suctioning
e. Prophylactic broad-spectrum intravenous antibiotics

58. You have been following a 72-year-old man admitted to the hospital with pneumonia. On the third day of his hospitalization you are called to the bedside by the nurse because of a heart rate of 150 beats/min. The nurse has already printed an ECG (see the following figure). The patient's current blood pressure is 118/89. He reports feeling weak and appears anxious but denies chest pain and does not appear to be confused or drowsy. What is the next best step in management of this patient?

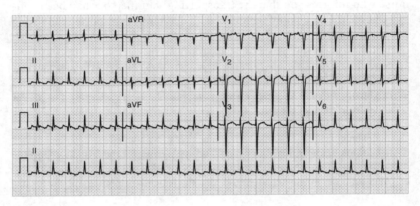

a. Administer IV beta-blocker such as metoprolol.
b. Administer IV dihydropyridine calcium-channel blocker such as nicardipine.
c. Arrange emergent electrical cardioversion.
d. Order STAT cardiac biomarkers including troponin levels.
e. Begin therapeutic IV heparin.

59. You are providing hospital care for a 36-year-old man who was admitted 2 days ago with an uncomplicated community-acquired pneumonia. When reviewing your patient's chart you notice the results of a normal abdominal ultrasound. You further note that there was no indication for an ultrasound and that it was never ordered. Further inquiry reveals that an ultrasound was ordered but has not yet been performed on a patient with the same last name in the next room. You discuss this with the charge nurse who informs you that the transporting staff member had been confused about the room number and had inadvertently transported the wrong patient to the ultrasound department who performed the procedure. Which of the following responses is most appropriate?

a. Since your patient did not suffer any harm, it is not necessary to inform him that the ultrasound was done unnecessarily.
b. Personally seek out the staff member responsible for transporting the patient and inform them of the error.
c. Inform your patient that he had an unnecessary procedure and apologize for the inconvenience.
d. In addition to informing your patient and apologizing for the mistake, report the error through the hospital's Patient Safety Network.
e. Write an order for the ultrasound so that the patient's insurance will pay for it.

60. A 42-year-old man was admitted to the hospital with pneumonia. On the third day of his hospitalization he becomes agitated and confused. He reports feeling "spiders" crawling on his skin. You note that he has a blood pressure of 172/94 mm Hg, heart rate of 107/min, and temperature of 38°C (100.4°F). With the exception of confusion, agitation, and tremor, the remainder of his physical examination is unchanged from earlier in the day. What is the best initial step in management of this patient?

a. Emergent noncontrast CT scan of the brain
b. Emergent administration of intravenous haloperidol
c. Emergent administration of intravenous lorazepam
d. Emergent administration of intravenous labetalol
e. Placement of physical restraints for patient safety

Hospital-Based Medicine

Answers

46. The answer is b. Although there are many causes of acute dyspnea in the hospitalized patient, the most likely etiology in this patient is pulmonary thromboembolism (PTE). In addition to the rapid onset of symptoms, the patient's risk factors for development of a venous thromboembolism (malignancy, bone fracture, and immobility) are suggestive of a PTE. Virchow triad predisposing to clot formation includes hypercoagulability, blood stasis, and endothelial injury. Specific risk factors for venous thromboembolism include recent surgery, trauma or pregnancy, prior thromboembolic event, immobility, malignancy, and a hypercoagulable state. Potential etiologies of the hypercoagulable state include prothrombin gene mutation, antiphospholipid antibody, Factor V Leiden mutation, hyperhomocysteinemia, and deficiencies in protein C, S, or antithrombin III. Assuming no absolute contraindication, the first-line therapy for a PTE is immediate anticoagulation. Because the majority of deaths from PTE occur within 1 hour of onset of symptoms, it would be inappropriate to withhold treatment until confirmatory testing (CT or V/Q scan) is completed. Evaluation of a V/Q scan (answer d) may be complicated by the likelihood that he has an abnormal chest x-ray given his history of lung cancer and thoracic radiation. In this circumstance, a CT pulmonary angiogram would be the preferred test.

Although a diagnosis of pneumonia could be considered (answer a) the rapidity of onset of symptoms, the lack of purulent sputum, and the clear lung fields make this diagnosis less likely than PE. There should be time to evaluate for pneumonia once the patient is stabilized. Answer c is incorrect because the patient likely has sinus tachycardia as a result of the PTE; sinus tachycardia will improve with treatment of the underlying cause. Although the patient may symptomatically improve in the short term with anxiolytic therapy (answer e), his low blood pressure may limit the use of benzodiazepines. If the patient were having an "anxiety attack" rather than a PE, the blood pressure would usually be elevated rather than depressed.

47. The answer is c. Pulseless electrical activity (PEA) is a common cause of cardiopulmonary arrest in the hospital setting. Etiologies of PEA that are potentially treatable include hypovolemia, hypoxia, hyperkalemia, severe acidosis, pulmonary embolism, cardiac tamponade, and tension pneumothorax. The loss of cardiac output results from decreased ventricular filling (hypovolemia, pulmonary embolism, cardiac tamponade, or tension pneumothorax) or electromechanical dissociation (hypoxia, hyperkalemia, or severe acidosis). Management of PEA arrest requires rapid establishment of vascular access, airway stabilization, and administration of IV fluids. Physical examination focuses on potential correctable etiologies. Electrical cardioversion will not benefit a patient in sinus rhythm. Similarly, cardiac pacing will not help, since the problem is not associated with severe bradycardia. Sudden pericardial tamponade is uncommon, but, if suspected (proper setting, jugular distension, low-voltage ECG), pericardiocentesis is performed. Rapid saline bolus is more likely to be effective and can be given immediately. If sepsis is suspected, broad-spectrum antibiotics would be appropriate, but antibiotic administration will not affect the immediate outcome of the cardiopulmonary arrest.

48. The answer is d. Many patients undergoing major noncardiac surgery are at risk for a perioperative cardiovascular event. The specific risk is related to patient and surgery-specific characteristics. Identification of increased risk provides the patient with information that helps them better understand the risks and benefits of surgery. The Revised Cardiac Risk Index (RCRI), also known as the Goldman Cardiac Risk Index, is a widely used tool to evaluate perioperative risk of fatal or nonfatal cardiovascular events following noncardiac surgeries. The components of the RCRI are (1) history of ischemic heart disease, (2) history of heart failure, (3) history of stroke, (4) insulin-dependent diabetes mellitus, and (5) preoperative serum creatinine > 2.0 mg/dL. This patient has diabetes but is not insulin-dependent, she has never had a stroke or congestive heart failure, and her creatinine is less than 2.0 mg/dL. Age is not a risk factor on the RCRI scale. Thus the risk factor placing her at highest risk for a major perioperative cardiovascular event is the history of ischemic heart disease.

49. The answer is b. This patient presents with an acute left middle cerebral artery stroke. Time is of the essence if thrombolytic therapy is to be beneficial. Intravenous thrombolytics may be administered up to 3 hours after the onset of symptoms. Recent studies have suggested expanding the window of opportunity to 4.5 hours. Fortunately, this patient was brought to the ED promptly. CT scan of the brain shows no evidence of bleed. CT evidence of ischemia may not become apparent until 48 to 72 hours.

A history of intracranial hemorrhage, recent surgery, bleeding diathesis, onset of symptoms greater than 3 to 4.5 hours prior to therapy, and unknown time of onset of symptoms are contraindications to thrombolytic therapy. This patient should be given intravenous tissue-type plasminogen activator (t-PA).

Anticoagulation in acute stroke (answer a) is not currently recommended. In most trials of anticoagulation, any benefit of therapy is matched by an increase in hemorrhagic transformation. Interferon-beta (answer c) is used to treat multiple sclerosis, not ischemic stroke. Emergent scanning with MRI (answer d) wastes precious time and is not always available. Patients with acute stroke often have mild elevation in cardiac biomarkers. Cardiac catheterization (answer e) is unnecessary, and may very well prove harmful in the setting of a stroke.

50. The answer is e. A handoff is the process of transferring information and responsibility for a patient to a different team. A signout is the process of transferring information about a patient until care is resumed by the original team at a later time. Many studies have shown that adverse events and patient safety errors occur with more frequency at the time of handoffs and signouts. Other studies have demonstrated that a structured handoff/ signout process can decrease the likelihood of these errors. Components of the structured process which have been shown to be efficacious include providing a written list of all patients with an estimate of illness severity, tasks to be performed by the cross-covering team, and contingency plans for changes in clinical status. Adding an addendum to the written history and physical does not provide specific guidance to the cross-covering team. It is better to provide a structured list of all your patients and not just a list of outstanding tests for one patient. Important laboratory tests should be followed up promptly and not wait until the next morning. Studies have also suggested that interactive sessions with few interruptions and a chance to review the written information and ask questions are more effective than providing written information alone.

51. The answer is b. Delirium is a common complication in the hospital setting. Delirium may be differentiated from dementia by its acute onset and waxing and waning mental state. Elderly patients, especially those with a history of dementia, and the severely ill are at greatest risk of developing delirium. Delirium may be precipitated by medications, postsurgical state, infection, or electrolyte imbalance. The management of delirium relies on nonpharmacologic approaches, including frequent reorientation, discontinuation of any unnecessary noxious stimuli (eg, urinary catheters, unnecessary oxygen delivery systems or telemetry monitors, and restraints), environmental modification to establish day/night sleep cycles, and discontinuation of unnecessary medications. This patient likely will continue to need pain control, but the dose of fentanyl should be minimized to the smallest effective dose. Benzodiazepines frequently induce a delirium and their continued use or escalation may impair recovery. Fluoroquinolones can worsen mental status in the elderly. Physical or chemical restraints actually impair recovery from delirium and should be used only as a last resort to prevent serious harm to self or others. A repeat urinalysis would provide no useful information since the original urine culture is still pending.

52. The answer is b. Inhibition of the renin-angiotensin-aldosterone system by either angiotensin converting enzyme inhibitors (ACEi) or angiotensin receptor blockers (ARB) has been proven to decrease mortality in patients with symptoms of congestive heart failure and a depressed ejection fraction. All patients with a history of congestive heart failure should be maintained on a beta-blocker and an ACEi or ARB. Most patients will require a diuretic for symptom control. Digitalis glycosides decrease rehospitalization rate but have not been shown to improve mortality. Thiazide diuretics are excellent medications for blood pressure control. Our patient, however, has well-controlled blood pressure. The patient is already on a selective beta-blocker and the addition of a nonselective beta-blocker is unlikely to be helpful. Spironolactone provides mortality benefit in patients with NYHA class III or IV heart failure. The patient in this scenario was able to walk two blocks before stopping and would be classified as NYHA class II.

53. The answer is d. This patient is septic, and immediate therapy should be directed at correcting her hemodynamic instability. Patients with sepsis require aggressive fluid resuscitation to compensate for capillary extravasation. This patient's vital signs suggest decreased effective circulating volume. Normal saline at 100 cc/h is insufficient volume replacement. The patient should be given a saline bolus of 2 L over 20 minutes, and then her blood pressure and clinical status should be reassessed. The elevated respiratory rate could be evidence of pulmonary edema or respiratory compensation for acidosis from decreased tissue perfusion. Even if the patient has evidence of pulmonary edema, fluid resuscitation remains the first intervention for hypotension from sepsis. She is more likely to die from hemodynamic collapse than from oxygenation issues related to pulmonary edema.

Stress doses of hydrocortisone and intravenous norepinephrine are both used in patients with shock refractory to volume resuscitation, but should be reserved until after the saline bolus. Vancomycin is a reasonable choice to cover enterococci, which can cause UTI-associated sepsis, but again would not address the immediate hemodynamic problem. If the patient does not improve, a central line (to measure filling pressures and mixed venous oxygen saturation) would allow the "early goal-directed" sepsis protocol to be used.

54. The answer is b. Empiric therapy for community-acquired pneumonia (CAP) includes either a respiratory fluoroquinolone or a third-generation cephalosporin plus a macrolide, the latter to cover for "atypical" pathogens. This would limit the correct answer options to a, b, or c. CAP can be caused by viruses, bacteria, fungi, or protozoa. The common bacterial causes of CAP include *Streptococcus pneumoniae, Mycoplasma pneumoniae, Haemophilus influenzae, Chlamydia pneumoniae,* and *Staphylococcus aureus.* Answer a is incorrect as our patient has an estimated creatinine clearance of 26 mL/min and an adjustment of the antibiotics based on renal function may be indicated depending on the specific drug that is selected. Furthermore, a cephalosporin would not cover *Mycoplasma* or *Chlamydia.* The patient in question has several risk factors for poor outcome (age, change in mental status, depressed glomerular filtration rate), so immediate discharge to home would be inappropriate (answer c). There is also a theoretical risk of worsening delirium from fluoroquinolones crossing the blood-brain barrier in patients at risk of delirium. The examination and chest x-ray do not suggest congestive heart failure, so treatment with a loop diuretic would not be efficacious. Inhaled bronchodilators do not improve outcomes in pneumonia and are used if the patient develops wheezing or other evidence of bronchospasm.

55. The answer is c. Bright red blood per rectum typically indicates a lower GI source of bleeding, although occasionally a high-output upper GI bleed may result in bright red blood. Diverticular bleeds can be massive. Although 80% resolve spontaneously, bleeding recurs in one-fourth of patients. Colonoscopy would be the diagnostic method of choice if diverticular bleed is suspected, but bleeding frequently stops before visualization occurs. With recurrent diverticular bleed, hemicolectomy may be necessary. Although nasogastric lavage has lost favor as a diagnostic maneuver, in this case, a negative lavage decreases the likelihood of a significant bleed from the stomach or esophagus. Neither internal hemorrhoids nor sessile colonic polyps usually results in hemodynamically significant acute bleeding. A Dieulafoy vessel is a large-caliber vessel close to the mucosal surface, most commonly located on the greater curvature of the stomach. Mallory-Weiss tears occur as a result of traumatic injury at the gastroesophageal junction from forceful vomiting and may lead to large-volume blood loss. Both of these lesions would be associated with evidence of upper GI bleeding.

56. The answer is a. The patient has electrocardiographic changes of hyperkalemia and is at risk of rapid deterioration. The usual ECG findings seen with hyperkalemia (in order of progressive risk of arrhythmia) include peaked T waves, prolongation of the PR interval, widening of the QRS segment, and loss of P waves. Progressive QRS widening with subsequent merger with the T wave produces a sine wave that precedes terminal ventricular fibrillation or asystole. Management of hyperkalemia frequently requires several interventions based on the rapidity of onset and duration of effect of the therapy. When there is ECG evidence of hyperkalemia, immediate administration of IV calcium to stabilize the cellular membrane is indicated. Acting almost immediately, the stabilizing effect of calcium will last 30 to 60 minutes, allowing time for other corrective measures to be taken. The calcium dose may be repeated if initial dosing does not reverse ECG changes, or if the implementation of other corrective measures is delayed. Following initial membrane stabilization with calcium, attention is then turned to other fast-acting therapies to decrease the serum potassium concentration. Insulin moves potassium into cells via insulin-dependent potassium/glucose cotransporter, but for rapid effect the insulin should be given intravenously. Unless the patient is hyperglycemic, IV glucose is also given to prevent hypoglycemia. The usual dose is 10 units of insulin and 25 g of IV glucose (one ampule of D50). Beta-agonists can also be used to drive potassium into cells. Bicarbonate therapy will cause the potassium to shift intracellularly via H^+/K^+ ion exchange as the body attempts to stabilize the pH. Given the risks associated with bicarbonate therapy, this therapy is usually reserved for patients who are significantly acidotic and are able to be effectively ventilated.

Each of these therapies has relatively rapid onset of action, but none changes the total body potassium content, and therefore they are bridge therapies until therapies to actually deplete potassium stores can be implemented. Loop diuretics and sodium polystyrene sulfonate (a potassium binder) will both reduce potassium stores in the body. Hemodialysis is utilized in refractory cases, or in chronic kidney disease patients who already have dialysis access. It is very reasonable to repeat the potassium if it may be a lab error (answer e). In the presence of electrocardiographic changes suggestive of severe hyperkalemia, however, you should "treat first and ask questions later."

57. The answer is a. Daily interruption of sedation ("sedation holiday") to assess readiness for extubation has been shown to decrease the risk of ventilator-acquired pneumonia (VAP). Oropharyngeal (rather than naso-pharyngeal) intubation, elevating the head of the bed (rather than keep-ing the patient flat), and subglottic secretion suctioning can also decrease VAP. Nasopharyngeal and gastrointestinal tract bacterial flora modulation via topical or oral antibiotics may also decrease VAP risk, although it is not routinely recommended. Prophylactic intravenous antibiotics are not recommended.

58. The answer is a. The patient has developed atrial flutter with a 2:1 conduction. Although supraventricular tachycardia (SVT) or ventricular tachycardia (VT) may occasionally present with a rate of 150/min, the most common cause of that particular heart rate in an elderly hospitalized patient is atrial flutter. The sawtooth pattern on the telemetry strip represents the circuitous atrial depolarization at an atrial rate of 300. Atrial fibrillation/flutter is more likely to develop in predisposed individuals when exposed to physiologic stress. Once atrial flutter or atrial fibrillation with rapid ventric-ular response has been diagnosed, the rate needs to be controlled. Although the patient has not yet decompensated, it is unlikely that an elderly heart will be able to maintain a rate of 150 for an extended period of time. Carotid massage, ocular pressure, or Valsalva maneuvers can be attempted to slow the heart rate, but medications are usually required. The first-line agents are AV nodal-blocking agents such as beta-blockers and non-dihydropyridine calcium-channel blockers (such as diltiazem). If patients do not respond to rate control, antiarrhythmic agents such as amiodarone can be employed. Dihydropyridine calcium-channel blockers (CCB) (answer b) may have a greater effect on blood pressure than heart rate, leading to hypotension. Immediate electrical cardioversion (answer c) is the treatment of choice for a patient with hypotension or evidence of end-organ hypoperfusion (confusion, chest pain, oliguria). Our patient, however, does not appear to have decompensated yet. Checking for lab evidence of myocardial isch-emia (answer d) is unlikely to be helpful at this time. Even if the patient has underlying coronary artery disease, elevated biochemical markers will not change the immediate management, that is, control of the ventricular rate. The patient may very well need to be anticoagulated (answer e) depending on the need for cardioversion and risk of cardioembolism (as derived from the CHADS2 score), but this will not take precedence over immediate rate control to decrease myocardial oxygen demand.

59. The answer is d. This patient suffered a medical error. Even though there was no harm to the patient, most physicians would feel that the ethical principle of truth-telling dictates that the patient should be informed. In addition to informing the patient and offering an apology, physicians have a responsibility to report this error to the institution. An institutional culture of patient safety facilitates the reporting of these types of errors in order to correct system issues which contributed to the error. Most hospitals have a formal reporting mechanism such as a Patient Safety Network. Simply informing the individual staff member is less likely to result in an institutional review and implementation of measures designed to decrease the likelihood of a similar error in the future. Writing an order for an ultrasound that was not indicated also violates the ethical principle of truth-telling.

60. The answer is c. This patient exhibits several symptoms suggestive of acute alcoholic withdrawal syndrome, including hypertension, tachycardia, fever, and delirium with hallucinations. An acute intracranial event will usually be associated with head trauma (subdural hematoma) or focal neurological abnormalities. In addition, radiographic imaging may be difficult to perform while the patient is acutely agitated. Haloperidol is commonly used to treat acute psychosis, but benzodiazepines are better in the setting of alcohol withdrawal. The patient's blood pressure will likely improve with administration of benzodiazepine and beta-blockade may be unnecessary. Physical restraints should only be used as a therapy "of last resort" and do not take the place of treating the underlying disorder.

Suggested Readings

1. Kasper DL, Fauci AS, Hauser SL, Longo DL, Jameson LJ, Loscalzo. *Harrison's Principles of Internal Medicine*, 19th ed. New York: McGraw-Hill; 2015. Chapters 9, 12e, 17e, 43, 97, 147, 264, 324 ,327, 473e.
2. Society of Hospital Medicine, Clinical topic webpage, available at: http://www.hospitalmedicine.org/Web/Quality_Innovation/Resources_by_Clinical_Topic/Web/Clinical_Topics/Clinical_Home.aspx.

3. Agency for Healthcare Research and Quality Patient Safety Network, available at: http://psnet.ahrq.gov/default.aspx), especially "Handoffs and signouts" and "Voluntary patient safety reporting (incident reporting)"
4. Surviving Sepsis Guidelines—Review and Update 2013, available at: http://pulmccm.org/2013/review-articles/surviving-sepsis-guidelines-2013-review-update/
5. Wachter RM. The hospitalist field turns 15: New opportunities and challenges. *J Hosp Med*. 2011;6:E1-4. doi: 10.1002/jhm.913.

Rheumatology

Questions

61. A 40-year-old woman complains of pain and swelling in both wrists and ankles for 7 weeks. She has several months of fatigue. Morning stiffness impairs her activities for approximately 2 hours. OTC naproxen provides temporary relief. On examination, the metacarpophalangeal (MCP) joints and wrists are warm and tender; there is slight tenderness to pressure over the ankles and metatarsophalangeal (MTP) joints as well. All other joints are normal. There is no alopecia, photosensitivity, kidney disease, or rash. Which of the following is correct?

a. The clinical picture suggests early rheumatoid arthritis (RA), and a rheumatoid factor and anti-cyclic citrullinated peptide (anti-CCP) should be obtained.
b. The prodrome of lethargy suggests chronic fatigue syndrome (CFS).
c. Lack of systemic symptoms suggests osteoarthritis.
d. X-rays of the hand are likely to show joint space narrowing and erosion.
e. An aggressive search for occult malignancy is indicated.

62. A 70-year-old man complains of fever and pain in his left knee. Several days ago, he suffered an abrasion of his knee while working in his garage. The knee is red, warm, and swollen. An arthrocentesis is performed, which shows 200,000 leukocytes/μL and a glucose of 20 mg/dL. No crystals are noted. Which of the following is the most important next step?

a. Gram stain and culture of joint fluid
b. Urethral culture
c. Uric acid level
d. Antinuclear antibody (ANA)
e. Antineutrophil cytoplasmic antibody (ANCA)

63. A 60-year-old woman complains of dry mouth and a gritty sensation in her eyes. She states it is sometimes difficult to speak for more than a few minutes. There is no history of diabetes mellitus or neurologic disease. The patient is on no medications. On examination, the buccal mucosa appears dry and the salivary glands are enlarged bilaterally. Which of the following best describes the pathophysiology of the condition?

a. Previous exposure to group A streptococcal organisms have stimulated an auto-immune response that leads to cross-reactivity between host and organism with tissue destruction and reduced tear and saliva production.
b. T cells infiltrate exocrine glands and B cells become hyper-reactive. Auto-antibodies ensue including anti-Ro/SSA and anti-La/SSB. Both pro- and anti-apoptotic messages are sent to ductal and acinar epithelial cells.
c. Activated T cells and monocytes accumulate in the skin leading to induration for unknown reasons. This infiltration leads to structural abnormalities in various tissues and organs hence a reduction in normal functioning. Anti-topoisomerase-I and anti-centromere autoantibodies are commonly present.
d. Immune complexes form and deposit in vessel walls. Vasoactive amines includ-ing histamine, bradykinin, and leukotrienes are released, and vessel permeability is increased. Complement activation occurs and mononuclear cells are attracted causing infiltration and decreased gland function.
e. Necrotizing vasculitis of small arteries and veins leads to granuloma formation and decreased exocrine function of salivary and lacrimal glands.

64. The patient in the previous question has read extensively on the Inter-net about her probable diagnosis and wonders if more testing can be done to confirm the diagnosis. She is aware of the Schirmer test (quantitative tear production test) and has already had that done by her optometrist. She is on cyclosporine eye drops with some improvement in the gritty eye symptoms. What more could be done at this point to further confirm the diagnosis?

a. Give a therapeutic trial of prednisone 20 mg/d for 1 month.
b. Obtain a detailed family history of rheumatologic conditions in first-degree family members.
c. Biopsy the patient's lip and check autoantibody levels in the serum.
d. Check IgG and IgM antibodies against mumps.
e. Diagnostic/therapeutic trial of hard candy, sugarless gum, and warm soaks to the parotid glands for 1 month.

65. A 40-year-old man complains of acute onset of exquisite pain and tenderness in the left ankle. There is no history of trauma. The patient is taking hydrochlorothiazide for hypertension. On examination, the ankle is very swollen and tender. There are no other physical examination abnormalities. Which of the following is the best next step in management?

a. Begin colchicine and broad-spectrum antibiotics.
b. Perform arthrocentesis.
c. Begin allopurinol if uric acid level is elevated.
d. Obtain ankle x-ray to rule out fracture.
e. Apply a splint or removable cast.

66. A 48-year-old Caucasian woman complains of joint pain and morning stiffness for 4 months. Examination reveals swelling of the wrists and MCPs as well as tenderness and joint effusion in both knees. The rheumatoid factor is positive, antibodies to cyclic citrullinated protein are present, and subcutaneous nodules are noted on the extensor surfaces of the forearm. Which of the following statements is correct?

a. Prednisone 60 mg/d should be started.
b. The patient should be evaluated for disease-modifying antirheumatic therapy.
c. A nonsteroidal anti-inflammatory drug (NSAID) should be added to aspirin.
d. The patient's prognosis is highly favorable.
e. The patient should receive a 3-month trial of full-dose NSAID before determining whether and/or what additional therapy is indicated.

67. The woman in the previous question is disturbed by her new diagnosis, not only because of the personal pain and suffering she may endure throughout the treatment of her lifelong condition, but also because she wonders about the implications for her four sons who are between the ages of 20 and 26 years. She requests information about the epidemiology and genetics of the condition. Choose the most accurate educational statement from the choices below.

a. This condition is rare and has no particular familial predilection so she can rest assured about her children.
b. This condition occurs in about 1% of the US population, is three times more common in women than men and increases in incidence with age. There is about a fourfold increase in the disease among first-degree family members and about 10% of affected individuals have a family member with the disease.
c. Ninety percent of patients with this disease are women of childbearing age; it affects all races although it is more prevalent in African-Americans.
d. This condition is seen worldwide on a sporadic basis. There are only 9 to 19 cases per million per year. This can affect people of all races.
e. This disease occurs in only 4 per 100,000 people in the United States. It usually occurs after the age of 50 and is slightly more common in women than men and slightly more common in whites than non-whites.

68. A 76-year-old man complains of a 1-year history of low back and buttock pain that worsens with walking and is relieved by sitting or bending forward. He has hypertension and takes hydrochlorothiazide but has otherwise been healthy. There is no history of back trauma, fever, or weight loss. On examination, the patient has a slightly stooped posture, pain on lumbar extension, and has a slightly wide based gait. Pedal pulses are normal and there are no femoral bruits. Examination of peripheral joints and skin is normal. What is the most likely cause for this patient's back and buttock pain?

a. Lumbar spinal stenosis
b. Herniated nucleus pulposus
c. Atherosclerotic peripheral vascular disease
d. Facet joint arthritis
e. Prostate cancer

69. A 22-year-old man develops the insidious onset of low back pain improved with exercise and worsened by rest. There is no history of diarrhea, conjunctivitis, urethritis, rash, or nail changes. On examination, the patient has loss of mobility with respect to lumbar flexion and extension. He has a kyphotic posture. Which test or group of tests would be most supportive of your suspected diagnosis?

a. MRI of the lumbosacral spine showing spinal compression fractures associated with bony destruction.

b. An elevated sedimentation rate, a mild anemia on CBC, positive HLA-B27 in blood and sclerosis of the sacroiliac joints on plain films of the back.

c. A positive rheumatoid factor, anti-CCP, and an elevated C-reactive protein level.

d. Lumbosacral x-rays showing vertebral joint space narrowing and osteophyte formation at various levels.

e. A colonoscopy with biopsy results consistent with Crohn disease.

70. A 20-year-old woman has developed low-grade fever, a malar rash, and arthralgias of the hands over several months. High titers of anti-DNA antibodies are noted, and complement levels are low. The patient's white blood cell (WBC) count is 3000/μL and platelet count is 90,000/μL. The patient is on no medications and has no signs of active infection. Which of the following statements is correct?

a. If glomerulonephritis, severe thrombocytopenia, or hemolytic anemia develops, high-dose glucocorticoid therapy would be indicated.

b. Central nervous system (CNS) symptoms will occur within 10 years.

c. The patient can be expected to develop Raynaud phenomenon when exposed to cold.

d. Joint deformities will likely occur.

e. The disease process described is an absolute contraindication to pregnancy.

71. A 45-year-old woman has pain in her fingers on exposure to cold, arthralgias, and difficulty swallowing solid food. She has a few telangiectasias over the chest but no erythema of the face or extensor surfaces. There is slight thickening of the skin over the hands, arms, and torso. What is the best diagnostic workup?

a. Rheumatoid factor and anti-CCP antibodies

b. Antinuclear, anti-Scl-70, and anticentromere antibodies

c. Creatine kinase (CK) and antisynthetase antibodies (such as anti-Jo-1)

d. BUN and creatinine

e. Reproduction of symptoms and findings by immersion of hands in cold water

72. A 20-year-old man complains of arthritis and eye irritation. He has a history of burning on urination. On examination, there is a joint effusion of the right knee and a rash of the glans penis. Which of the following is correct?

a. *Neisseria gonorrhoeae* is likely to be cultured from the glans penis.
b. The patient is likely to be rheumatoid factor-positive.
c. An infectious process of the gastrointestinal (GI) tract may precipitate this disease.
d. An ANA is very likely to be positive.
e. CK will be elevated.

73. A 22-year-old man presents to your office with complaint of right knee pain and swelling for the past 2 weeks. Although uncomfortable, it has not prevented ambulation. He denies any fevers or night sweats. He has had four sexual partners over the past 6 months but denies dysuria or urethral discharge. With prompting, the patient recalls a rash on his arm accompanied by fever after a trip to upstate New York to attend a music festival 1 month ago. He felt the rash was interesting, and took a picture which he saved to his smartphone (shown in figure below). Which of the following would be the most appropriate next step in the management of this disease?

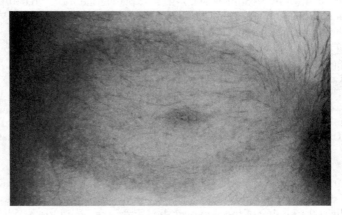

Reproduced, with permission, from Wolff K, et al. *Fitzpatrick's Color Atlas & Synopsis of Clinical Dermatology*. 5th ed. New York, NY: McGraw-Hill Education, 2005. Figure 22-63.

a. Urethral swab and empiric treatment for *Chlamydia*
b. Empiric therapy with doxycycline while awaiting the results of Lyme antibody titers
c. Western blot testing for Lyme disease
d. Empiric corticosteroids
e. Testing for rheumatoid factor and anti-CCP

74. A 75-year-old man complains of headache. On one occasion he transiently lost vision in his right eye. He also complains of aching in the shoulders and neck, particularly in the morning. There are no focal neurologic findings. Carotid pulses are normal without bruits. Laboratory data show a mild anemia. Erythrocyte sedimentation rate (ESR) is 85. Which of the following is the best approach to management?

a. Begin glucocorticoid therapy and arrange for temporal artery biopsy.
b. Schedule temporal artery biopsy and begin corticosteroids based on biopsy results and clinical course.
c. Schedule carotid angiography.
d. Follow ESR and consider further studies if it remains elevated.
e. Start aspirin and defer any invasive studies unless further symptoms develop.

75. A 53-year-old woman presents with pain in the fingers bilaterally. Examination reveals inflammation of the synovium of multiple distal interphalangeal (DIP) and proximal interphalangeal (PIP) joints. Larger joints are spared. Skin examination reveals this lesion (see figure). What is the most likely diagnosis?

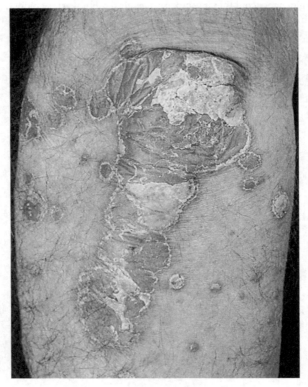

Reproduced, with permission, from Wolff K, et al. *Fitzpatrick's Color Atlas & Synopsis of Clinical Dermatology.* 6th ed. New York, NY: McGraw-Hill Education, 2009. Figure 3-3.

a. Hemochromatosis
b. Rheumatoid arthritis
c. Osteoarthritis
d. Systemic lupus erythematosus (SLE)
e. Psoriatic arthritis

76. A 65-year-old man develops the onset of severe right knee pain over 24 hours. The knee is red, swollen, and tender. The patient does not have fever or systemic symptoms; he has never had severe joint pain before. Plain film of the knee shows linear calcification of the articular cartilage without destructive change. Definitive diagnosis is best made by which of the following?

a. Serum uric acid
b. Serum calcium
c. Arthrocentesis and identification of positively birefringent rhomboid crystals
d. Rheumatoid factor
e. ANA

77. A 35-year-old woman complains of aching all over. She sleeps poorly and all her muscles and joints hurt. Her symptoms have progressed over several years. She reports that she is desperate because pain and weakness often cause her to drop things. Physical examination shows multiple points of tenderness over the neck, shoulders, elbows, and wrists. There is no joint swelling or deformity. A complete blood count and ESR are normal. Rheumatoid factor is negative. Which of the following is the best therapeutic option in this patient?

a. Graded aerobic exercise
b. Prednisone
c. Weekly methotrexate
d. Hydroxychloroquine
e. An NSAID

78. A 38-year-old man has pain and stiffness in his right knee. This began 2 weeks ago after he fell while skiing. On two occasions he had the sense that his knee was locked in a semiflexed position for a few seconds. He has noted a popping sensation when he bends his knee. On examination there is tenderness over the medial joint line of the knee. Marked flexion and extension of the knee are painful. The Lachman test (anterior displacement of the lower leg with the knee at 20 degree of flexion) and the anterior drawer test are negative. What is the most likely diagnosis?

a. Medial meniscus tear
b. Osteoarthritis
c. Anterior cruciate ligament tear
d. Chondromalacia patellae
e. Lumbosacral radiculopathy

79. Over the past 6 weeks a 35-year-old nurse has developed progressive difficulty getting out of chairs and climbing stairs. She can no longer get in and out of the bathtub. She has no muscle pain and takes no regular medications. She does not use alcohol and does not smoke cigarettes. On examination she has a purplish rash that involves both eyelids. There is weakness of the proximal leg muscles. Neurological examination is normal. What is the best next diagnostic test?

a. Vitamin B_{12} level
b. Chest x-ray
c. HLA B27
d. MRI scan of the lumbar spine
e. CK

80. A previously healthy and active 72-year-old woman presents to your office with a complaint of stiffness and pain in her neck and shoulders. The symptoms are much worse in the morning and improve throughout the day. The pain affects the soft tissues and does not appear localized to the shoulder or hip joints. She denies headache or jaw claudication. Physical examination is unrevealing; there is no inflammatory synovitis, muscle tenderness, or skin rash. Muscle strength is normal in the deltoid and iliopsoas muscle groups. She has normal range of motion of the shoulder and hip joints. Laboratory studies reveal an elevated ESR of 92 mm/h and a mild normocytic anemia. Which of the following is the best next step in management of this patient?

a. Empiric trial of prednisone 15 mg daily
b. Graded exercise regimen
c. MRI of bilateral shoulders
d. Trapezius muscle biopsy
e. Temporal artery biopsy

81. A 28-year-old woman presents to her primary care physician with a 3-month history of fatigue. Her medical history includes severe acne. She has had three uncomplicated vaginal deliveries and has healthy children aged 5, 3, and 2 years. Questioning reveals that she develops an erythematous rash upon minimal sun exposure, and has heavy menstrual periods despite being on oral contraceptives for the past 2 years. For the past 6 months, she has taken minocycline for acne. Physical examination reveals small joint effusions and tenderness to palpation of the knees bilaterally. Laboratory testing reveals a normocytic anemia, thrombocytopenia, mild hyperbilirubinemia, and a marked elevation in her ANA titer. Which of the following statements best characterizes this patient's illness?

a. Her anemia is due to bone marrow suppression from chronic disease.
b. Her anemia is due to iron deficiency.
c. Minocycline should be discontinued.
d. Anti-histone antibodies are likely to be negative.
e. The likelihood of this patient developing venous thromboembolism is comparable to the general population.

82. A 42-year-old African-American woman presents to the clinic with a 4-week history of nonproductive cough, progressive dyspnea on exertion, and joint pain. During this time she has developed night sweats and moderate fatigue. She was born in the United States and denies travel outside the country, homelessness, or incarceration. Review of systems highlights the fact that she recently visited an optometrist secondary to blurred vision, but a change in glasses did not improve the symptom. A 5-lb unintentional weight loss is noted in her chart since her last clinic visit 3 months ago. Current vital signs include BP 110/68, HR 88, RR 22, and oxygen saturation 95% on room air. Her lungs are clear, but she has mild peripheral lymphadenopathy, with bilateral supraclavicular and axillary nodes up to 2 cm in size. The nodes are rubbery and nontender. A chest radiograph performed in your office indicates bilateral hilar lymphadenopathy, with a small area of infiltrate in the right upper lobe. Of the following, which is the best next step in management of this patient?

a. Place a tuberculin skin test to assess for active tuberculosis (TB) infection.
b. Arrange for biopsy of a lymph node.
c. Arrange for repeat chest x-ray in 3 months.
d. Begin empiric anti-tuberculous therapy.
e. Begin empiric corticosteroids.

83. A 32-year-old Japanese woman has a long history of recurrent aphthous oral ulcers. In the past 2 months she has had recurrent genital ulcers. She now presents with a red painful eye that was diagnosed as anterior uveitis. What is the most likely diagnosis?

a. Herpes simplex
b. HIV infection
c. Behçet disease
d. Diabetes mellitus
e. Systemic lupus erythematosus

84. A 53-year-old man presents with arthritis, cough, hemoptysis, and bloody nasal discharge. Urinalysis reveals 4+ proteinuria, RBCs, and RBC casts. Chest x-ray shows several bilateral cavitary nodules. CT scan of chest is shown in the figure below. Antineutrophil cytoplasmic antibody (ANCA) titers are positive in a cytoplasmic pattern. Antiproteinase 3 (PR3) antibodies are present, but antimyeloperoxidase (MPO) antibodies are absent. Which of the following is the most likely diagnosis?

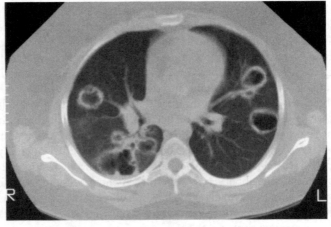

Reproduced, with permission, from Fauci A, et al. *Harrison's Principles of Internal Medicine*. 17th ed. New York, NY: McGraw-Hill Education, 2008. Figure 319-3.

a. Behçet disease
b. Sarcoidosis
c. Granulomatosis with polyangiitis (Wegener granulomatosis)
d. Henoch-Schönlein purpura
e. Classic polyarteritis nodosa

85. A 50-year-old white woman presents with aching and stiffness in the trunk, hip, and shoulders. There is widespread muscle pain after mild exertion. Symptoms are worse in the morning and improve during the day. They are also worsened by stress. The patient is always tired and exhausted. She has trouble sleeping at night. On examination, joints are normal. ESR is normal, and Lyme antibody and HIV test are negative. The patient has multiple tender points to palpation on physical examination. She asks about the best treatment option for her condition. After telling her it is still under investigation, which is the most accurate next statement?

a. Tricyclic antidepressants have proven to be the single most effective medication for the disorder.
b. Given the fact that lack of restorative sleep has been determined to exacerbate the condition, the use of sleep-inducing medications such as zolpidem has been instrumental in the treatment.
c. Low urinary cortisol in these patients has been noted; hence beginning long term, low dose prednisone has been effective in relieving symptoms.
d. Chronic opiates are the first line of treatment for this debilitating condition.
e. A multidisciplinary approach is most effective including treatment of any depression, physical therapy, an exercise program, support group attendance, and possibly the use of acetaminophen, gabapentin or similar medications as needed.

86. A 35-year-old right-handed construction worker presents with complaints of nocturnal numbness and pain involving the right hand. Symptoms wake him and are then relieved by shaking his hand. There is some atrophy of the thenar eminence. Tinel sign is positive. What is the best advice for this patient?

a. Always ensure he has a firm grip on his equipment while working on the construction site as this may relieve pressure on the median nerve.
b. Apply ice to his wrist each evening after performing his usual work.
c. Wear a wrist splint at night as initial therapy prior to considering surgery.
d. Refer the patient to physical therapy for exercises to alleviate the pain.
e. He should take a methylprednisolone taper pack for anti-inflammatory action.

87. A 35-year-old man who has been incarcerated for 3 years develops slowly progressive back pain eventually accompanied by fatigue, intermittent fevers, night sweats, weight loss, and pain in the right foot that progresses to weakness of the right leg. His WBC count and platelet count are normal but he has a normochromic, normocytic anemia. Renal and hepatic functions are normal. What is the most likely diagnosis?

a. Multiple myeloma
b. Acute myeloid leukemia (AML)
c. Spinal tuberculosis (Pott disease)
d. Transverse myelitis
e. Spondyloarthropathy

Questions 88 to 91

Select the most probable diagnosis for each patient. Each lettered option may be used once, more than once, or not at all.

a. Churg-Strauss syndrome
b. Cryoglobulinemic vasculitis.
c. Temporal arteritis
d. Granulomatosis with polyangiitis (Wegener granulomatosis)
e. Takayasu arteritis
f. Polyarteritis nodosa
g. Henoch-Schönlein purpura

88. A 78-year-old man presents with a 2-month history of fever and intermittent abdominal pain. He develops peritoneal signs and at laparotomy is found to have an area of infarcted bowel. Biopsy shows inflammation of small- to medium-sized muscular arteries.

89. An elderly male presents with pain in his shoulders and hips. Temporal arteries are tender to palpation. ESR is 105 mm/L.

90. A 45-year-old man has wheezing for several weeks and now presents with severe tingling of the hands and feet. There is wasting of the intrinsic muscles of the hands and loss of sensation in the feet. WBC is 13,000 with 28% eosinophils.

91. A 42-year-old woman with hepatitis C develops fatigue, joint aches, and palpable purplish spots on her legs. Serum creatinine is 2.1 mg/dL and a 24-hour urine protein is 750 mg.

Questions 92 to 95

Match each description with the appropriate disease. Each lettered option may be used once, more than once, or not at all.

a. Acromegaly
b. Hemochromatosis
c. Hemophilia
d. Charcot arthropathy
e. Reactive arthritis (Reiter syndrome)
f. Whipple disease

92. A 52-year-old man has a 5-year history of intermittent wrist pain and swelling, as well as lower back pain and stiffness. He presents with the complaint of diarrhea and weight loss for the past 3 months.

93. A 67-year-old man presents with pain in the small joints of the hands bilaterally. The pain is worse after prolonged activity. He is noted to be well tanned, and has nontender hepatomegaly.

94. A 33-year-old male sex worker presents with knee pain. Examination reveals bilateral conjunctivitis and a tense effusion and joint tenderness in the right knee.

95. A 62-year-old diabetic presents with burning pain of the right foot 3 weeks after an inversion injury of the ankle. Examination reveals flat arches and decreased proprioception bilaterally.

Rheumatology

Answers

61. The answer is a. The clinical picture of symmetrical swelling and tenderness of the MCP and wrist joints (as well as corresponding joints in the lower extremities) lasting longer than 6 weeks strongly suggests RA. Rheumatoid factor, an immunoglobulin directed against the Fc portion of IgG, is positive in about two-thirds of cases and may be present early in the disease. Anti-CCP antibodies are more specific (95% vs 80% for rheumatoid factor) and should be obtained as well. The history of lethargy or fatigue is a common prodrome of RA. The inflammatory joint changes on examination are not consistent with CFS; furthermore, patients with CFS typically report fatigue existing for many years. The MCP-wrist distribution of joint symptoms makes osteoarthritis very unlikely. The x-ray changes described are characteristic of RA, but would occur later in the course of the disease. Although arthritis can occasionally be a manifestation of hematologic malignancies and, rarely, other malignancies, the only indicated screening would be a complete history and physical examination along with a CBC.

62. The answer is a. The clinical and laboratory picture suggests acute septic arthritis. The most important first step is to determine the etiologic agent of the infection. *Staphylococcus aureus* is the most likely agent in this setting, and antibiotics with potent anti-Staph effect are usually started empirically while awaiting the culture results. Synovial leukocyte counts in gout typically range between 2000/µL and 50,000/µL; in addition, serum uric acid levels are often normal in acute gout. In the absence of negatively birefringent crystals in the synovial fluid, a uric acid level will not be helpful. There are no symptoms suggesting connective tissue disease, and synovial fluid cell count in lupus is generally in the 5000 to10,000 range (rather than the septic range, as in this patient). *Neisseria gonorrhoeae* can cause septic arthritis but is more common in men under age 35. Urethral culture in the absence of urethral discharge would not be helpful. ANCAs are present in certain vasculitides. There is no indication of systemic vasculitis in this patient.

63. The answer is b. The pathogenesis of Sjögren syndrome is briefly described in the answer. This process leads to lymphocytic infiltration and destruction of lacrimal and salivary glands. The clinical evaluation often includes the Schirmer test, which assesses tear production by measuring the amount of wetness on a piece of filter paper placed in the lower eyelid for 5 minutes. Each of the other answers describe the pathophysiology of another rheumatologic condition, Answer a describes post-streptococcal autoimmune response; answer c describes systemic sclerosis; answer d describes vasculitis in general; and answer e describes the pathogenesis of granulomatosis with polyangiitis (Wegener granulomatosis).

64. The answer is c. Labial biopsy can be performed to look for characteristic lymphocytic infiltration if the diagnosis is uncertain and to rule out other pathologic conditions. The specific antibodies to test for include the anti-Ro/SSA and anti-La/SSB, which are part of the international diagnostic criteria for Sjögren syndrome. Mumps can cause bilateral parotid swelling but would not involve the eyes. Systemic steroids such as prednisone are not typically used in Sjögren syndrome unless symptoms are severe and include a vasculitic component. Warm compresses, hard candy, and gum can all help with the xerostomia (dry mouth) symptoms, but a therapeutic trial would not definitively confirm or deny the diagnosis for this educated patient.

65. The answer is b. The sudden onset and severity of this monoarticular arthritis suggests acute gouty arthritis, especially in a patient on diuretic therapy. However, an arthrocentesis is indicated in the first episode to document gout by demonstrating needle-shaped, negatively birefringent crystals and to rule out other diagnoses such as infection. The level of serum uric acid during an episode of acute gouty arthritis may actually fall. Therefore, a normal serum uric acid does not exclude a diagnosis of gout. For most patients with acute gout, NSAIDs are the treatment of choice. Colchicine is also effective but causes nausea and diarrhea. Systemic corticosteroids can be used if NSAIDs are contraindicated. Antibiotics should not be started for suspected septic arthritis before an arthrocentesis is performed. Treatment for hyperuricemia should not be initiated in the setting of an acute attack of gouty arthritis. Long-term goals of management are to control hyperuricemia, prevent further attacks, and prevent joint damage. Long-term prophylaxis with allopurinol or febuxostat is considered for repeated attacks of acute arthritis, urolithiasis, or formation of tophaceous deposits. X-ray of the ankle would likely be inconclusive in this patient with no trauma history. In addition, the x-ray changes of tophaceous gout take years to develop. In the absence of trauma, there is no indication for immobilization.

66. The answer is b. The patient has more than four of the required signs or symptoms of RA, including morning stiffness, swelling of the wrist or MCP joints, simultaneous swelling of joints on both sides of body, subcutaneous nodules, and positive rheumatoid factor. Subcutaneous nodules and anti-CCP antibodies are poor prognostic signs for the activity of the disease, and disease-modifying antirheumatic drugs (DMARDs) such as methotrexate, hydroxychloroquine, sulfasalazine, leflunomide, anti-TNF agents, or a combination of these drugs should be instituted. Methotrexate is a cornerstone of most disease-modifying regimens, to which other agents are often added. High-dose corticosteroids, however, should be avoided. Use of anti-inflammatory doses of both aspirin and nonsteroidals together is not desirable because it will increase the risk of side effects. Given the aggressive nature of this woman's RA and negative prognostic signs, use of DMARDs is indicated. Significant joint damage has been shown by MRI to occur quite early in the course of disease.

67. The answer is b. Patient education about their disease, its implications on their future, and the risk that family members will develop the disease is an important part of the practice of medicine. Given the ready availability of health information on the Internet, much of which is incorrect or distorted by special interest or fringe groups, practicing clinicians must be prepared to share factual information in a nonjudgmental fashion and to help their patients understand the sometimes complex mathematical and clinical concepts involved. Answer b provides these facts about RA, but it would still be necessary to explain the concepts in laymen's terms depending on the educational level of the patient. Answer a was simply an incorrect distractor since many rheumatologic conditions have a genetic predisposition component of some sort. Answer c describes the epidemiology of SLE; d describes that of systemic sclerosis and e describes polymyalgia rheumatica (PMR).

68. The answer is a. Lumbar spinal stenosis is a frequent cause of back pain in the elderly. Patients typically have pain that radiates into the buttocks (and sometimes thighs) and is aggravated by walking and by lumbar extension. Decreased vibratory sensation and a wide based gait may also be seen. Narrowing of the spinal canal is usually caused by age-related degenerative changes. A randomized controlled trial demonstrated that surgery was more effective than medical therapy in the relief of symptoms for patients with lumbar spinal stenosis. Symptoms often recur several years after surgery.

Disc herniation and facet joint arthropathy usually cause unilateral radicular symptoms. Leg pain associated with walking can also be caused by vascular disease, but the symptoms often are unilateral and usually occur in the distal leg. Normal pedal pulses and the classic history make vascular claudication an unlikely diagnosis in this patient. The bone pain of metastatic cancer is rarely positional and is usually unremitting, causing pain both day and night.

69. The answer is b. As indicated in the question, insidious back pain occurring in a young male and improving with exercise suggests one of the spondyloarthropathies—ankylosing spondylitis, reactive arthritis (formerly termed Reiter syndrome), psoriatic arthritis, or enteropathic arthritis. In the absence of symptoms or findings to suggest one of the other conditions, laboratory tests that show a mild anemia, a positive HLA-B27 (present in 90% of patients with ankylosing spondylitis), an elevated sedimentation rate, and symmetrical sacroiliitis on x-ray would all be very supportive of the diagnosis of ankylosing spondylitis. The prognosis in ankylosing spondylitis is generally good, with only 6% dying of the disease itself. While pulmonary fibrosis and restrictive lung disease can occur, they are rarely a cause of death (cervical fracture, heart block, and amyloidosis are leading causes of death as a result of ankylosing spondylitis). The MRI described in answer a would be more suggestive of spinal tuberculosis (Pott disease) or metastatic cancer. Rheumatoid factor is negative in all the spondyloarthropathies as would be the anti-CCP test, although the C-reactive protein level could be elevated in any inflammatory condition. Joint space narrowing and osteophytes are the hallmarks of osteoarthritis which would be unusual in a young man. While Crohn disease can cause an enteropathic arthritis, which may precede the GI manifestations, this diagnosis is far less likely in this case than ankylosing spondylitis.

70. The answer is a. The combination of fever, malar rash, and arthritis suggests SLE, and the patient's thrombocytopenia, leukopenia, and positive antibody to native DNA provide more than four criteria for a definitive diagnosis. Other criteria for the diagnosis of lupus include discoid rash, photosensitivity, oral ulcers, serositis, renal disorders (proteinuria or cellular casts), and neurologic disorder (seizures or psychosis). High-dose corticosteroids would be indicated for severe or life-threatening complications of lupus such as described in answer a. The arthritis in SLE is nondeforming. Patients with SLE have an unpredictable course. Few patients develop all signs or symptoms. Neuropsychiatric disease occurs at some time in about half of all SLE patients and Raynaud phenomenon in about 25%. Pregnancy is relatively safe in women with SLE who have controlled disease and are on less than 10 mg of prednisone.

71. The answer is b. The symptoms of Raynaud phenomenon, arthralgia, and dysphagia point toward the diagnosis of scleroderma. Scleroderma, or systemic sclerosis, is characterized by a systemic vasculopathy of small- and medium-sized vessels, excessive collagen deposition in tissues, and an abnormal immune system. It is an uncommon multisystem disease affecting women more often than men. There are two variants of scleroderma— a limited type (previously known as CREST syndrome) and a more severe, diffuse disease. Antinuclear antibodies are almost universal. Anti-Scl-70 (also known as anti-topoisomerase-1) antibody occurs in only 30% of patients with diffuse disease, but a positive test is highly specific. Anti-centromere antibodies are more often positive in limited disease. Rheumatoid factor is nonspecific and present in 20% of patients with scleroderma. Elevated CK and anti-Jo-1 antibodies are expected in an inflammatory myositis such as polymyositis. Skin thickening similar to scleroderma can be seen in nephrogenic systemic fibrosis (NSF), a progressive condition that occurs in patients with stage 5 chronic kidney disease, but NSF almost always follows gadolinium administration for an MR scan. Reproduction of Raynaud phenomena is nonspecific and is not recommended as an office test.

72. The answer is c. Reactive arthritis (formerly termed Reiter syndrome) is a reactive polyarthritis that develops several weeks after an infection such as nongonococcal urethritis (NGU) or GI infection caused by *Yersinia enterocolitica*, *Campylobacter jejuni*, or *Salmonella* or *Shigella* species. Occasionally the classic triad of oligoarticular arthritis, conjunctivitis, and urethritis is seen. The disease is most common among young men and is associated with the histocompatibility antigen, HLA-B27. Reactive arthritis is the only HLA-B27-associated disease NOT characterized by sacroiliitis. Circinate balanitis is a painless red rash on the glans penis that occurs in 25% to 40% of patients with reactive arthritis. Keratoderma blenorrhagicum (a rash on the palms and soles indistinguishable from papular psoriasis) may be seen as well. Gonorrhea rarely precipitates reactive arthritis, and a negative urethral culture would be expected. ANA and rheumatoid factor are usually negative. CK would be elevated in polymyositis or dermatomyositis but not in reactive arthritis.

73. The answer is b. The patient in question has Lyme disease. Lyme disease is caused by infection with the spirochete *Borrelia burgdorferi*, transmitted by the bite of the *Ixodes* tick. In the United States, most cases are reported in the Northeast and North-central parts of the country. The majority of patients develop a characteristic rash (erythema migrans) which slowly expands over days before resolving. As the spirochete disseminates, patients can develop aseptic meningitis, nerve palsies, and cardiac conduction abnormalities. Patients will frequently develop a migratory monoarticular arthritis that can recur intermittently for months to years. Eventually, the infection causes destructive large-joint monoarticular arthritis, often of the knee or hip. The diagnosis of Lyme disease is difficult if erythema migrans (EM) is not present. With the documentation of EM and a history consistent with Lyme disease (high suspicion), a patient can be treated empirically with antibiotics. This patient's presentation with the accompanying arthritis complaints indicates disseminated disease which justifies obtaining Lyme titers and empiric therapy while awaiting the result. Western blot testing for Lyme disease is a confirmatory test performed only after an initial ELISA test has returned positive or equivocal. For very low-probability patients, neither titers nor empiric therapy are recommended. Although the patient may benefit from STD testing and treatment after his attendance to the music festival (answer a), the rash shown is not consistent with *Chlamydia*-induced reactive arthritis. As the pathogenesis of Lyme disease is fundamentally one of infection rather than immune dysregulation, empiric steroid therapy would not be indicated (answer d). It would be highly unusual for RA (answer e) to present as primarily knee involvement in this demographic, and RA would not account for the associated rash.

74. The answer is a. Headache and transient unilateral visual loss (amaurosis fugax) in this elderly patient with PMR symptoms suggest a diagnosis of temporal arteritis. The ESR is high in almost all cases. Temporal arteritis occurs most commonly in patients older than 55 years and is highly associated with PMR. However, only about 25% of patients with PMR have giant

cell arteritis. Older patients who complain of diffuse myalgias and joint stiffness, particularly of the shoulders and hips, should be evaluated for PMR
with an ESR. Unilateral visual changes or even permanent visual loss may
occur abruptly in patients with temporal arteritis. Biopsy results should not
delay initiation of corticosteroid therapy. Biopsies may show vasculitis even
after 14 days of glucocorticoid therapy. Delay risks permanent loss of sight.
Once an episode of loss of vision occurs, workup must proceed as quickly
as possible. Treatment for temporal arteritis requires relatively high doses
of steroids, beginning with prednisone at 40 to 80 mg/d for about 1 month
with subsequent tapering. Aspirin should be added because it decreases
the risks of vascular occlusions but is not sufficient alone. The treatment
for PMR without concomitant temporal arteritis requires lower doses of
steroids, in the range of 10 to 20 mg/d of prednisone. Carotid disease can
cause amaurosis fugax but would not account for the headache, PMR, or
the elevated sedimentation rate.

75. The answer is e. The patient has psoriatic arthritis. Psoriatic arthritis is an immune-mediated arthritis affecting up to 30% of patients with
psoriasis. Although psoriasis usually precedes the development of arthritis, occasionally the joint symptoms come first. Classic manifestations
include involvement of the DIP joints, presence of dactylitis ("sausage
digit"), and of course the presence of psoriasis of the skin. Joint involvement patterns are variable, however, and can mimic RA or can affect
primarily the axial skeleton. Nail changes, including pitting, horizontal
ridging, onycholysis, dystrophic hyperkeratosis, and yellowish discoloration are common. The diagnosis is primarily clinical, although radiographic evidence of "pencil in cup" deformity of the DIP joint may lend
additional weight to the diagnosis. Immunosuppression is required to
prevent deformation of the joints, either with methotrexate- or TNF-
alpha-antagonist-based therapy. Although hemochromatosis can cause
joint involvement, it typically mimics the noninflammatory presentation
of osteoarthritis, often with involvement of the second and third MCP
joints (an unusual pattern in primary osteoarthritis). The cardinal skin
manifestation of hemochromatosis is diffuse hyperpigmentation, leading to the colloquial description of "bronze diabetes." RA could cause the
joint manifestations described here, but would not cause hyperkeratotic
skin lesions. RA classically affects the MCP and spares the DIP joints.
Osteoarthritis will not present with polyarticular synovitis or a psoriatic
plaque. SLE can mimic many diseases, but discoid lupus lesions typically

have an atrophic center with erythematous scaly edge, as opposed to the uniformly thick scale seen in psoriasis.

76. The answer is c. Acute monoarticular arthritis in association with linear calcification of the cartilage of the knee (chondrocalcinosis) suggests the diagnosis of pseudogout, a form of calcium pyrophosphate dihydrate deposition (CPPDD) disease. In its acute manifestation, the disease resembles gout. Positively birefringent crystals (looking blue when parallel to the axis of the red compensator on a polarizing microscope) can be demonstrated in joint fluid, although careful search is sometimes necessary. Serum uric acid and calcium levels are normal, as are rheumatoid factor and ANA. Pseudogout is about half as common as gout, but becomes more common after the age of 65. CPPDD disease is diagnosed in symptomatic patients by characteristic x-ray findings and crystals in synovial fluid. Pseudogout is treated with NSAIDs, colchicine, or steroids. Arthrocentesis and drainage with intra-articular steroid administration is also an effective treatment. Linear calcifications or chondrocalcinosis are often found in the joints of elderly patients who do not have symptomatic joint problems; such patients do not require treatment.

77. The answer is a. The patient's multiple tender points, associated sleep disturbance, and lack of joint or muscle findings make fibromyalgia a likely diagnosis. Patients with fibromyalgia often report dropping things due to pain and weakness, but objective muscle weakness is not present on examination. The diagnosis hinges on the presence of multiple tender points in the absence of any other disease likely to cause musculoskeletal symptoms. CBC and ESR are characteristically normal. Cognitive behavioral therapy and graded aerobic exercise programs have been demonstrated to relieve symptoms. Tricyclic antidepressants are considered if medication is needed and may help restore sleep. Cyclobenzaprine is a next step medication. If both of those fail, then a trial of gabapentin, pregabalin, or duloxetine can be undertaken. Aspirin, other anti-inflammatory drugs (including corticosteroids), and DMARDs (such as methotrexate or hydroxychloroquine) are not helpful, nor are simple stretching/flexibility exercises. Of note, rheumatoid factor and ANAs occur in a small number of normal individuals. They are more frequent in women and increase in frequency with age. It is not uncommon for an individual with fibromyalgia and an incidentally positive RF or ANA to be misdiagnosed as having collagen vascular disease. Therefore, it is necessary to be careful to separate subjective tenderness on examination from objective musculoskeletal findings and to assiduously search for other criteria before diagnosing RA, SLE, or other collagen vascular disease.

78. The answer is a. This patient has a medial meniscus tear. This may occur after trauma, but sometimes occurs spontaneously. Patients complain of pain, stiffness, and a popping sensation. A sensation of locking is very characteristic. On examination patients frequently have tenderness at the joint line and pain on flexion and extension. Routine x-rays are usually negative and the diagnosis is made by MRI scanning. Osteoarthritis usually occurs in patients older than age 50 unless the patient is very obese. OA pain typically comes on gradually, and physical examination may reveal patellofemoral crepitance. An anterior cruciate tear usually results from a twisting injury. It is a common injury in female soccer and basketball players. Frequently a large effusion occurs acutely. Chondromalacia patellae (also called patellofemoral pain syndrome) is a common problem in runners. The pain typically worsens when the patient walks downstairs. The physical examination demonstrates lateral displacement of the patella with knee extension. Pathology in the back and hip may be referred to the knee, but is not associated with physical examination abnormalities localized to the knee.

79. The answer is e. This woman has dermatomyositis, which typically affects patients aged 40 to 50 who present with progressive proximal myopathy and complain of difficulty arising from chairs, climbing stairs, and getting out of the bathtub. About half of patients with dermatomyositis have the classic heliotrope rash. Gottron papules (red to purple papules over extensor surfaces of joints, especially of the hands) are pathognomonic if present. Lung involvement is common, but (unlike genetic muscular dystrophy) cardiac involvement is rare. Almost all patients have an elevated CK. Patients may have the anemia of chronic disease, which is normocytic. The electromyography (EMG) is characteristically abnormal with muscle fibrillations, spontaneous discharges, and sharp waves. In a small percentage of patients, the EMG may be normal. Muscle biopsy is usually diagnostic. High-dose oral corticosteroids are the treatment of choice. Some patients require the addition of methotrexate or azathioprine. Only 25% of patients are cured and most will develop a chronic condition with significant morbidity. Vitamin B_{12} deficiency causes distal sensory findings (rather than this patient's proximal motor findings) and would not account for the heliotrope rash. Imaging studies of the lumbar spine would not focus on the primary process, although MRI scanning of the thigh musculature can be a useful study. HLA B27 is diagnostically useful in the spondyloarthropathies such as ankylosing spondylitis; this patient has no back pain or morning stiffness to suggest this diagnosis.

80. The answer is a. The patient has PMR. A relatively common disease of the elderly, PMR presents as morning stiffness and pain in the shoulders, neck, and hip girdle. Diagnosis is mainly clinical; improvement of symptoms throughout the day and an absence of joint findings on physical examination provide clues to the diagnosis. Most patients have a markedly elevated ESR. PMR overlaps with giant cell (temporal) arteritis, so it is worthwhile to ask about symptoms of headache or jaw claudication. In the absence of symptoms or signs of temporal arteritis, no additional testing is indicated, and the diagnosis is presumptively confirmed by prompt response to moderate dose steroids (10-20 mg prednisone per day). Patients with occult temporal arteritis will not usually respond to modest doses of prednisone. Caution must be taken in tapering the steroids as patients with PMR frequently relapse upon discontinuation of treatment. A graded exercise regimen (answer b) would be an appropriate treatment option for fibromyalgia, but fibromyalgia rarely begins at age 72 and does not cause elevation of the ESR. MRI of the upper torso may show inflammation of the bursa and shoulder joint synovium, but this patient does not have localized tenderness in these structures. Muscle biopsy (answer d) is indicated in polymyositis or inclusion body myositis, but this patient does not have muscle weakness. Temporal artery biopsy (answer e) should be performed in patients suspected of having giant cell arteritis. Our patient, however, denies symptoms consistent with arterial involvement. If the patient does not respond to treatment with modest dose steroids, stronger consideration should be given to "blind" temporal artery biopsy.

81. The answer is c. This patient likely has drug-induced lupus erythematosus. Minocycline is one of many medications implicated. Other common offenders include procainamide, hydralazine, propylthiouracil, carbamazepine, phenytoin, and isoniazid. Stopping the offending agent is essential and will lead to resolution of the disease in weeks to months. Renal and CNS disease are uncommon in drug-induced lupus; usually skin and joint manifestations predominate. In this patient, immune-mediated hemolysis is the most likely cause of the anemia. Although depressed erythropoiesis from anemia of chronic disease (answer a) can contribute to the patient's low hemoglobin, the elevated bilirubin suggests hemolysis. Likewise, despite the heavy periods from her thrombocytopenia, long-standing iron deficiency anemia (answer b) will cause a low MCV (microcytic anemia). Anti-histone antibodies (answer d) are very common in drug-induced lupus. Answer e is incorrect as patients with lupus (drug-induced or otherwise) have a higher rate of clot formation and may suffer from antiphospholipid antibody syndrome. Although not directly related to venous thromboembolism, long-standing inflammation with lupus accelerates the rate of atherosclerosis, predisposing to arterial occlusive disease over time.

82. The answer is b. This patient presents with a likely diagnosis of sarcoidosis. The differential diagnosis includes TB (made less likely by her paucity of risk factors) and lymphoma. Sarcoidosis affects the lung in over 90% of patients. Although any organ can be affected by sarcoidosis, skin and eye are often involved. Joint involvement occurs in 10% to 20% of patients, usually affecting knees and ankles. The acute arthritis (often associated with hilar lymphadenopathy) is usually self-limited, but the chronic arthritis can be destructive. The diagnosis of sarcoidosis is made through a combination of clinical and pathologic findings. Although there are several other reasonable "best next" approaches to this patient (including clarification of the x-ray findings with a CT scan, performing additional blood work such as a blood count, hemoglobin, peripheral smear, and angiotensin converting enzyme [ACE] level), biopsy is necessary to establish the diagnosis. Although ACE level is elevated in 30% to 80% of patients with sarcoidosis, its relatively low sensitivity and specificity prevent this test from replacing the need for pathologic tissue diagnosis. TB skin testing (TST) is an imperfect approach to diagnosis in the setting of concern for active TB. Some patients exhibit anergy with active TB, leading to a false-negative skin test. Many patients will have a positive skin test that reflects latent TB, atypical mycobacterium exposure, or prior BCG vaccination. If active TB is suspected, sputum smears and cultures with patient isolation would be a more appropriate choice than skin testing, although the TST may be a part of that workup. Additionally, answer a is incorrect because the test itself does not assess "active" infection. Although many patients with asymptomatic sarcoidosis can be managed with conservative therapy and close follow-up (answer c), the diagnosis must be crystallized first. This patient is not asymptomatic; eye, joint, and lung involvement would likely require active treatment. Beginning empiric anti-tuberculous drugs may be an appropriate step (answer d) in the management of active TB, but the patient's negative risk factors for TB and the presence of bilateral hilar lymphadenopathy (unusual in TB except for those cases associated with AIDS) argue against empiric therapy. Steroids may very well be used in this patient (answer e) if the diagnosis of sarcoidosis is established, but other etiologies such as lymphoma and TB must be ruled out first.

83. The answer is c. This patient has classic Behçet disease, which occurs more commonly in Asians. Behçet disease is a multisystem disorder that usually presents with recurrent oral and genital ulcers. One-fourth of patients develop superficial or deep vein thrombophlebitis. Iritis, uveitis, and nondeforming arthritis are common. Blindness, aseptic meningitis, and CNS vasculitis may occur. Rare complications include pulmonary artery aneurysms and GI inflammation which may lead to perforation. Mucocutaneous lesions are usually treated with topical corticosteroids. Immunosuppressive therapy is recommended for patients with threatened blindness or CNS disease. The oral lesions of herpes simplex infection occur over the lips; anterior uveitis would be very uncommon. The mucocutaneous lesions of HIV infection are usually caused by *Candida* and are easily distinguishable from aphthous ulcers. Neither diabetes nor lupus would cause genital ulcers or anterior uveitis.

84. The answer is c. Granulomatosis with polyangiitis (Wegener granulomatosis) is a granulomatous vasculitis of small- and medium-sized arteries and veins. It affects the lungs, sinuses, nasopharynx, and kidneys, where it causes a focal and segmental glomerulonephritis. Cavitary lung nodules are caused by ischemic necrosis from arterial occlusion. Other organs can also be damaged, including the skin, eyes, and nervous system. Most patients with the disease develop antibodies to certain proteins in the cytoplasm of neutrophils, called ANCAs. The most common ANCA staining pattern seen in WG is cytoplasmic, C-ANCA. The C-ANCA pattern is usually caused by antibodies to proteinase-3. A perinuclear pattern, P-ANCA, is sometimes seen. P-ANCA is usually caused by antibodies to myeloperoxidase. Behçet disease is not associated with ANCA positivity. Sarcoidosis may involve the upper respiratory tract (20%), but it does not cause bloody nasal discharge, cavitary lung disease, or glomerulonephritis. Henoch-Schönlein purpura and classic polyarteritis do not involve the upper airways and rarely affect the lungs.

85. The answer is e. As discussed in the question, fibromyalgia is a very common disorder, particularly in middle-aged women, characterized by diffuse musculoskeletal pain, fatigue, and nonrestorative sleep. The American

College of Rheumatology has established diagnostic criteria for the disease, which include a history of widespread pain in association with 11 of 18 specific tender point sites. In this patient with very characteristic signs and symptoms, including the identification of 11 specific trigger points, the diagnosis is evident. Patients with fibromyalgia have an increased lifetime incidence of psychiatric disorders, particularly depression and panic disorder. However, there is convincing evidence that fibromyalgia is a disease of abnormal central nervous pain processing associated with amplification of nociceptive stimuli. This suggests that lower thresholds for noxious stimuli are caused by a CNS abnormality of as yet undetermined etiology. Tricyclic antidepressants can provide some relief in some patients but are not the single most effective medication. It is true that fibromyalgia patients have been found to lack restorative sleep in general; however, the use of sleep-inducing medications such as zolpidem is not specifically recommended. Low urinary cortisol in these patients has indeed been noted, however, there is no evidence that using steroids is helpful. Opiates are to be avoided. Some authorities recommend trials of other medications including cyclobenzaprine, gabapentin, pregabalin, or duloxetine. As described, a multidisciplinary approach is the most effective treatment and must be tailored to the individual patient.

86. The answer is c. Carpal tunnel syndrome results from median nerve entrapment and is frequently associated with excessive use of the wrist. The process can be associated with thickening of connective tissue, as in acromegaly, or with deposition of amyloid. It also occurs in hypothyroidism, RA, and diabetes mellitus. As in this patient, numbness is frequently worse at night and is relieved by shaking the hand. Atrophy of the abductor pollicis brevis as evidenced by thenar wasting is a sign of advanced disease and an indication for surgery. Tinel sign (paresthesia induced in the median nerve distribution by tapping on the volar aspect of the wrist) is characteristic but not specific. A reasonable first approach is to recommend a wrist splint at night or throughout 24 hours as initial therapy. If symptoms persist or worsen, it is typical to obtain nerve conduction velocity/EMG testing followed by carpal tunnel release surgery. The other options listed have not been proven to be effective in the condition.

87. The answer is c. Back pain is one of the most common diagnoses one encounters in medical practice. When it is accompanied by systemic symptoms of fever and night sweats and eventually neurologic deficits one must consider spinal tuberculosis (Pott disease) or a bacterial diskitis. Any patient diagnosed with TB should also be checked for HIV infection. This patient's 3 years of living in jail increased his risk of developing TB. Multiple myeloma certainly can present with back pain and bone pain but it is usually a disease of older people with the median age at onset of 66. It is often associated with renal dysfunction. AML does share the symptoms of fatigue and weight loss although joint and bone pain is less common. Most patients with AML present with symptoms related to their pancytopenia and this patient was reported to have a normal WBC count. This is also a disease of older patients generally with the median age of onset of 65. Transverse myelitis typically has a clearly defined sensory level, bilateral symptoms and autonomic symptoms including bladder dysfunction, symptoms which are not mentioned with regard to the patient in question. Spondyloarthropathy would be more likely if there was an emphasis on sacroiliitis, possible association with inflammatory bowel disease, HLA B-27 positivity, a positive family history, and other possible criteria that are not mentioned in this question.

88 to 91. The answers are 88-f, 89-c, 90-a, 91-b. The large vessel vasculitides include temporal (giant cell) arteritis and Takayasu arteritis. Temporal arteritis (question 89) typically occurs in older patients and is accompanied by aching in the shoulders and hips, jaw claudication, and a markedly elevated ESR. Takayasu arteritis, a granulomatous inflammation of the aorta and its main branches, typically occurs in young women. Symptoms are attributed to local vascular occlusion and may produce arm or leg claudication. Systemic symptoms of arthralgia, fatigue, malaise, anorexia, and weight loss may precede the vascular symptoms. Surgery may be necessary to correct occlusive lesions.

The patient in question 88 has classic polyarteritis nodosa. It is a multisystem necrotizing medium-size vessel vasculitis that, prior to the use of steroids and cyclophosphamide, was uniformly fatal. Patients commonly present with signs of vascular insufficiency in the involved organs. Abdominal involvement is common. In 30% of patients, antecedent hepatitis B virus infection can be demonstrated; immune complexes containing the virus have been found and are likely pathogenic.

Small-vessel vasculitides include granulomatosis with polyangiitis (Wegener), microscopic polyangiitis, the Churg-Strauss syndrome, Henoch-Schönlein purpura, and cryoglobulinemic vasculitis. Granulomatosis with polyangiitis usually involves the sinuses, lungs, and kidneys. Chest x-ray may reveal cavities, infiltrates, or nodules. Many patients also develop glomerulonephritis which may result in acute renal failure. On biopsy, the vasculitis is necrotizing and granulomatous. Microscopic polyangiitis is a multisystem necrotizing vasculitis that typically results in glomerulonephritis, pulmonary hemorrhage, and fever. Lung biopsy shows inflammation of capillaries. Patients may also have mononeuritis multiplex and palpable purpura. Classic polyarteritis nodosa rarely involves the lungs.

The Churg-Strauss syndrome (question 90) is characterized by wheezing, fever, eosinophilia, and systemic vasculitis that may involve the peripheral nerves, central nervous system, heart, kidneys, or GI tract. Henoch-Schönlein purpura primarily occurs in children and presents with palpable purpura, arthritis, and glomerulonephritis. One-third of affected children will have a glomerulonephritis which occasionally results in renal failure. Cryoglobulinemia (question 91) can be associated with a small-vessel vasculitis. Patients typically present with palpable purpura, arthritis, and glomerulonephritis. Cryoglobulinemia is often associated with hepatitis C.

92 to 95.   The answers are 92-f, 93-b, 94-e, 95-d. Many joint and musculo-skeletal disorders are associated with broader systemic disease.

Acromegaly results from the overproduction of growth hormone from the anterior pituitary. Over time, this causes the disorganized growth of cartilage in the joint, with widening of the joint space. This disorganized cartilage is predisposed to ulceration and destruction. With destruction of the excess cartilage, ligament laxity can occur. The clinical presentation involves joint pain with activity, joint laxity, and crepitus. Additional findings include coarsening of facial features, enlargement of the hands and feet, and carpal tunnel syndrome. Patients may also complain of Raynaud phenomenon.

Hemochromatosis (question 93) is an abnormality of iron absorption. Although iron deposition can affect any organ, up to 40% of patients with hemochromatosis develop joint abnormalities. The patient typically will note pain in the small joints of the hands with activity, although other joints can be involved. Often bilateral second and third MCP joints are affected early in the disease course. As in pseudogout and acromegaly, chondrocalcinosis may be present radiographically. Clues to this diagnosis include skin hyperpigmentation and liver or pancreatic dysfunction. Ferritin level and transferrin saturation (iron level divided by total iron binding capacity) will be elevated. Appropriate management of hemochromatosis with phlebotomy does not usually reverse the joint symptoms.

Hemophilia can induce arthritic changes because of recurrent bleeding into a joint. After bleeding into the joint (usually a large joint such as the knee), blood is slowly resorbed over a period of weeks. With recurrent bleeding episodes, the joint becomes chronically inflamed and swollen. Flexion deformities can lead to severe limitation of function.

Charcot arthropathy (question 95) occurs with the loss of innervation to the joint. In the absence of neurologic input, normal muscle responses that attenuate the wear and damage on a joint are lost. Over time, the joint loses articular cartilage. Additionally, there may be an increase in blood flow and bone resorption in the affected limb, leading to increased risk of bone fractures and injury. Patients may present after an injury from relatively minor trauma, and the degree of pain may be less than anticipated because of the neuropathy. Diabetes mellitus is the most common cause of neuropathic joint.

Reactive arthritis, formerly termed Reiter syndrome, (question 94) is an immune-mediated event typically triggered by an infectious agent. Enteric pathogens such as *Campylobacter, Salmonella,* and *Shigella* can trigger the syndrome, as can *Chlamydia trachomatis* genital infections. Classically the disease presents with urethritis, conjunctivitis, and arthritis. Unlike enteric pathogen-triggered disease, chlamydial-triggered reactive arthritis usually occurs in men. The arthritis is usually asymmetric and involves the lower extremities. In spite of obvious joint effusion and intense inflammation in the synovial fluid, culture of synovial fluid will be negative.

Whipple disease (question 92) is an uncommon chronic bacterial infection caused by the organism *Tropheryma whipplei*. Although classically recognized by the development of a malabsorption syndrome, in the majority of patients arthritis precedes the GI symptoms by years. The arthritis is migratory, intermittent, and of relatively short duration (hours to days). Antimicrobial treatment can be curative.

Suggested Readings

1. Kasper DL, Fauci AS, Hauser SL, Longo DL, Jameson LJ, Loscalzo J. *Harrison's Principles of Internal Medicine*, 19th ed. New York: McGraw-Hill; 2015. Chapters 22, 378, 380, 382, 384, 385, 393, 394, 395, 396.
2. Lawry GV. *Systematic Musculoskeletal Examinations*. New York: McGraw-Hill; 2012. Chapters 3, 4, 5. ISBN 978-0-07-174521-5.

3. Imboden JB, Hellmann DB, Stone JH. *Current Diagnosis & Treatment: Rheumatology.* 3rd ed. New York: McGraw-Hill; 2013. Chapters 2, 3, 4, 5, 6. ISBN 978-0-07-163805-0.
4. Rheumatology Best Practices website available at: http://www.cleveland-clinicmeded.com/online/rhr-best-practices/
5. Rheumatology guidelines (American College of Rheumatology) available at: https://www.rheumatology.org/Practice/Clinical/Guidelines/Clinical_Practice_Guidelines/
6. Tsokos GC. Systemic lupus erythematosus. *N Engl J Med.* 2011;365: 2110-2121.
7. Vaglio A, Buzio C, Zwerina J. Eosinophilic granulomatosis with polyangiitis (Churg-Strauss): State of the art. *Allergy.* 2013;68:261-273.
8. Khanna PP, Gladue HS, Singh MK, et al. Treatment of acute gout: A systematic review. *Semin Arthritis Rheum.* 2014;44:31-38.

Pulmonary Disease

Questions

96. A 50-year-old patient with long-standing chronic obstructive lung disease develops the insidious onset of aching in the distal extremities, particularly the wrists bilaterally. He reports a 10-lb weight loss. The skin over the wrists is warm and erythematous. There is bilateral clubbing. Plain film of the forearms reveals bilateral periosteal thickening, but no joint abnormality. Which of the following is the most appropriate management of this patient?

a. Start vancomycin.
b. Obtain chest x-ray.
c. Aspirate both wrists.
d. Begin methotrexate therapy.
e. Obtain erythrocyte sedimentation rate.

97. A 63-year-old man who has been previously healthy is admitted to the hospital with a 2-day history of cough, rigors, fever, and right-sided pleuritic chest pain. Chest x-ray shows consolidation of the right lower lobe (RLL) and a free-flowing right pleural effusion. Thoracentesis is performed, and the pleural fluid has the following characteristics:

Cell count = 1110/mm^3
Glucose = 75 mg/dL (serum glucose = 85 mg/dL)
Protein = 4.0 g/dL (serum protein = 7.0 g/dL)
LDH = 400 U/L (serum LDH = 200 U/L, normal = 100 – 200 U/L)
pH = 7.35

What is the pathogenesis of the pleural effusion?

a. Increase in hydrostatic pressure
b. Decrease in oncotic pressure
c. Increased permeability of visceral pleural membrane capillaries
d. Bacterial infection in the pleural space
e. Hemorrhage into the pleural space

98. A 40-year-old alcoholic develops cough and fever. Sputum is fetid and examination reveals crackles in the right base. Chest x-ray, shown below, shows an air-fluid level in the superior segment of the right lower lobe. Which of the following is the most likely etiologic agent?

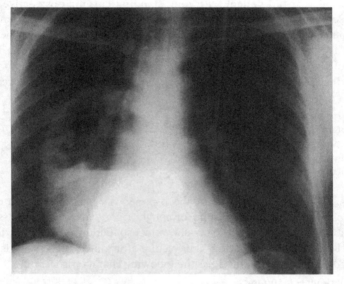

Reproduced, with permission, from Fauci A, et al. *Harrison's Principles of Internal Medicine*. 17th ed. New York, NY: McGraw-Hill Education, 2008.

a. *Streptococcus pneumoniae*
b. *Haemophilus influenzae*
c. *Legionella pneumophila*
d. Anaerobes
e. *Mycoplasma pneumoniae*

99. A previously healthy 18-year-old high school student suddenly develops left-sided pleuritic chest pain and dyspnea while at the senior prom. In the emergency room examination reveals BP = 110/60 mm Hg, P = 110 beats/min, respiratory rate = 36 breaths/min, T = 37°C (98°F). There are hyperresonance to percussion, decreased tactile fremitus, and absent breath sounds over the left chest anteriorly. Chest x-ray is as shown.

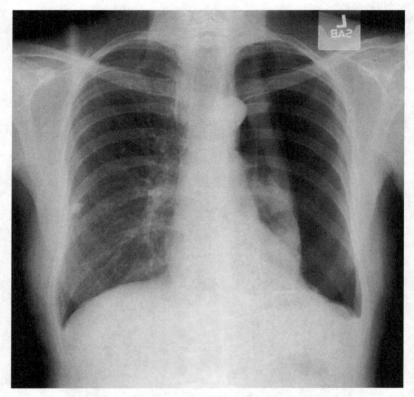

Reproduced, with permission, from Stead L, Stead SM, Kaufman M. *First Aid Radiology for the Wards*. New York: McGraw-Hill Education, 2009. Figure 2-28.

What is the most likely etiology of this patient's condition?

a. Infection of the lung parenchyma
b. Malignant neoplasm of the pleura
c. Rib fracture
d. Rupture of a subpleural apical bleb
e. Anxiety

100. A 70-year-old man with chronic obstructive lung disease requires 2 L/min of nasal O_2 to treat his hypoxia, which is sometimes associated with angina. The patient develops pleuritic chest pain, fever, and purulent sputum. While using his oxygen at an increased flow of 5 L/min, he becomes stuporous and develops a respiratory acidosis with CO_2 retention and worsening hypoxia. What would be the most appropriate next step in the management of this patient?

a. Stop oxygen
b. Begin medroxyprogesterone
c. Intubate and begin mechanical ventilation
d. Treat with antibiotics and observe on the general medicine ward for 24 hours
e. Begin sodium bicarbonate

101. A 34-year-old black woman presents to your office with symptoms of cough, dyspnea, and fatigue. Physical examination shows cervical lymphadenopathy and hepatomegaly. Spleen tip is palpable. Her chest radiograph is shown below. Which of the following is the best approach in establishing a diagnosis?

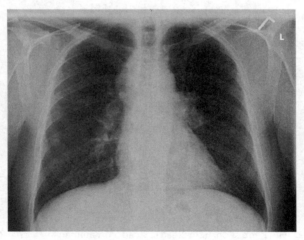

Reproduced, with permission, from Fauci A, et al. *Harrison's Principles of Internal Medicine.* 17th ed. New York, NY: McGraw-Hill Education, 2008.

a. Open lung biopsy
b. Liver biopsy
c. Bronchoscopy and transbronchial lung biopsy
d. Mediastinoscopic lymph node biopsy
e. Serum angiotensin-converting enzyme (ACE) level

102. A 64-year-old woman presents with 6 weeks of fatigue, dyspnea, and night sweats. She has lost 11 lb. She has no history of trauma, has never had surgery, and takes no medications. Chest x-ray reveals a large right-sided pleural effusion. Thoracentesis yields pleural fluid that appears milky. Pleural fluid triglyceride level is 500 mg/dL. Which of the following disorders is most likely in this patient?

a. Lymphoma
b. Congestive heart failure
c. Pulmonary embolism
d. Pneumonia
e. Systemic lupus erythematosus

103. A 25-year-old man presents to the clinic for evaluation of infertility. He has a lifelong history of a productive cough and recurrent pulmonary infections. On his review of symptoms he has indicated chronic problems with abdominal pain, diarrhea, and difficulty gaining weight. He also has diabetes mellitus. His chest x-ray suggests bronchiectasis. Which is the most likely diagnosis?

a. Chronic obstructive pulmonary disease (COPD)
b. Immunoglobulin deficiency
c. Cystic fibrosis
d. Whipple disease
e. Asthma

104. A 62-year-old automobile service worker presents with gradually worsening exertional dyspnea over the preceding several months. Recently, he has noticed right pleuritic chest pain. He has hypertension, well controlled on amlodipine 5 mg/d. He takes no other medications. He has never noticed cough or wheezing while at work. He worked for 15 years in construction and demolition and for 20 years thereafter in the service department of an automotive dealership. He denies fever, chills, or night sweats. On physical examination, he is in no respiratory distress but has right basilar dullness. His finger oximetry reads 96% on room air. Chest x-ray reveals a moderate right pleural effusion and lateral pleural thickening on both sides. Thoracentesis shows reddish fluid, which on formal analysis is an exudate with 45,000 RBCs/hpf. Cytology is negative. What is the most likely explanation for this patient's symptoms?

a. Drug-induced interstitial lung disease
b. Infection due to *Mycobacterium tuberculosis*
c. Hypersensitivity pneumonitis due to thermophilic actinomycetes
d. Occupational asthma due to isocyanates
e. Asbestos exposure

105. A 40-year-old man without a significant medical history comes to the emergency room with a 3-day history of fever and shaking chills, and a 15-minute episode of rigor. He also reports a cough productive of yellow-green sputum, anorexia, and the development of right-sided pleuritic chest pain. Shortness of breath has been present for the past 12 hours. Chest x-ray reveals a consolidated right middle lobe infiltrate, and CBC shows an elevated neutrophil count with many band forms present. Which feature would most strongly support inpatient admission and IV antibiotic treatment for this patient?

a. Recent exposure to a family member with influenza
b. Respiratory rate of 36/min
c. Recent sexual exposure to an HIV-positive patient
d. Purulent sputum with gram-positive diplococci on Gram stain
e. Signs of consolidation (bronchial breath sounds, egophony) on physical examination

106. A 57-year-old man is admitted to the hospital because of acute shortness of breath several days after a 12-hour transcontinental air flight. Findings on physical examination are normal except for tachypnea and tachycardia. He does not have edema or popliteal tenderness. An electrocardiogram (ECG) reveals sinus tachycardia but is otherwise normal. Which of the following statements is correct?

a. A normal D-dimer level excludes pulmonary embolus
b. If there is no contraindication to anticoagulation, full-dose heparin or enoxaparin should be started pending further testing
c. Normal findings on examination of the lower extremities make pulmonary embolism unlikely
d. Early treatment of pulmonary embolism has little effect on overall mortality
e. A normal lower extremity venous Doppler study will rule out a pulmonary embolus

107. A 40-year-old woman has had increasing fatigue and shortness of breath for 6 months. Physical examination reveals normal vital signs and a resting O_2 saturation of 97%. Her lungs are clear without rales or wheezing. Cardiac examination shows a prominent pulmonary component of the second heart sound (P_2) and a soft systolic murmur at the left sternal border that varies with respiration. Her neck veins show a prominent v wave. Chest x-ray shows right ventricular hypertrophy and enlargement of the central pulmonary arteries. What is the best next step in establishing a diagnosis in this patient?

a. Echocardiogram
b. Spirometry with measurement of diffusing capacity of carbon monoxide
c. Exercise stress test
d. Alpha-1 antitrypsin level
e. Right heart catheterization

108. A 65-year-old man with mild congestive heart failure is scheduled to receive total hip replacement. He has no other underlying diseases and no history of hypertension, recent surgery, or bleeding disorder. Which of the following is the best approach to prevention of pulmonary embolus in this patient?

a. Aspirin 75 mg/d
b. Aspirin 325 mg/d
c. Enoxaparin 30 mg subcutaneously bid
d. Early ambulation
e. Graded compression elastic stockings

109. An obese 50-year-old woman complains of insomnia, daytime sleepiness, and fatigue. During a sleep study she is found to have recurrent episodes of arterial desaturation—about 30 events per hour—with evidence of obstructive apnea. Which of the following is the treatment of choice for this patient?

a. Nasal continuous positive airway pressure
b. Uvulopalatopharyngoplasty
c. Hypocaloric diet
d. Tracheostomy
e. Oxygen via nasal cannula

110. A 42-year-old woman comes to the hospital with 3 days of fever, nausea, vomiting, and right-sided flank pain. On examination she appears ill and has right costovertebral angle tenderness. Urinalysis is positive for leukocyte esterase, and microscopic examination of urine reveals numerous white blood cells and gram-negative rods. She is admitted with a diagnosis of pyelonephritis and is begun on IV ceftriaxone. Blood cultures subsequently are positive for *Escherichia coli* sensitive to ceftriaxone. She initially improves, but on the third hospital day complains of severe dyspnea that is not relieved by the administration of oxygen. On examination that day she appears ill and has tachypnea, tachycardia, labored breathing, cyanosis, and diffuse rales. Arterial blood gases (ABGs) drawn while on a 100% nonrebreathing mask show pH = 7.45, partial pressure of oxygen (Po_2) = 45, and partial pressure of carbon dioxide (Pco_2) = 38. Chest x-ray is as shown. An emergency echocardiogram shows normal left ventricular ejection fraction and no evidence of elevated left atrial pressures. What is the best treatment for this condition?

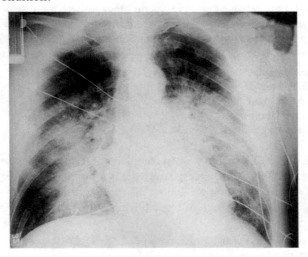

Reproduced, with permission, from Kasper DL, et al. *Harrison's Principles of Internal Medicine.* 16th ed. New York, NY: McGraw-Hill Education, 2005:1497.

a. Broadening antibiotic coverage with an anti-pseudomonal penicillin
b. Addition of vancomycin to cover for methicillin-resistant *Staphylococcus aureus* (MRSA)
c. IV corticosteroids
d. Mechanical ventilation with low tidal volumes and positive end-expiratory pressure (PEEP)
e. IV furosemide

111. A 60-year-old man has had a chronic cough with clear sputum production for over 5 years. He has smoked one pack of cigarettes per day for 40 years and continues to do so. Chest x-ray shows hyperinflation without infiltrates. Arterial blood gases show pH of 7.38, Pco_2 of 40 mm Hg, Po_2 of 65 mm Hg, and O_2 saturation of 93%. Spirometry shows an FEV_1/FVC of 45% without bronchodilator response. Which of the following is the most important treatment modality for this patient?

a. Oral corticosteroids
b. Home oxygen
c. Broad-spectrum antibiotics
d. Smoking cessation program
e. Oral theophylline

112. A 57-year-old man presents with hemoptysis and generalized weakness. His symptoms began with small-volume hemoptysis 4 weeks ago. Over the past 2 weeks, he has become weak and feels "out of it." His appetite has diminished, and he has lost 10 lb of weight. He has a 45-pack-year history of cigarette smoking. Physical examination is unremarkable. Laboratory studies reveal a mild anemia and a serum sodium value of 118 mEq/L. Chest x-ray shows a 5-cm left mid-lung field mass with widening of the mediastinum suggesting mediastinal lymphadenopathy. MR scan of the brain is unremarkable. What is the most likely cause of his symptoms?

a. Bronchial carcinoid
b. Adenocarcinoma of the lung
c. Small cell carcinoma of the lung
d. Lung abscess
e. Pulmonary aspergilloma

113. A 42-year-old woman presents with gradually worsening dyspnea over the preceding 6 months. She has a mild nonproductive cough. She previously had been diagnosed with systemic sclerosis (scleroderma) but her skin thickening has been stable. She controls her Raynaud syndrome with amlodipine and her esophageal reflux with daily omeprazole. She has no renal disease or hypertension. On physical examination, her RR is 22/min and resting O_2 saturation is 92%. She has thickened, hide-bound skin on the face, torso, and abdomen. Lung examination shows mild "Velcro" rales in the bases bilaterally. Neck veins are flat. Cardiac examination is normal with normal P_2 and no lift or heave. Chest x-ray shows increased interstitial lung markings and a normal heart size. What is the most important next step in evaluating this patient's dyspnea?

a. Arterial blood gas
b. 2D echocardiogram
c. Measurement of autoantibodies including anti-topoisomerase-1 (anti-Scl-70) antibodies
d. Barium swallow to detect microaspiration
e. Noncontrast high-resolution CT scan (HRCT) of chest

114. A 30-year-old quadriplegic man presents to the emergency room with fever, dyspnea, and cough. He has a chronic indwelling Foley catheter. Recurrent urinary tract infections have been a problem for a number of years. He has been on therapy to suppress the urinary tract infections. On examination, the patient has a temperature of 38°C (100.4°F), HR 88, and BP 126/76. Mild wheezing is audible over both lungs. A diffuse erythematous rash is noted. The chest x-ray shows diffuse alveolar infiltrates. The CBC reveals a WBC of 13,500, with 50% segmented cells, 30% lymphocytes, and 20% eosinophils. Which of the following is the most likely diagnosis?

a. Sepsis with acute respiratory distress syndrome (ARDS) secondary to urinary tract infection
b. Health care-related pneumonia
c. Drug reaction to one of his medications
d. Acute exacerbation of COPD
e. Lymphocytic interstitial pneumonitis

115. A 35-year-old woman complains of slowly progressive dyspnea. Her history is otherwise negative, and there is no cough, sputum production, pleuritic chest pain, or thrombophlebitis. She has taken appetite suppressants at different times. Physical examination reveals jugular venous distention, a palpable right ventricular lift, and a loud P_2 heart sound. Chest x-ray shows clear lung fields. Oxygen saturation is 94%. ECG shows right axis deviation. A perfusion lung scan is normal, with no segmental deficits. Which of the following is the most likely diagnosis?

a. Pulmonary arterial hypertension
b. Recurrent pulmonary emboli
c. Right-to-left cardiac shunt
d. Interstitial lung disease
e. Left ventricular diastolic dysfunction

116. A 60-year-old obese man complains of excessive daytime sleepiness. He has been in good health except for mild hypertension. He drinks alcohol in moderation. The patient's wife states that he snores at night and awakens frequently. Examination of the oropharynx is normal. Which of the following studies is most appropriate?

a. Electroencephalogram (EEG) to assess sleep patterns
b. Ventilation pattern to detect apnea
c. Arterial O_2 saturation
d. Study of muscles of respiration during sleep
e. Polysomnography

Questions 117 and 118 pertain to the following scenario.

A 19-year-old college student is being evaluated in the Student Health Center for asthma that she has had since childhood. She states that she had been asymptomatic during high school, but since arriving at college she has had episodes of wheezing three or four times per week. In addition she has awakened at night with wheezing twice in the past month. She occasionally used an inhaler in middle school. She currently is not taking any medicines.

117. How would you classify her asthma?

a. Asymptomatic
b. Mild intermittent
c. Mild persistent
d. Moderate persistent
e. Severe persistent

118. What therapy would you recommend at this time?

a. Short-acting beta-agonist on an "as-needed" basis
b. Daily low-dose inhaled corticosteroid and short-acting beta-agonist on an "as-needed" basis
c. A combination inhaled corticosteroid and a PRN short-acting beta agonist
d. Oral corticosteroid and short-acting beta-agonist on an "as-needed" basis
e. A leukotriene inhibitor

119. A 55-year-old woman with long-standing chronic obstructive lung disease and episodes of acute bronchitis complains of increasing sputum production, which now occurs on a daily basis. Sputum is thick, and daily sputum production has dramatically increased over several months. There are flecks of blood in the sputum. The patient has lost 8 lb. Fever and chills are absent, and sputum cultures have not revealed specific pathogens. Chest x-ray and CT chest are shown in the following figures. Which of the following is the most likely cause of the patient's symptoms?

a. Pulmonary tuberculosis
b. Exacerbation of chronic bronchitis
c. Bronchiectasis
d. Anaerobic lung abscess
e. Carcinoma of the lung

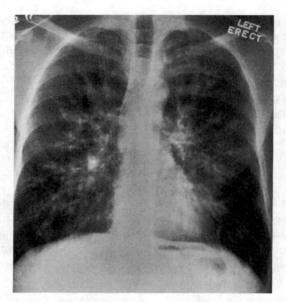

Reproduced, with permission, from Chen M, et al. *Basic Radiology*. New York, NY: McGraw-Hill Education, 2004.

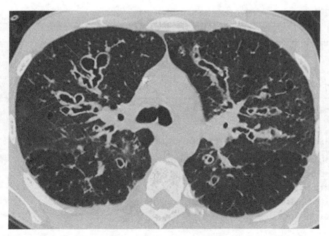

Reproduced, with permission, from Fauci A, et al. *Harrison's Principles of Internal Medicine*. 17th ed. New York, NY: McGraw-Hill Education, 2008.

120. A 20-year-old fireman comes to the emergency room complaining of headache and dizziness after putting out a garage fire. He does not complain of shortness of breath, and the arterial blood gas shows a normal Po_2. There is no cyanosis. Which of the following is the best first step in the management of this patient?

a. Assess for methemoglobinemia
b. Obtain ECG
c. Obtain carboxyhemoglobin level
d. Obtain CT scan of head
e. Evaluate for anemia

121. A 45-year-old woman with rheumatoid arthritis is seen for dyspnea on exertion that has occurred over the past 3 to 4 months. She has not noticed cough or fever and has had no associated orthopnea, paroxysmal dyspnea, edema, or chest pain. She has hypertension. Regular medications include lisinopril and methotrexate. She has smoked a package of cigarettes daily since age 20. Results of pulmonary function tests (PFTs) are shown in the table.

	Results	Predicted	% Predicted
Before Bronchodilators			
FEV_1	1.60 L	2.85 L	56%
FVC	1.94 L	3.53 L	55%
FEV_1/FVC	82%	84%	99%
After Bronchodilators			
FEV_1	1.62 L	2.85 L	57%
FVC	1.96 L	3.53 L	55%
FEV_1/FVC	84%	84%	100%

Abbreviation: FVC, forced vital capacity.

What is the correct interpretation of her PFTs?

a. Obstructive lung disease, not responsive to bronchodilators
b. Obstructive lung disease, responsive to bronchodilators
c. Restrictive lung disease
d. Mixed obstructive and restrictive lung disease
e. Small airways disease

122. A 56-year-old woman presents with cough for the past 2 months and streak hemoptysis for the past 3 days. She denies dyspnea on exertion. She has smoked 2 packs of cigarettes a day for the past 35 years. She is otherwise healthy and has not lost weight. Physical examination is normal. Chest x-ray reveals a shaggy 3-cm nodule in the right mid-lung field. Transthoracic needle biopsy shows a squamous cell carcinoma. PET/CT scan confirms the hypermetabolic 3-cm nodule and shows a 1.5-cm ipsilateral hilar lymph node. Mediastinal lymphadenopathy, intraparenchymal metastases, pleural effusion, and distant metastases are absent. Spirometry is normal. What is the best management option for this patient?

a. Surgical lobectomy
b. Radiation therapy
c. Combination chemotherapy
d. Endobronchial brachytherapy
e. Await development of symptoms such as pain or hemoptysis, then palliative radiation therapy or chemotherapy

123. A 43-year-old woman complains of gradually worsening dyspnea over the past year. She smokes 1 pack of cigarettes a day. She is trying to "cut back," because her father, also a smoker, died at age 52 of emphysema. She works as an equestrian riding instructor, often with exposure to animals and hay, but has not noticed exacerbation of symptoms while at work. She has three healthy children, one of whom has childhood asthma. On examination, she is comfortable at rest. Her O_2 saturation is 93%. She has no basilar crackles or wheezing, but her breath sounds are distant. Chest x-ray shows hyperexpansion especially prominent in the lung bases. Spirometry reveals FEV_1 of 46% of predicted but near normal forced vital capacity (FVC). The ratio of FEV_1 to FVC is 52%. In addition to advice about smoking cessation, what study would be most important to obtain?

a. Sweat chloride
b. Diffusing capacity of carbon monoxide
c. High-resolution CT scan of the chest
d. Serum alpha-1 antitrypsin level
e. Hypersensitivity pneumonitis serology panel

124. A 69-year-old woman presents with complaint of chronic cough. She is a former smoker, but quit over 20 years ago. She is healthy except for hypertension, for which she takes amlodipine; she is on no other medications. The cough has been present for 6 months. She produces scant clear sputum in the morning and denies hemoptysis or weight loss. The cough is more prominent at night. It is not exacerbated by exercise or cold exposure. There is no exposure history to potential lung toxins. She denies runny nose, nasal allergies, or postnasal drip. She has occasional heartburn, promptly relieved by two tablets of calcium carbonate. Physical examination and PA/lateral chest x-ray are normal. What is the next best step in the evaluation of this patient?

a. Therapeutic trial of proton-pump inhibitor (PPI)
b. Bronchoscopy
c. CT scan of chest
d. Spirometry
e. Therapeutic trial of nasal corticosteroid and systemic decongestant

125. A 25-year-old healthy medical student celebrates the end of his third year with a camping and climbing trip to Colorado. He has a mild headache after flying to Denver; the next day he drives to a cabin at 10,000 ft, and the following day climbs to 13,500 ft with friends. During the climb, he becomes unduly short of breath and develops a cough productive of blood tinged sputum. He is evacuated to a clinic, where he is disoriented and in respiratory distress. His room air O_2 saturation is 79%. His neck veins are flat and cardiac examination is normal except for tachycardia. He has bilateral crackles. What statement best characterizes this patient's medical condition?

a. Echocardiogram will show decreased left ventricular contractility
b. He is at risk of recurrence if he climbs at high altitude again
c. Nifedipine is the most important immediate treatment
d. Young age and physical fitness are protective factors
e. Acetazolamide is useful in preventing recurrence of this condition

126. A 62-year-old man seeks your advice for management of his COPD. He is a former 60-pack-year smoker, but stopped smoking 3 years ago. He uses inhaled albuterol when he feels particularly short of breath. He has noticed mild peripheral edema. He has diabetes mellitus, hypertension, and peripheral vascular disease. For these conditions he takes metformin, hydrochlorothiazide (HCTZ), lisinopril, and cilostazol. Physical examination reveals a thin man who appears older than his stated age. His BP is 136/78, HR is 88, and RR is 18. Room air O_2 saturation is 85%. He has distant breath sounds, but no rales, rhonchi, or wheezes. What treatment is most important in his overall health status?

a. Long-acting bronchodilator such as tiotropium or salmeterol
b. Inhaled corticosteroids
c. Continuous oxygen to keep O_2 saturation 90% or above
d. Pulmonary rehabilitation
e. Antibiotics promptly at time of purulent exacerbation

127. A 57-year-old man presents with gradually worsening dyspnea on exertion for the past 6 months. He has a 40-pack-year history of tobacco use. He has noted a minimally productive cough, worse in the mornings, for the past 2 years. He is otherwise healthy, without hypertension, hypercholesterolemia, or diabetes mellitus. On physical examination, he is comfortable at rest. His room air oximeter reading is 93%. His neck veins are flat and his cardiac examination is normal. He has no basilar crackles, but breath sounds are distant bilaterally. Chest x-ray shows hyperexpansion without evidence of cardiomegaly or pulmonary congestion. What is the most important next step in staging this patient's illness?

a. Arterial blood gas
b. CT scan of chest
c. Exercise tolerance test with measurement of maximum oxygen consumption
d. Echocardiogram with estimation of RV pressures
e. Spirometry

Questions 128 to 130

Match the patient described with the type of pleural effusion. Each lettered option may be used once, more than once, or not at all.

a. Unilateral effusion, turbid, cell count 90,000 (95% polymorphonuclear cells), protein 4.5 g/dL (serum protein 5.2), LDH 255 U/L (serum LDH 290), pH 6.84, glucose 20 mg/dL. Culture and Gram stain pending.
b. Bilateral effusions, straw colored, cell count 150 (20% polys, 35% lymphocytes, 45% mesothelial cells), protein 1.4 g/L (serum protein 5.4), LDH 66 U/L (serum LDH 175), pH 7.42, glucose 100 mg/dL.
c. Bilateral effusions, slightly turbid, cell count 980 (10% polys, 30% lymphocytes, 60% mesothelial cells), protein 3.9 g/L (serum 3.8), LDH 225 U/L (serum 240), pH 7.52, glucose 5 mg/dL.
d. Bilateral effusions, straw colored, cell count 4200 (100% lymphocytes), protein 3 g/dL (serum 5.0), LDH 560 U/L (serum 450), pH 7.27, glucose 77 mg/dL.
e. Right-sided effusion, bloody, white cell count 1200 (15% polys, 5% lymphocytes, 80% "reactive" mesothelial cells), RBC 130,000, protein 4.2 g/L (serum 4.6), LDH 560 U/L (serum 226), pH 6.90, glucose 120 mg/dL.
f. Left-sided effusion, turbid, cell count 54,000 (92% polys, 8% lymphocytes), protein 5.2 g/L (serum 5.2), LDH 400 U/L (serum 200), pH 3.02, glucose 40 mg/dL.
g. Left-sided effusion, straw colored, cell count 2000 (80% polys, 10% lymphocytes, 10% mesothelial cells), protein 2.0 (serum 4.8), LDH 158 (serum 220), pH 7.52, Gram stain negative, amylase 32,000.

128. A 52-year-old alcoholic man develops left chest pain after repeated bouts of vomiting. On presentation he is diaphoretic with fever of 101.5, heart rate 126, and BP 84/52. There are crackles and moderate dullness at the left base. The right lung is clear. He has subcutaneous emphysema over the left supraclavicular area.

129. A 72-year-old woman is admitted from the nursing home with fever and cough. Physical examination shows right basilar crackles and moderate dullness. CXR shows RLL pneumonia with moderate pleural effusion. She is treated with vancomycin and levofloxacin but remains febrile. Her shortness of breath worsens, and a follow-up chest x-ray shows enlarging pleural effusion.

130. A 52-year-old woman is admitted with abdominal pain and hypertriglyceridemia. Amylase is elevated, and she is treated for pancreatitis with
IV fluids and narcotics. Over the next several days she becomes more short
of breath; left basilar dullness develops.

Questions 131 to 134

Match the chest x-ray letter (see pages 104-106) with the most likely clinical description. Each lettered option may be used once, more than once, or
not at all.

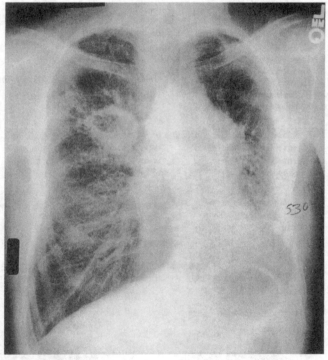

a

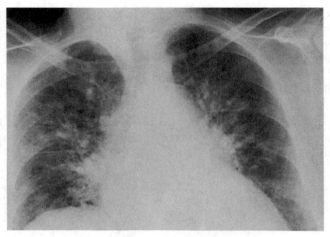

b

Reproduced, with permission, from Cheitlin MD, Sokolow M, McIlroy MB: *Clinical Cardiology*, 6th ed. Originally published by Appleton & Lange. Copyright © 1993 by The McGraw-Hill Companies, Inc.

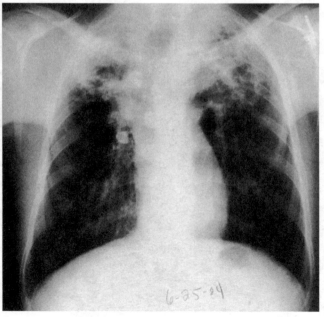

c

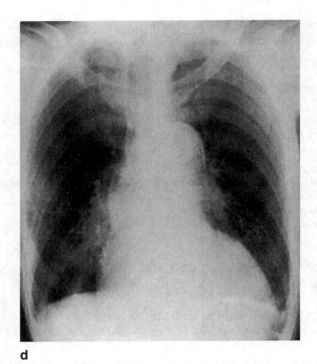

d

Reproduced, with permission, from Chen M, et al. *Basic Radiology*. New York, NY: McGraw-Hill Education, 2004.

131. A 60-year-old man develops fever, chills, and productive cough while in the hospital after surgery. There is increased tactile fremitus in the right mid-lung field. Sputum Gram stain shows few squamous cells, many polys, and gram-positive cocci in clusters.

132. A 45-year-old man with known coronary artery disease develops shortness of breath and awakens gasping for breath at night. Bibasilar crackles are present.

133. An 85-year-old man, newly arrived from Vietnam, has been complaining of productive cough and night sweats for more than 3 months. There are upper lobe crackles bilaterally.

134. A 50-year-old woman has had long-standing hypertension that is poorly controlled. Physical examination shows the PMI to be displaced to the sixth intercostal space. An S4 gallop is present.

Questions 135 to 137

For each scenario below, match the primary mechanism of action of the asthma medications prescribed. Each answer can be used once, more than once, or not at all.

a. Inhibits synthesis of cytokines
b. Relaxes bronchial smooth muscle by activating beta-adrenergic receptors
c. Blocks muscarinic receptors and inhibits bronchoconstriction
d. Inhibits phosphodiesterase
e. Blocks leukotriene receptors
f. Prevents mast cell degranulation

135. A 20-year-old athlete with exercise-induced asthma inhales cromolyn before participating in the 100-m hurdles event.

136. A 34-year-old asthmatic is admitted to hospital with severe exacerbation of asthma and is prescribed oral prednisone.

137. A 28-year-old asthmatic with moderate persistent asthma is prescribed montelukast.

Questions 138 and 139

For each set of patients below, select the most likely diagnosis. Each lettered option may be used once, more than once, or not at all.

a. Lymphangioleiomyomatosis
b. Bronchoalveolar carcinoma of the lung
c. Silicosis
d. Eosinophilic pneumonia
e. Cystic fibrosis
f. Asbestosis

138. A 20-year-old man has a cough and history of bronchitis with thick greenish sputum. There is no history of cigarette smoking. The patient has also been treated for abdominal cramping and malabsorption.

139. A 40-year-old construction worker has noted increasing shortness of breath and cough over many years. On physical examination bilateral inspiratory crackles are heard. Chest x-ray shows egg shell calcifications in hilar adenopathy and bilateral small nodular interstitial markings in the upper lobes.

Questions 140 to 142

For each of the clinical situations below, select the most likely diagnosis. Each lettered option may be used once, more than once, or not at all.

a. Tuberculosis
b. Lung cancer
c. Bronchiectasis
d. Idiopathic pulmonary fibrosis
e. Asbestosis
f. Histoplasmosis

140. A 32-year-old man has cough with yellow, blood-tinged sputum. He also has a history of night sweats and a 10-lb weight loss. The patient was born in India. On physical examination there is dullness to percussion above both clavicles. Chest x-ray shows bilateral upper lobe infiltrates with cavity formation.

141. A 55-year-old woman who is a heavy cigarette smoker complains of cough with small amounts of bright red blood. She has also noted loss of appetite and a 12-lb weight loss. A 3-cm pulmonary nodule with shaggy margins is seen on chest x-ray.

142. A 65-year-old who is retiring from work as a plumber has complained of a dry cough. He has also had some shortness of breath on walking. On physical examination there are bilateral crackling rales at both lung bases. Bilateral clubbing is also noted. On chest x-ray, bilateral linear infiltrates are seen at the lung bases. Pleural scarring is noted on CT scan.

Pulmonary Disease

Answers

96. The answer is b. The clinical picture suggests hypertrophic osteoarthropathy. This process, the pathogenesis of which is unknown, is characterized by clubbing of digits, periosteal new bone formation, and arthritis. Hypertrophic osteoarthropathy is associated with intrathoracic malignancy, suppurative lung disease, and congenital heart problems. Treatment is directed at the underlying disease process. While x-rays may suggest osteomyelitis, the process is usually bilateral and easily distinguishable from osteomyelitis. The first step in evaluation of this patient is to obtain a chest x-ray looking for lung infection and carcinoma.

The process is periarticular, not articular; so septic arthritis, treated with parenteral antibiotics, would not be a consideration. Although there is warmth over the wrists, the clubbing and periosteal changes would not be seen in rheumatoid arthritis, so wrist aspiration and methotrexate therapy would not address the underlying problem. An elevated sedimentation rate could be seen in neoplasm, infection, and inflammatory arthritis and would therefore be of little diagnostic value.

97. The answer is c. Clinical conditions associated with either an increase in hydrostatic pressure (such as congestive heart failure) or a decrease in oncotic pressure (such as nephrotic syndrome) are associated with transudative pleural effusions. This patient's pleural fluid is exudative by all three of the Light criteria: pleural fluid/serum protein ratio is greater than 0.5, pleural fluid LDH/serum LDH ratio is greater than 0.6, and pleural fluid LDH is greater than two-thirds the upper limits of the normal serum LDH. The most likely explanation for an exudative pleural effusion in the setting of an acute pneumonia is a parapneumonic effusion. Parapneumonic effusions occur in about 40% of patients with bacterial pneumonia. Parapneumonic effusions are exudative due to the fact that there is increased permeability of the visceral pleural membrane capillaries, and interstitial fluid moves across the visceral pleura into the pleural space. Parapneumonic effusions may be simple or complicated. Simple parapneumonic effusions are sterile and free flowing. If bacteria invade the pleural space, neutrophils move into the pleural space and anaerobic metabolism of glucose results in a low pleural fluid pH (<7.20) and glucose (<60). The characteristics of this patient's pleural fluid suggest that bacterial invasion of the pleural space has not occurred, and that this is a simple parapneumonic effusion. Hemorrhage into the pleural space occurs with trauma, cancer, and pulmonary embolism, but rarely with pneumonia.

98. The answer is d. The chest x-ray shows a lung abscess in the right lower lobe with an air-fluid level. This is characteristic of an anaerobic infection. These are usually associated with a period of loss of consciousness and/or with poor oral hygiene. The location of the infiltrate suggests aspiration, also making anaerobic infection most likely. The superior segment of the right lower lobe is the segment most likely to develop aspiration pneumonia. Treatment of lung abscess with single-agent clindamycin for 4 to 6 weeks is usually curative. Lung abscess indicates a necrotizing process, which is uncommon with the "typical" bacterial pathogens pneumococci and *H influenzae*, and very rare in the usually patchy "atypical" pneumonias caused by *Legionella* and *Mycoplasma*.

99. The answer is d. This patient's chest x-ray shows a pneumothorax, which is a collection of air in the pleural space. Patients with pneumothorax usually complain of sudden onset of dyspnea and unilateral pleuritic chest pain. Examination of the chest shows hyperresonance to percussion, decreased tactile fremitus, and decreased or absent breast sounds over the affected lung. Sometimes a pleural defect can act as a one-way valve and a tension pneumothorax can occur. This results in hypotension, tracheal deviation, and jugular venous distention, and requires urgent relief of the pneumothorax, usually with a chest tube. As in this patient, spontaneous pneumothorax may occur due to rupture of congenital subpleural apical blebs. This condition is usually seen in tall thin males under the age of 25. Pneumothorax may also be caused by trauma (especially with gunshot wounds and trauma causing rib fractures), following thoracentesis or with mechanical ventilation. Occasionally pneumothorax is seen in pneumonia (especially with *Pneumocystis jiroveci* and *S aureus*) and with lung cancer. All of these etiologies are unlikely in this patient who has been previously healthy. Pleural neoplasm usually causes a bloody pleural effusion, not pneumothorax. Patients who have pneumothorax often appear anxious, but anxiety is a result of the pain and dyspnea and is not the etiology.

100. The answer is c. This patient presents with severe COPD and hypoxemia. Chronic CO_2 retention has blunted his hypercarbic drive to breathe; he is dependent on mild hypoxia to stimulate respiration. Delivery of high oxygen concentration has decreased his hypoxic drive, with resulting acute respiratory acidosis and CO_2 narcosis. However, stopping the oxygen will result in severe hypoxemia. Of the choices listed, the initiation of mechanical ventilation is the only acceptable choice. If the patient's mental status were better, noninvasive ventilation (BiPAP) might be considered. Medroxyprogesterone has only a mild stimulatory effect on the respiratory center, and is not appropriate therapy in this case. Antibiotics and inhaled bronchodilators are appropriate treatments for COPD exacerbation but would not manage this patient's acute hypercarbic respiratory failure. The patient has declared a deteriorating course. Continuing to monitor his status on the general medicine ward might be fatal. This patient has respiratory (not metabolic) acidosis. Bicarbonate plays a minimal role in this acidosis. The correct therapy is to improve the patient's ventilation.

101. The answer is c. Sarcoidosis is a systemic illness of unknown etiology. There is a higher prevalence in female patients and in the African-American population. Most patients have respiratory symptoms, including cough and dyspnea. Hilar and peripheral lymphadenopathy is common, and 20% to 30% of patients have hepatosplenomegaly. The chest x-ray shows symmetrical hilar lymphadenopathy. The diagnostic method of choice is fiberoptic bronchoscopy with endobronchial and transbronchial biopsies, which will show a mononuclear cell granulomatous inflammatory process. While liver and mediastinal lymph node biopsies are often positive, bronchoscopy is a safer and less invasive procedure. ACE levels are elevated in two-thirds of patients; since an elevated ACE value is common in other granulomatous diseases, it is not specific enough to exclude alternative diagnoses. Open-lung biopsy is more invasive and would only be considered if fiberoptic bronchoscopy failed to yield a diagnosis.

102. The answer is a. This patient has a chylothorax. In chylothorax, the pleural fluid appears milky and has a triglyceride level over 110 mg/dL. Chylothorax occurs when chyle accumulates in the pleural space due to disruption of the thoracic duct. This is most often due to traumatic or surgical injury to the thoracic duct. In this patient without trauma or recent surgery, a mediastinal tumor (such as lymphoma) would be most likely. Chylous pleural effusions are usually exudative. Pulmonary embolism, systemic lupus, and pneumonia may all be associated with pleural effusions, but pleural effusions associated with these conditions are not chylous. Congestive heart failure is a very rare cause of chylous pleural effusion, but would be much less likely than lymphoma.

103. The answer is c. Patients with cystic fibrosis are now surviving into adulthood. The median survival exceeds age 40. Most cases are diagnosed in childhood; however, because of variable penetration of the genetic defect, approximately 7% are not found until the patient is an adult. Most male patients (>95%) are azoospermic. Chronic pulmonary infections occur, and bronchiectasis frequently develops. Diabetes mellitus and gastrointestinal problems indicate pancreatic insufficiency. This patient should have sweat chloride measurement; if abnormal (sweat Cl above 70 mEq/L), cystic fibrosis transmembrane conductance regulator (CFTR) mutation analysis should be ordered. COPD or emphysema at this age would be unusual unless the patient were deficient in alpha-1 antitrypsin. Immunoglobulin deficiencies can cause recurrent sinopulmonary infections but would not cause malabsorption or infertility. Whipple disease causes malabsorption but not the pulmonary manifestations or infertility; it would be vanishingly rare in a young patient. Asthma would not cause the abdominal symptoms, diabetes, or changes of bronchiectasis.

104. The answer is e. Occupational lung disease is an important branch of pulmonology, and new inhaled workplace toxins are being described every year. A detailed occupational history and knowledge of potential culprits are, therefore, critical in patients with unexplained lung disease. Exposure to asbestos in demolition, automobile servicing, or ship building industries is suggestive of asbestos-related disease; bilateral pleural thickening (often calcified, a finding especially evident on CT scan) indicates prior asbestos exposure. Occasionally, the pleural involvement is associated with a pleural effusion (often with an elevated red cell count) called benign asbestos pleural effusion (BAPE). "Benign" distinguishes this syndrome from malignant effusions due to lung cancer or mesothelioma, both of which occur with increased frequency in asbestosis. Progressive debility from an interstitial lung disease (ILD) (which worsens even after asbestos exposure has ceased) may occur in asbestosis, but this patient's physical examination and chest x-ray do not suggest interstitial disease.

Medications, especially nitrofurantoin and cancer chemotherapeutic agents, can cause interstitial lung disease, but amlodipine has not been reported to do so. Tuberculosis (TB) occurs with increased frequency in silicosis, not in asbestosis. Although TB can cause a bloody pleural effusion, this patient does not have the systemic symptoms that usually accompany TB. Hypersensitivity pneumonitis is an important cause of occupational lung disease, but it is caused by exposure to organic materials such as thermophilic actinomycetes (farmer's lung). In addition, hypersensitivity pneumonitis usually causes acute symptoms (including fever) at time of exposure. Occupational asthma is an important category, since continued exposure can lead to irreversible changes. Isocyanates in automobile paints are an important cause of occupational asthma, but the symptoms are usually more acute and associated with wheezing on physical examination. Hypersensitivity pneumonitis and occupational asthma do not cause pleural disease.

105. The answer is b. Because of the development of effective oral antibiotics (respiratory fluoroquinolones, extended spectrum macrolides), many patients with community-acquired pneumonia (CAP) can be managed as an outpatient as long as compliance and close follow-up are assured. The CURB-65 score is a validated instrument for determining if inpatient admission (either observation or full admission) is indicated. Factors predicting increased severity of infection include confusion, urea above 19 mg/dL, respiratory rate above 30, BP below 90 systolic (or 60 diastolic), and age 65 or above. If more than one of these factors is present, hospitalization should be considered.

This patient's presentation (lobar pneumonia, pleuritic pain, purulent sputum) suggests pneumococcal pneumonia. The pneumococcus is the commonest organism isolated from patients with CAP. Fortunately, *S pneumoniae* is almost always sensitive to oral antibiotics such as clarithromycin/azithromycin and the respiratory fluoroquinolones. A Gram stain suggestive of pneumococci would therefore only confirm the clinical diagnosis. Exposure to influenza is an important historical finding. Patients with influenza often have a prodrome (upper respiratory symptoms, myalgias, prostrating weakness), but influenza would not cause a lobar infiltrate. *Staphylococcus aureus* pneumonia can sometimes follow influenza. Acute lobar pneumonia, even in an HIV-positive patient, is usually due to the pneumococcus and can often be treated as an outpatient. *Pneumocystis jiroveci* pneumonia is usually insidious in onset, causes diffuse parenchymal infiltrates, and does not cause pleurisy or pleural effusion. Physical examination signs of consolidation confirm the CXR finding of a lobar pneumonia (as opposed to a patchy bronchopneumonia) and would simply affirm the importance of coverage for classic bacterial pathogens (ie, pneumococci, *H influenzae*). Atypical pneumonias (due to *Mycoplasma, Chlamydia,* or *Legionella*) are usually patchy and do not usually cause pleural effusion. Currently recommended treatment regimens for CAP cover both typical and atypical pathogens.

106. The answer is b. The clinical situation strongly suggests pulmonary embolism. In greater than 80% of cases, pulmonary emboli arise from deep venous thrombosis (DVT) of the lower extremities, but a normal lower extremity Doppler does not exclude the diagnosis. DVTs often begin in the calf, where they rarely if ever cause clinically significant pulmonary embolic disease. However, thromboses that begin below the knee frequently "grow," or propagate, above the knee; clots that dislodge from above the knee cause clinically significant pulmonary emboli. Untreated pulmonary embolism is associated with a 30% mortality rate. Interestingly, only about 50% of patients with DVT of the lower extremities have clinical findings of swelling, warmth, erythema, pain, or palpable "cord." When a clot does dislodge from the deep venous system and travels into the pulmonary vasculature, the most common clinical findings are tachypnea and tachycardia; chest pain is less likely and usually indicates pulmonary infarction. The ABG is usually abnormal, and a high percentage of patients exhibit low P_{CO_2} with respiratory alkalosis, and a widening of the alveolar-arterial oxygen gradient. The ECG usually shows sinus tachycardia, but atrial fibrillation or the classic S1Q3T3 (prominent S wave in lead I, Q wave and inverted T wave in lead III) may be seen. Initial treatment for suspected pulmonary embolic disease includes prompt hospitalization and institution of IV heparin or therapeutic dose subcutaneous low-molecular-weight heparin. It is particularly important to make an early diagnosis of pulmonary embolus, as intervention can decrease the mortality rate from 30% down to 5%. A normal D-dimer level helps exclude pulmonary embolus in the low-risk setting. This patient, however, has a high pretest probability of PE; further testing (CT pulmonary angiogram, V/Q lung scan) must be done to exclude this important diagnosis.

107. The answer is a. This patient likely has primary pulmonary hypertension. Echocardiogram is a reliable noninvasive test to confirm the clinical suspicion. Once pulmonary hypertension is confirmed, secondary causes (pulmonary or congenital heart disease) should be ruled out. These are unlikely in this patient without clinical or radiographic evidence of chronic pulmonary disease. Once pulmonary hypertension is confirmed by echocardiography and secondary causes ruled out, patients should undergo right heart catheterization with measurement of pulmonary vascular resistance in response to various pulmonary vasodilators. Treatment choices have expanded in recent years; endothelin-1 receptor antagonists (such as bosentan), phosphodiesterase-5 inhibitors (such as sildenafil), and in severe cases, infused prostanoids are effective treatments. In refractory cases, heart-lung transplantation (with its considerable risks) may be necessary.

Spirometry is useful in defining obstructive or restrictive lung disease. Spirometry will be normal in pulmonary hypertension. Exercise stress testing in this patient will show a nonspecific decline in exercise tolerance; it is diagnostically useful when ischemic heart disease is a consideration. Measurement of alpha-1 antitrypsin would be indicated if this young woman had obstructive lung disease, but none of her clinical features point in this direction. If COPD were causing her symptoms, O_2 desaturation or radiographic evidence of hyperexpansion would be expected.

108. The answer is c. Effective prophylaxis against DVT in the high-risk setting (eg, after major orthopedic surgery of the hip or knee) requires pharmacologic treatment with unfractionated heparin, low-molecular-weight heparin, fondaparinux, therapeutic doses of warfarin, apixaban, or rivaroxaban. These treatments, when given at approved dosages and time intervals, decrease the risk of radiographic DVT by over 50%; dosage guidelines should be carefully followed. Aspirin alone is not as effective in prevention of pulmonary embolus. Early ambulation, sequential compression devices, and elastic stockings provide some additional benefit, but are not adequate in themselves in this high-risk situation.

109. The answer is a. This patient with multiple episodes of desaturation has obstructive sleep apnea (OSA). In OSA, upper airway muscle tone decreases as the patient achieves deep stages (stages 3 and 4) of sleep; the soft palate falls against the base of the tongue, leading to obstruction of air flow and snoring. Microawakening occurs, leading to improvement in muscle tone but at the cost of shallow unrefreshing sleep. This leads to daytime somnolence (due to sleep deprivation), hypertension (due to hyper-adrenergic state), and even cor pulmonale and chronic hypercarbia (due to hypoxia). At present fewer than five apneic episodes per hour are considered normal. The severity of sleep apnea is graded using the apnea/hypopnea index. Mild sleep apnea is 5 to 15 events per hour; moderate sleep apnea is 16 to 30; and severe apnea is greater than 30 events per hour.

Continuous positive airway pressure (CPAP) is the recommended therapy. Weight loss is often helpful and should be recommended as well. However, weight loss alone will take significant time and may not be sufficient. Surgical uvulopalatopharyngoplasty, when applied to unselected patients, is effective in less than 50%. A trial of CPAP is indicated before surgical therapy. Tracheostomy is a treatment of last resort in severe and refractory sleep apnea; it does provide immediate relief of the upper airway obstruction. Oxygen alone is less effective than CPAP because it does not prevent interruption of airflow.

110. The answer is d. This woman has ARDS. This condition is characterized by acute onset of hypoxemia refractory to oxygen administration, poor lung compliance, and pulmonary edema that is noncardiogenic. Diagnosis is confirmed by a Po_2/FIO_2 ratio of less than 200, diffuse alveolar infiltrates on chest x-ray, and exclusion of cardiogenic pulmonary edema, usually with an echocardiogram. ARDS is often precipitated by sepsis, aspiration, or severe trauma and can be seen postpartum. This patient has a classic clinical presentation, CXR and Po_2/FIO_2 ratio (her ratio is 45/1.0 = 45). ARDS is not due to continued bacteremia or secondary bacterial infection, and therefore changing antibiotics will not be effective. Though this condition mimics cardiogenic pulmonary edema, pulmonary capillary wedge pressures are not elevated and diuretics are not effective. The pathogenesis of ARDS is thought to be diffuse endothelial injury related to the underlying event. Interestingly, clinical trials have not established efficacy of corticosteroids. The mainstay of treatment is mechanical ventilation with low tidal volumes and PEEP. Even with this treatment and supportive therapy, mortality is 30% to 40%.

111. The answer is d. This patient's chronic cough, hyperinflated lungs, abnormal PFTs, and smoking history are all consistent with chronic bronchitis. A smoking cessation program can decrease the rate of lung deterioration and is successful in as many as 40% of patients, particularly when the physician gives a strong antismoking message and uses both counseling and nicotine replacement. Continuous low-flow oxygen becomes beneficial when resting arterial oxygen saturation falls below 88%. Inhaled beta-agonists such as albuterol or anticholinergics such as ipratropium or tiotropium are the cornerstones of symptomatic therapy but do not prevent progression of airways obstruction if the patient continues to smoke. Antibiotics are indicated only for acute exacerbations of chronic lung disease, which present with fever, change in sputum color or amount, and increasing shortness of breath. Oral corticosteroids are helpful in acute exacerbations, but their side-effect profile precludes chronic use. Theophylline is a fourth-line treatment in COPD.

112. The answer is c. Hyponatremia in association with a lung mass usually indicates small cell lung cancer (SCLC) with inappropriate antidiuretic hormone (ADH) production by the tumor. About 10% of lung cancers present with a paraneoplastic syndrome. Tumors producing ADH or adrenocorticotropic hormone (ACTH) are overwhelmingly SCLCs, which arise from hormonally active neuroendocrine cells. SCLC is a rapidly growing neoplasm; early mediastinal involvement, as in this case, is common. Tumor staging for SCLC differs from non-small cell cancers. SCLCs are simply classified as limited (confined to one hemithorax) or extensive. Limited tumors are usually managed with combination radiation and chemotherapy, with approximately 20% cure rate. Extensive tumors are treated with palliative chemotherapy alone; durable remissions are rare. Surgery is not curative in SCLC.

Bronchial carcinoids are usually benign. Although they can produce ACTH, mediastinal involvement and hyponatremia would not be expected. Adenocarcinoma of the lung, although common, rarely causes a paraneoplastic syndrome. Localized benign lung infections (especially lung abscess) can cause syndrome of inappropriate antidiuretic hormone (SIADH), but would not account for this patient's mediastinal adenopathy. Lung abscess usually causes fever and fetid sputum. Pulmonary aspergilloma (a fungus ball growing in an old cavitary lesion) can cause hemoptysis but not this patient's hyponatremia or mediastinal lymphadenopathy.

113. The answer is e. This patient has interstitial lung disease (ILD) due to her systemic sclerosis. Over 75% of patients will have CT evidence of ILD. Now that scleroderma renal crisis can be managed with ACE inhibitors, ILD is the most common disease-related cause of death in scleroderma. The two most important studies for the diagnosis of ILD are spirometry with measurement of diffusion capacity of carbon monoxide (DLCO) and high-resolution CT scan. The latter will show reticular interstitial thickening and subpleural microblebs. Advanced cases will show thickened fibrotic bands with parenchymal destruction known as honeycombing.

Treatment of connective tissue disease associated ILD is unsatisfactory, but cyclophosphamide will slow progression in some patients. In addition to systemic sclerosis, ILD is an important potential complication of polymyositis/ dermatomyositis, rheumatoid arthritis, and occasionally systemic lupus.

An arterial blood gas study would probably show alveolar hyperventilation (ie, low Pco_2) with a widened alveolar-arterial oxygen gradient but would not give specific information as to cause and prognosis. In most cases, finger oxygen saturation measurements provide sufficient information. Pulmonary hypertension can be detected with 2D echocardiogram according to the degree of tricuspid regurgitation. Pulmonary hypertension can be an important complication of connective tissue disease (especially limited scleroderma but sometimes diffuse scleroderma as well). You would expect, however, a loud P_2 and evidence of central pulmonary artery enlargement on CXR. In addition, Velcro rales and increased interstitial markings are not seen in uncomplicated pulmonary hypertension. Autoantibodies are usually found in systemic sclerosis, but the diagnosis is already established. The titer of anti-Scl-70 antibodies does not correlate with disease activity; so once the diagnosis is established, serial measurement of autoantibodies is not necessary. Aspiration due to esophageal dysmotility can complicate scleroderma, but usually causes intermittent exacerbations associated with sputum production, fever, and alveolar infiltrates, none of which has characterized this patient's course.

114. The answer is c. Clues to this diagnosis are recurrent urinary tract infections and the use of suppressive therapy to control these infections. Nitrofurantoin is commonly used for this purpose. Nitrofurantoin can cause an acute hypersensitivity pneumonitis. This condition can progress to a chronic alveolitis with pulmonary fibrosis. The presenting symptoms are fever, chills, cough, and bronchospasm. In addition, the patient may experience arthralgias, myalgias, and an erythematous rash. The chest x-ray will show interstitial or alveolar infiltrates. CBC often shows leukocytosis with a high percentage of eosinophils. The treatment is to discontinue the nitrofurantoin, and to begin corticosteroids. Sepsis secondary to a urinary tract infection and health care-related pneumonia might be considered. However, these would not present with a diffuse erythroderma or eosinophilia. Acute bacterial infections cause a neutrophilic leukocytosis; eosinophils are usually undetectable owing to the stress effect of catecholamines and cortisol. COPD rarely presents in a 30-year-old. Lymphocytic interstitial pneumonia is a rare disease and would cause interstitial rather than alveolar infiltrates. Lung biopsy to establish the diagnosis of an interstitial lung disease would be considered only after the potentially offending drug had been discontinued.

115. The answer is a. Although a difficult diagnosis to make, pulmonary arterial hypertension (PAH) is the most likely diagnosis in this young woman who has used appetite suppressants. Pulmonary arterial hypertension (also known as primary pulmonary hypertension) has been associated with fenfluramine-type appetite suppressants. The predominant symptom is dyspnea, which is usually not apparent until the disease has advanced. When physical findings, chest x-ray, or echocardiography suggest pulmonary hypertension, recurrent pulmonary emboli must be ruled out. In this case, a normal perfusion lung scan makes pulmonary angiography unnecessary. Right-to-left cardiac shunts cause hypoxia (oxygen desaturation) that characteristically does not improve with oxygen supplementation. Restrictive lung disease should be ruled out with pulmonary function testing but is unlikely with a normal chest x-ray. An echocardiogram will show right ventricular enlargement and a reduction in the left ventricle size consistent with right ventricular pressure overload. Left ventricular dysfunction can cause pulmonary edema but not pulmonary hypertension.

116. The answer is e. With the history of daytime sleepiness and snoring at night, the patient requires evaluation for obstructive sleep apnea syndrome. Frequent awakenings are actually more suggestive of central sleep apnea. Polysomnography is required to assess which type of sleep apnea syndrome is present. EEG variables are recorded to identify various stages of sleep. Arterial oxygen saturation is monitored by finger or ear oximetry. Heart rate is monitored. The respiratory pattern is monitored to detect apnea and whether it is central or obstructive. Outpatient sleep monitoring with oxygen saturation studies alone might identify multiple episodes of desaturation, but negative results would not rule out a sleep apnea syndrome. Overnight oximetry alone can be used in some patients when the index of suspicion for obstructive sleep apnea is low. Polysomnography includes all of these and is the best choice. In addition, "split-night" testing allows for titration of the CPAP to the most effective tolerated level.

117 and 118. The answers are 117 c and 118 b. Almost all experts now classify asthma on the basis of severity. Mild intermittent asthma is classified as having wheezing less than 2 days per week and awakening with wheezing less than 2 nights per month. Mild persistent asthma (which this patient has) is diagnosed when the patient has wheezing more than 2 days per week but less than daily, and awakens with symptoms more than 2 nights per month. Moderate persistent asthma is diagnosed when the patient has daily symptoms and awakens with wheezing more than once per week. Severe persistent asthma is diagnosed in patients who have almost continual symptoms.

This classification system also directs therapy. A short-acting inhaled beta-agonist is recommended for all phases of asthma. This "rescue inhaler" is to be used on an as-needed (PRN) basis. No daily medications are recommended for mild intermittent asthma. In mild persistent asthma, a daily low-dose inhaled corticosteroid is added. A low to medium dose inhaled corticosteroid is combined with a long-acting inhaled beta-agonist in moderate persistent asthma. Severe persistent asthma is usually treated with a high-dose inhaled corticosteroid combined with a long-acting beta-agonist. Patients with this degree of asthma also are often treated with other agents such as leukotriene inhibitors, cromolyn, or oral steroids.

119. The answer is c. While symptoms such as sputum production and cough are nonspecific, particularly in a patient with known chronic lung disease, the high volume of daily sputum production suggests bronchiectasis. In this process, an abnormal and permanent dilatation of bronchi occurs as the muscular and elastic components of the bronchi are damaged. Clearance of secretions becomes a major problem, contributing to a cycle of bronchial inflammation and further destruction. High-resolution CT scan, the diagnostic test of choice for this disease, shows prominent dilated bronchi and the signet ring sign of a dilated bronchus adjacent to a pulmonary artery. This CT scan picture is pathognomonic for bronchiectasis. Tuberculosis usually causes upper lobe cavitary disease. COPD causes hyperexpansion, upper lobe bullae, and nonspecific bronchial wall thickening. CT scan in anaerobic lung abscess would show an air-fluid level, usually within a shaggy inflammatory infiltrate. This CT scan shows no nodule or mass to suggest lung cancer.

120. The answer is c. With symptoms of headache and dizziness in a fireman, the diagnosis of carbon monoxide poisoning must be addressed quickly. A venous or arterial measure of carboxyhemoglobin must first be obtained, if possible, before oxygen therapy is begun. The use of supplementary oxygen prior to obtaining the test may be a confounding factor in interpreting blood levels. Oxygen or even hyperbaric oxygen is given after blood for carboxyhemoglobin is drawn. Methemoglobinemia causes cyanosis, which is not present in this patient. ECG is unlikely to be abnormal in this young healthy patient without chest pain. Central nervous system imaging would not be indicated, and there are no diagnostic patterns that are specific to carbon monoxide poisoning. Anemia might cause dizziness, but the symptom would not occur as acutely as in this case.

121. The answer is c. Restrictive lung disease is characterized spirometrically by a normal FEV_1/FVC ratio. The FEV_1 is decreased in proportion to the FVC. In obstructive lung disease the FEV_1 is selectively decreased, so that the FEV_1/FVC ratio is decreased. When interpreting spirometry, look first at the FEV_1/FVC ratio. If this is normal, and the FVC is low, the patient has a restrictive defect. If the FEV_1/FVC ratio is low (less than 75%), the patient has an obstructive defect. In patients with an obstructive defect, low FVC indicates a mixed obstructive/restrictive pattern. Restrictive lung disease is seen with interstitial lung disease and can be associated with collagen vascular disease such as rheumatoid arthritis and medications such as methotrexate. Bronchodilator response is determined by looking at the change in the FEV_1 after the administration of a bronchodilator. A positive bronchodilator response is judged as an increase in the FEV_1 of 9% or more than 200 mL.

122. The answer is a. This patient has stage IIB non-small cell lung cancer (NSCLC) and should be considered for surgical resection with curative intent. As a general rule, patients with stages I and II lung cancer are surgical candidates unless other medical contraindications or severe COPD are present. Adjuvant chemotherapy is often recommended in stage II disease, but surgery is the curative modality with the best track record. Patients with stage I lung cancer have tumors less than 5 cm in size localized to the lung. Stage II cancers are larger than 5 cm or associated with ipsilateral peribronchial or hilar lymph node involvement. Mediastinal lymph node involvement, pleural effusion, or distant metastases generally preclude curative surgery. These patients, however, may respond to radiation and/or chemotherapy.

Although some patients have achieved long-term remission after radiation therapy, it is less effective than surgical resection. Combination chemotherapy can prolong life expectancy in selected patients but is not considered curative. Endobronchial radiation therapy (brachytherapy) can palliate intractable hemoptysis or bronchial obstruction but is not curative; survival in NSCLC after brachytherapy averages 6 months. "Watchful waiting" would be inappropriate in this patient with potentially curable disease.

123. The answer is d. This woman has COPD (chronic symptoms, obstructive defect on spirometry) at age younger than 45. Early-onset symptoms, even in a smoker, coupled with a positive family history, should raise the possibility of alpha-1 antitrypsin (AAT) deficiency, and a serum AAT level should be ordered. If it is low, a phenotype assay will confirm the abnormal gene product. AAT deficiency tends to cause more prominent alveolar destruction in the lower lung zones, as opposed to usual smoker's emphysema, which has upper lobe predominance. Diagnosing AAT deficiency would be important for her family members. In addition, infusion of pooled human AAT, although quite expensive, can raise AAT levels and probably slows progression of the disease.

Cystic fibrosis, which is diagnosed by the sweat chloride level, can present with lung disease in adulthood. However, this woman's lack of cough and sputum production, as well as her normal fertility, makes this a less likely diagnosis than AAT deficiency. Diffusing capacity will be low in any cause of emphysema, and CT scanning will confirm bullous changes, but neither is recommended in the routine management of COPD. High-resolution CT scanning is used in the diagnosis of interstitial, not obstructive, lung disease. This woman has a history of exposure to organic compounds known to cause hypersensitivity pneumonitis, but her lack of symptoms during or soon after exposure, as well as the absence of patchy infiltrates on CXR, makes this diagnosis less likely. Many agricultural workers have immunoprecipitins to thermophilic actinomycetes. In the absence of convincing history, these results are nonspecific.

124. The answer is a. Chronic cough is a common problem encountered in ambulatory practice. Although patients are often worried about serious disease such as lung cancer, emphysema, or tuberculosis, these dire diagnoses are rare in the absence of a compatible history and chest x-ray. The commonest causes are (1) acid reflux (with inflammation of the larynx and trachea); (2) postnasal drip syndrome; (3) cough-variant asthma; and (4) drug-induced cough due to angiotensin-converting enzyme inhibitors (ACEIs). Extensive testing such as CT scanning, bronchoscopy, or esophageal pH monitoring is not recommended. The practitioner should make the best diagnosis on the basis of initial data, and then institute a therapeutic trial, understanding that a response often takes weeks or months. This patient's nocturnal symptoms and occasional postprandial reflux (patients often do not have severe symptoms of gastroesophageal reflux disease [GERD]) would direct you toward a trial of a PPI. If she had allergic symptoms or cobblestoning of the posterior pharynx, a trial of nasal steroids/decongestants would be reasonable. Childhood asthma, intermittent wheezing, or exacerbation of symptoms with exercise or cold exposure would direct you toward a therapeutic trial of bronchodilators. Spirometry is usually normal unless the patient is having symptoms at the time of examination; methacholine challenge can be employed in selected patients. Amlodipine does not cause drug-induced cough. If the patient does not respond to high-dose PPIs, other therapeutic trials might be instituted.

125. The answer is b. This young man is suffering from high-altitude pulmonary edema (HAPE), a life-threatening condition. It is the commonest nontraumatic cause of death in high-altitude climbers. Susceptible persons have increased pulmonary vasoconstriction in response to hypoxia; this damages capillary endothelium and leads to exudation of fluid into the alveoli. Patients with HAPE are at significant risk of recurrence. The cornerstone of treatment is oxygen administration and/or descent to lower altitude, where the Po_2 is higher. HAPE is a form of noncardiogenic pulmonary edema; left ventricular function is normal. Although nifedipine decreases pulmonary vascular tone and is a useful adjunct, relief of hypoxia is a much more important aspect of treatment. Rapid ascent, sleeping at high altitude, and individual susceptibility are important risk factors; interestingly, youth and physical conditioning are not protective (perhaps because young people have vigorous pulmonary vascular reactivity). Acetazolamide (a carbonic anhydrase inhibitor) is useful in prevention of acute mountain sickness (which causes malaise and headache) but not of HAPE. Nifedipine has some prophylactic value.

126. The answer is c. Oxygen treatment (as close to 24 h/d as possible) is the one active treatment modality that has been shown to decrease mortality in COPD. Interestingly, it decreases the incidence of sudden death. This effect is presumably due to the beneficial effect of oxygen on cor pulmonale and right heart strain. It is important to emphasize to the patient that they should use the oxygen continuously, not just at times of increased dyspnea. Several treatments (inhaled corticosteroids, long-acting bronchodilators) are symptomatically useful and may slow progression of functional loss but have not been shown to prolong life. Pulmonary rehabilitation can increase functional status but does not improve parameters such as FEV_1 or mortality. The number of exacerbations is an important determinant of functional decline in COPD, but preventing them is difficult. Prompt antibiotic treatment of purulent exacerbations decreases the rate of hospitalization but has not been proven to affect mortality. Methods to slow progression of COPD are important research topics, as COPD is approaching cerebrovascular disease as the third leading cause of death in the United States.

127. The answer is e. The Global initiative for chronic Obstructive Lung Disease (GOLD) guidelines recommends the use of spirometric values to standardize the diagnosis and staging of COPD. The diagnosis emphasizes a compatible history and evidence of fixed or incompletely reversible airway obstruction as demonstrated by a ratio of FEV_1 to FVC less than 70%. Restrictive lung disease causes a proportional decline in both FEV_1 and FVC; so the ratio of the two will remain normal. The stage of COPD is then determined by the decrease in FEV_1 (see the below table).

Stage I	FEV1 above 80% predicted
Stage II	FEV1 50%-80% predicted
Stage III	FEV1 30%-50% predicted
Stage IV	FEV1 less than 30% predicted (or chronic respiratory failure)

None of the other tests is recommended in the routine staging or management of COPD. Reliable finger oximeters have replaced ABGs as a means of checking for O_2 desaturation. An elevated serum bicarbonate on a chemistry profile may indicate metabolic compensation for a chronic respiratory acidosis; sometimes (but not routinely) ABGs will be necessary to precisely quantify the degree of CO_2 retention. Chest CT will demonstrate bullous changes in patients with emphysema but is not part of routine patient care. Patients with COPD will usually have limitation of exercise tolerance, but this can be estimated and followed by clinical history. Echocardiogram can confirm pulmonary hypertension (often indicative of cor pulmonale) in patients with clinical evidence of RV dysfunction but again is not necessary in the routine case. Giving O_2 for relief of hypoxia is the best way of preventing mortality from cor pulmonale in these patients.

128 to 130. The answers are 128-f, 129-a, 130-g. The first step in determining the cause of a pleural effusion is to categorize it as either a transudate or exudate. Transudative effusions are caused by alteration in Starling forces (usually elevated hydrostatic pressure as in CHF or low plasma oncotic pressure as in hypoalbuminemia). The relatively low pleural fluid protein value means that capillary permeability is normal and that only small molecules (ie, salt and water) can leak out. Exudative effusions occur when an inflammatory (or neoplastic) process allows large molecules to enter the pleural space. According to the Light criteria, exudative effusions have one of the following characteristics: pleural fluid protein to serum protein ratio greater than 0.5, pleural fluid LDH to serum LDH ratio greater than 0.6, or pleural fluid LDH more than two-thirds the normal upper limit for serum.

The alcoholic patient with repetitive nausea and vomiting has ruptured his esophagus (Boerhaave syndrome). Gastric contents enter the left pleural space and cause an inflammatory (ie, exudative) effusion. The very low pH is a tip-off that gastric acid is present and will distinguish Boerhaave syndrome from the more usual empyema.

The elderly woman with pneumonia has developed empyema, a bacterial infection of the pleural space. Empyema is characterized by a very high white cell count, turbid fluid, and pH less than 7.2. Antibiotics alone will not cure empyema. Pleural fluid drainage, either with a chest tube (if the effusion is free flowing) or surgical drainage (if the fluid is loculated), is necessary to fully eradicate the infection.

The patient with abdominal pain has developed a pleural effusion resulting from pancreatitis. Many peripancreatic effusions simply occur in response to nearby inflammation of the pancreas (so-called sympathetic effusion). Occasionally, as in this case, a pancreaticopleural fistula will form leading to an exudate with very high amylase level. Such effusions often require chest tube drainage. Almost all effusions resulting from pancreatitis are left-sided exudates.

The pleural fluid in answer b (bilateral transudative fluid) suggests congestive heart failure. Answer c is characteristic of rheumatoid arthritis, with a chronic exudate, very low glucose, and high LDH in the absence of infection. Answer d suggests tuberculosis (exudative effusion with high lymphocyte count). A unilateral bloody effusion with atypical mesothelial cells (choice e) raises concern for mesothelioma.

131 to 134. The answers are 131-a, 132-b, 133-c, 134-d. The 60-year-old man has developed nosocomial pneumonia. Sputum showing gram-positive cocci in clusters is most likely *Staphylococcus aureus*. Chest x-ray (answer a) shows a necrotizing pneumonia characteristic of this infection. Cavities develop when necrotic lung tissue is discharged into airways. Cavities greater than 2 cm are described as lung abscesses.

The 45-year-old with shortness of breath and paroxysmal nocturnal dyspnea has congestive heart failure. Chest x-ray (answer b) shows signs of congestive heart failure, including cardiomegaly, bilateral infiltrates, and cephalization. Cephalization occurs when long-standing venous hypertension causes the upper lobe vessels to become more prominent owing to redistribution of pulmonary blood flow. When pulmonary edema becomes severe, fluid extends out from both hila in a bat-wing distribution.

The elderly Vietnamese patient with fever and night sweats has pulmonary tuberculosis (answer c). This x-ray shows characteristic changes of tuberculosis, including extensive apical and upper lobe scarring. When the lung is involved with tuberculosis, the range of abnormalities is broad. Cavitary infiltrates in the posterior apical segments are very common. Mass lesions, interstitial infiltrates, and noncavitary infiltrates also occur.

The woman with long-standing hypertension has chest x-ray (answer d), with evidence for left ventricular hypertrophy. The cardiac silhouette is enlarged and takes on a boot-shaped configuration.

135 to 137.   The answers are 135-f, 136-a, 137-e. A variety of medications used in the treatment of asthma have different mechanisms of action. In moderate or severe asthma, combining agents with different effects can improve response rates. Beta-agonists, the most commonly prescribed, are short acting and relax bronchial smooth muscle by stimulating beta-2 adrenergic receptors. Corticosteroids, both inhaled and oral, work by inhibition of cytokine synthesis. Ipratropium, another inhaled medication, blocks muscarinic receptors in bronchial smooth muscle. Muscarinic receptors are responsible for bronchoconstriction. Theophylline and other methylxanthines (including caffeine) cause bronchodilation by the inhibition of phosphodiesterase, thus increasing cyclic AMP. Cromolyn inhibits the degranulation of mast cells. It is only indicated for prophylaxis use, such as in exercise-induced asthma or before certain occupational exposures. Leukotriene inhibitors, such as montelukast and zafirlukast, block leukotriene receptors.

138 and 139.   The answers are 138-e, 139-c. The 20-year-old man has evidence of chronic airway infection not associated with cigarette smoking. Cystic fibrosis is a multisystem disease with signs and symptoms usually beginning in childhood. However, 7% of patients are diagnosed as adults. This is an autosomal recessive disease with a gene mutation on chromosome 7. In addition to respiratory tract infection, there are intestinal complications and exocrine pancreatic insufficiency. This results in malabsorption with bulky stools.

The 40-year-old construction worker provides an example of environmental lung disease. Silicosis is caused by the inhalation of crystalline silica. Occupations typically at risk include cement workers and sandblasters. These workers should be provided with respiratory protection such as a respirator. Usually, a latency period of 10 to 15 years from first exposure is required for the disease process to become evident. Asbestosis, another occupational lung disease, affects lower lobes (rather than the predominantly upper lobe involvement of silicosis). Asbestosis causes pleural disease, whereas silicosis causes lymphadenopathy.

Lymphangioleiomyomatosis is a rare progressive cystic lung disease that occurs exclusively in young women; spontaneous pneumothorax is common. Bronchoalveolar carcinoma (a subtype of adenocarcinoma of the lung) may present as a nonresolving infiltrate, often with air bronchograms due to alveolar filling by the malignant cells. Eosinophilic pneumonia causes a "reverse pulmonary edema" pattern with peripheral infiltrates; it responds to corticosteroids.

140 to 142. The answers are 140-a, 141-b, 142-e. The 32-year-old man has signs and symptoms of chronic tuberculosis. The disease presents with productive cough, hemoptysis, and weight loss. Night sweats are particularly characteristic of tuberculosis. Chronic cavitary disease usually involves the upper lobes.

The woman who is a heavy cigarette smoker is most likely to have primary lung cancer. The symptom of hemoptysis in association with weight loss and loss of appetite is particularly concerning. A pulmonary nodule greater than 3 cm is most often malignant, and the shaggy border of the lesion also suggests malignancy. Metastases to the lung are more sharply defined and are usually multiple.

Asbestosis is a risk for those such as construction workers, shipbuilders, and plumbers who may have long-standing history of exposure to asbestos-containing materials. Symptoms are usually subtle and include an annoying dry cough and dyspnea on exertion. Asbestosis on chest x-ray produces a linear interstitial process at the lung bases. Pleural fibrosis and pleural plaques may also be noted, especially on CT scan.

Bronchiectasis is associated with chronic productive cough and often hemoptysis; chest x-ray shows "train-track" pattern from peribronchial thickening. Idiopathic pulmonary fibrosis causes dry "Velcro" rales, clubbing and interstitial thickening on chest x-ray; unlike asbestosis, it does not cause pleural disease. Chronic pulmonary histoplasmosis can resemble tuberculosis; exposure history (Mississippi or Ohio valleys) will help in the differential diagnosis.

Suggested Readings

1. Kasper DL, Fauci AS, Hauser SL, Longo SL, Jameson JL, Loscalzo J. *Harrison's Principles of Internal Medicine*, 19th ed. New York: McGraw-Hill; 2015. Chapters 47e, 153, 305, 309, 311, 314, 316, 319, 322.
2. Asthma diagnosis and treatment guidelines. National Asthma Education and Prevention Program, Third Expert Panel on the Diagnosis and Management of Asthma. Expert Panel Report. Guidelines for the Diagnosis and Management of Asthma. Bethesda (MD): National Heart, Lung, and Blood Institute (US); 2007 Aug. available at: http://www.ncbi.nlm.nih.gov/books/NBK7232/
3. American College of Chest Physicians. Clinical Guidelines and Resources available at: http://www.chestnet.org/Guidelines-and-Resources
4. CDC Tuberculosis Webpage available at: http://www.cdc.gov/tb/
5. Pellegrino R, Viegi G, Brusasco V, et al. Interpretative strategies for lung function tests. *Eur Respir J.* 2005;26:948-068. doi:10.1183/09031936.05.00035205
6. Light RW. Pleural effusion. *N Engl J Med.* 2002;346:1971-1977.

Cardiology

Questions

143. A 60-year-old male patient is receiving aspirin, atorvastatin, isosorbide mononitrate, and a beta-blocker for chronic stable angina. He presents to the ER with episodes of unusually severe and long-lasting anginal chest pain each day over the past 3 days. His ECG and cardiac enzymes are normal. Which of the following is the best course of action?

a. Admit the patient and add intravenous digoxin
b. Admit the patient and begin low-molecular-weight (LMW) heparin and clopidogrel
c. Admit the patient for thrombolytic therapy
d. Admit the patient for observation with no change in medication
e. Increase the doses of current medications and follow closely as an outpatient

144. A 54-year-old man presents after a syncopal episode. The patient has no recollection of the event; according to bystanders, he awakened about 45 seconds after he "fell out." The patient has a history of bipolar disorder managed with quetiapine. He recently had an episode of prostatitis treated with ciprofloxacin. His other medications include lisinopril and hydrochlorothiazide (HCTZ) for hypertension and cyclobenzaprine and a hydrocodone/acetaminophen combination pill for low back pain. On examination, the patient is alert and oriented. Neurological examination is nonfocal. Cardiac examination is unremarkable, without murmur, gallop, or jugular distention. ECG shows nonspecific ST and T wave changes and a prolonged QT interval (QTc of 540 milliseconds). What is the best initial management approach?

a. Admit the patient for telemetry, check serum electrolytes including potassium and magnesium levels, and withhold all medications
b. Admit for permanent implantable cardioverter-defibrillator (ICD)
c. Admit and begin amiodarone infusion
d. Refer for genetic counseling
e. Admit for coronary angiography

145. A 15-year-old student presents to your office on the advice of his football coach. The patient started playing football this year and suffered a syncopal episode at practice yesterday. He reports that he was sprinting with the rest of the team and became light-headed. He lost consciousness and fell to the ground, regaining consciousness within 1 or 2 minutes. He has had no prior episodes of syncope. The patient is adopted and family history is unavailable. Physical examination reveals a systolic murmur heard at the left lower sternal border and apex. There is no midsystolic click. Arising from squatting to the standing position and Valsalva maneuver increases the intensity of the murmur. ECG reveals sinus rhythm with evidence of left ventricular hypertrophy (LVH). PR and QT intervals are normal. What is the likely pathogenesis of this patient's murmur?

a. Hypertrophy of the septum causes dynamic obstruction of blood flow in the aortic outflow tract. Decrease in ventricular volume makes the outflow obstruction more severe.

b. Scarring and calcification from congenitally bicuspid aortic valve obstructs aortic outflow.

c. Congenitally stenotic pulmonary valve occludes blood flow to the lungs during systole, leading to syncope.

d. Floppy mitral leaflets billow back into the left atrium during systole, leading to mitral regurgitation. Decrease in ventricular volume increases the degree of prolapse.

e. Normal flow across the pulmonary valve is accentuated by anxiety or exercise.

146. An 82-year-old white woman is admitted to the hospital for observation after presenting to the emergency department with syncope. After being placed on a cardiac monitor in the ER, the rhythm strip (shown in the following figure) was recorded. There is no history of cardiac disease, diabetes, or hypertension. With prompting, the patient discloses several prior episodes of transient dizziness and one episode of brief syncope in the past. Physical examination is unremarkable. Which of the following is the best plan of care?

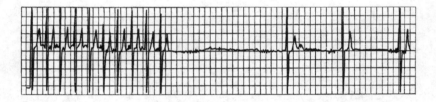

a. Reassurance. This is a benign condition, and no direct therapy is needed.
b. Reassurance. The patient may not drive until she is symptom-free, but otherwise no direct therapy is needed.
c. Nuclear cardiac stress testing; treatment depending on results.
d. Begin therapy with clopidogrel.
e. Arrange placement of a permanent pacemaker.

147. One month after hospital discharge for documented myocardial infarction, a 65-year-old man returns to your office concerned about low-grade fever and chest pain. He describes the chest pain as sharp, worse on deep inspiration, and better when sitting up. He denies shortness of breath; his lungs are clear to auscultation. On cardiac examination you hear a soft, scratchy sound both in mid-systole and in mid-diastole. ECG is shown in the following figure. Which therapy is most likely to be effective in relieving his chest pain?

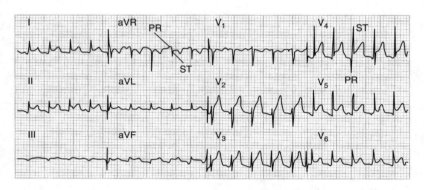

a. An antibiotic
b. Warfarin
c. An anti-inflammatory agent
d. Nitrates
e. An anxiolytic

148. A 55-year-old man presents with gradually increasing shortness of breath and leg swelling over the past month. He has also noticed orthopnea and paroxysmal nocturnal dyspnea. He takes simvastatin for hypercholesterolemia and hydrochlorothiazide for hypertension. Blood pressure is 140/90 mm Hg; there is mild jugular venous distension, soft bibasilar crackles, an S_3 gallop, and minimal pedal edema. An echocardiogram shows left ventricular ejection fraction (LVEF) of 40% without segmental wall-motion abnormality. The patient desires to keep medications to a minimum. What change in his management would you recommend at this time?

a. Add spironolactone
b. Add an ACE inhibitor and a beta-blocker
c. Add digoxin
d. Add a calcium-channel blocker
e. Arrange for implantable cardioverter-defibrillator placement

149. A 34-year-old woman is referred by an OB-GYN colleague for the onset of fatigue and dyspnea on exertion 1 month after her second vaginal delivery. Physical examination reveals a laterally displaced PMI, elevated jugular venous pressure, and pitting lower extremity edema. Echocardiogram shows systolic dysfunction with an ejection fraction (EF) of 30%. Which statement most accurately describes her condition?

a. This condition may occur unexpectedly years after pregnancy and delivery
b. Her chance of eventual recovery is 50%
c. The condition is idiosyncratic; her risk of recurrence with a future pregnancy is no greater than average
d. This condition will require a different therapeutic approach than the typical dilated cardiomyopathy
e. Diagnosis will require endomyocardial biopsy

150. A 55-year-old man is admitted to the hospital because of an episode of chest pain. The patient has medical history of chronic obstructive pulmonary disease (COPD), peripheral vascular disease with claudication, hypertension, hypercholesterolemia, and severe osteoarthritis of the knees. On admission his BMI is 40, there is bilateral wheezing, and cardiac examination reveals a grade 1/6 early systolic murmur at the upper left sternal border without radiation. Blood pressure readings are consistently 140/90 to 150/100. Cardiac enzymes are normal. A resting ECG shows left ventricular hypertrophy with secondary ST-T-wave changes ("LVH with strain"). Risk assessment according to the TIMI protocol indicates an intermediate risk of coronary artery disease. Which cardiac stress test would be most appropriate for this patient?

a. Exercise ECG stress test
b. Exercise nuclear stress test
c. Pharmacologic nuclear stress test with adenosine
d. Pharmacologic nuclear stress test with dipyridamole
e. Pharmacologic echo stress test with dobutamine

151. A 75-year-old patient presents to the ER after a syncopal episode. He is now alert and in retrospect describes occasional substernal chest pressure and shortness of breath on exertion. His blood pressure is 110/80 mm Hg and lungs have a few bibasilar rales. Which auscultatory finding would best explain his findings?

a. A harsh systolic crescendo-decrescendo murmur heard best at the upper right sternal border
b. A diastolic decrescendo murmur heard at the mid-left sternal border
c. A holosystolic murmur heard best at the apex with radiation to the axilla
d. A midsystolic click
e. A leathery two-component rub over the precordium

152. A 72-year-old man presents with shortness of breath that awakens him at night. He is unable to walk more than one city-block before stopping to catch his breath. Physical examination findings include normal blood pressure, bilateral basilar rales, and neck vein distention. The patient has diabetes and a known history of congestive heart failure. His last echocardiogram revealed a left ventricular ejection fraction of 25% with hypokinetic areas at the apex and inferior wall. The patient has been compliant with his medications, including an ACE inhibitor, beta-blocker, a loop diuretic, metformin, and glipizide. What is the most likely etiology for the patient's heart failure?

a. Toxic/metabolic
b. Infiltrative
c. Ischemic
d. Valvular
e. Infectious

153. A 72-year-old man comes to the office with intermittent symptoms of dyspnea on exertion, palpitations, and cough occasionally productive of blood. On cardiac auscultation, a low-pitched diastolic rumbling murmur is faintly heard at the apex. What is the most likely cause of the murmur?

a. Rheumatic fever as a youth
b. Long-standing hypertension
c. A silent MI within the past year
d. A congenital anomaly
e. Anemia from chronic blood loss

154. A 21-year-old man presents in the emergency room with new onset of slurred speech and right hemiparesis. On auscultation the patient has a systolic murmur at the pulmonic region with a diastolic rumble along the left sternal border. The second heart sound is split and fixed relative to respiration. What is the likely cause of patient's symptom?

a. Ventricular septal defect
b. Atrial septal defect (ASD)
c. Patent ductus arteriosus
d. Aortic insufficiency
e. Coarctation of the aorta

155. A 52-year-old woman returns for yearly follow-up of mitral valve prolapse (MVP). She is asymptomatic; she jogs daily without undue shortness of breath. She takes metoprolol 25 mg bid because of previous palpitations and occasional nonexertional chest pain. These symptoms are well-controlled. Physical examination shows normal vital signs with BP 126/72. Lungs are clear and neck veins flat. Auscultation shows a midsystolic click followed by a 3/6 blowing systolic murmur that radiates to the axilla. Her echocardiogram, however, shows deterioration of LV function, with ejection fraction dropping from 65% to 50%. The LV has dilated, with LV end-systolic diameter rising from 35 to 45 mm (normal 28±7). Transesophageal echocardiogram (TEE) confirms the mitral valve prolapse and LV dilation; the TEE shows evidence of severe mitral regurgitation. What is the best next recommendation for management of her valvular abnormality?

a. Begin lisinopril 10 mg daily
b. Begin digoxin 0.125 mg daily
c. Emphasize endocarditis prophylaxis with antibiotics before dental procedures, and continue yearly follow-up
d. Refer for mitral valve repair
e. Refer for ICD implantation

156. A 30-year-old woman presents with a chief complaints of palpitations. She has no other cardiac symptoms. A 24-hour Holter monitor shows occasional unifocal premature ventricular contractions and premature atrial contractions (PACs). An echocardiogram is normal, with left ventricular ejection fraction greater than 60%. Which of the following is the best management for this patient?

a. Anxiolytic agent
b. Beta-blocker therapy
c. Digoxin
d. Quinidine
e. Reassurance, no medication

157. An active 78-year-old woman with hypertension presents with a new left hemiparesis. Cardiac monitoring reveals atrial fibrillation. She had been in sinus rhythm 3 months ago. She takes a beta-blocker for her blood pressure. Aside from blood pressure and heart rate control, which of the following is appropriate?

a. ICD and permanent pacemaker
b. Immediate direct-current cardioversion
c. Aspirin 81 mg daily
d. Antiplatelet therapy plus warfarin with a target INR of 1.5
e. Warfarin with a target INR of 2.0 to 3.0

158. A 64-year-old man with type 2 diabetes mellitus and well-controlled hypertension presents for evaluation of self-detected irregular heartbeat. He takes lisinopril 10 mg daily and metformin 850 mg bid. He has no symptoms of heart failure or hyperthyroidism. He has been admitted with binge drinking of alcohol many times in past years. Physical examination shows an irregularly irregular heart rhythm at 84/min, normal neck veins, and clear lung fields. Apex impulse is normal (within the midclavicular line); no gallops or murmurs are noted. ECG is shown in the following figure. Echocardiogram shows normal systolic LV function, mild diastolic dysfunction, mild LV hypertrophy, and no valvular abnormalities. What is the best approach to prevention of cardiogenic embolism in this patient?

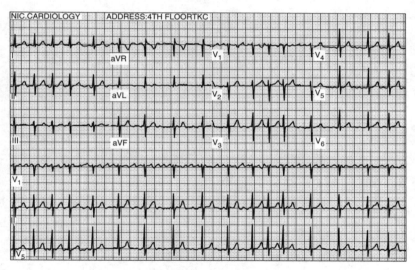

Reproduced, with permission, from Fuster V, Walsh RA, Harrington RA. *Hurst's the Heart*. 13th ed. New York: McGraw-Hill Education, 2011. Figure 40-1.

a. Aspirin 81 mg daily
b. Clopidogrel 75 mg daily
c. Warfarin adjusted to INR of 2-3
d. Apixaban 5 mg bid
e. Amiodarone 200 mg bid to convert him into normal sinus rhythm (NSR)

159. A 67-year-old man presents to your office after community ultrasound screening revealed an aortic aneurysm measuring 3.0 × 3.5 cm. Physical examination confirms a palpable, pulsatile, nontender abdominal mass just above the umbilicus. The patient's medical conditions include hypertension, hyperlipidemia, and tobacco use. What is the best recommendation for the patient to consider?

a. Watchful waiting is the best course until the first onset of abdominal pain
b. Surgery is indicated now except for the excess operative risk represented by the patient's hypertension and tobacco use
c. Serial follow-up with ultrasound, CT, or MRI is indicated, with the major determinant for surgery being aneurysmal size greater than 5.5 cm
d. Serial follow-up with ultrasound, CT, or MRI is indicated, with the major determinant for surgery being involvement of a renal artery
e. Unlike stents in coronary artery disease, endovascular stent grafts have proven unsuccessful in the management of abdominal aneurysms

160. An otherwise asymptomatic 65-year-old man with diabetes presents to the ER with a sports-related right shoulder injury. His heart rate is noted to be irregular, and ECG is obtained (shown in the following figure). Which of the following is the best immediate therapy?

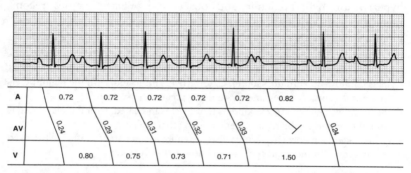

Reproduced, with permission, from Fuster V, Walsh RA, Harrington RA. *Hurst's the Heart*. 13th ed. New York: McGraw-Hill Education, 2011. Figure 43-5.

a. Atropine
b. Isoproterenol
c. Pacemaker placement
d. Electrical cardioversion
e. Observation

161. A woman with known mitral valve prolapse is admitted with a 2-week history of fever and chills. The patient had received oral levofloxacin without improvement. On examination, the patient appears moderately ill with T 38.3°C (100.9°F) and BP 152/68. No splinter hemorrhages or conjunctival petechiae are noted. Cardiac examination shows a harsh 3/6 systolic ejection murmur radiating to the carotids but also a new soft diastolic decrescendo murmur at the left sternal border. CBC reveals WBC of 13,200 with neutrophilic predominance; 5 to 10 RBC/hpf are seen on microscopic urinalysis. Three sets of blood cultures are positive for *Staphylococcus aureus* (sensitive to methicillin). Transthoracic echocardiogram reveals an 8-mm mobile mass on the posterior leaflet of the mitral valve. What development in this case would be an indication for surgical replacement of the damaged mitral valve?

a. An 8-mm vegetation is already indication for surgery
b. History of penicillin allergy
c. Presence of immune-mediated glomerulonephritis
d. History of intravenous substance abuse
e. The development of pulmonary edema

162. A 70-year-old woman has been healthy except for hypertension treated with a thiazide diuretic. She presents with sudden onset of a severe, tearing chest pain, which radiates to the back and is associated with dyspnea and diaphoresis. Blood pressure is 210/94. Lung auscultation reveals bilateral basilar rales. A faint murmur of aortic insufficiency is heard. The brain-natriuretic peptide (BNP) level is elevated at 550 pg/mL (normal <100). ECG shows nonspecific ST-T changes. Chest x-ray (CXR) suggests a widened mediastinum. Which of the following choices represents the best initial management?

a. IV furosemide plus IV loading dose of digoxin
b. Percutaneous coronary intervention with consideration of angioplasty and/or stenting
c. Blood cultures and rapid initiation of vancomycin plus gentamicin, followed by echocardiography
d. IV beta-blocker to control heart rate, IV nitroprusside to control blood pressure, transesophageal echocardiogram, and emergency thoracic surgery consultation
e. IV heparin followed by CT pulmonary angiography

163. A 55-year-old African-American woman presents to the ER with lethargy and blood pressure of 250/150. Her family members indicate that she was complaining of severe headache and visual disturbance earlier in the day. They report a history of asthma, for which she has used an inhaled corticosteroid and a long-acting beta-agonist as well as PRN albuterol. On physical examination, retinal hemorrhages are present. Neurological examination reveals that she responds briefly to verbal commands; no focal weakness is present. Serum creatinine is normal. Which of the following is the best approach?

a. Intravenous labetalol therapy
b. Continuous-infusion nicardipine
c. Clonidine by mouth to lower blood pressure
d. Nifedipine sublingually to lower blood pressure
e. Intravenous furosemide

164. A 73-year-old man with history of hypertension and osteoarthritis is evaluated for gradually increasing dyspnea over the preceding 6 weeks. He takes metoprolol for hypertension and naproxen for the arthritis. He has occasionally awakened in the night with mild dyspnea relieved by sitting up but has not noticed edema. Physical examination shows BP of 148/94, HR 96, and RR 16. O_2 saturation is 92%. Neck veins show the jugular column 7 cm above the sternal angle. Lung examination reveals mild basilar crackles but no wheezing. Cardiac examination shows sustained apex impulse, S_4 gallop, and no murmur. There is no peripheral edema. ECG shows stable left ventricular hypertrophy; no Q waves are seen. Chest x-ray shows increased interstitial markings and some cephalization of flow to the upper lobe vessels. The cardiac silhouette is boot-shaped, but there is no definite cardiomegaly. Echocardiogram shows left ventricular hypertrophy and LV ejection fraction of 55% (normal 50%-70%). What is the likely pathogenesis of this patient's dyspnea?

a. Increased metabolic demands leading to high-output heart failure (HF)
b. Occult coronary artery disease with dyspnea as an angina equivalent
c. Impaired diastolic relaxation and filling
d. Interstitial lung disease (ILD) mimicking pulmonary vascular congestion
e. Failure of oxygen-carrying capacity due to anemia

165. A 36-year-old man presents with the sensation of a racing heart. His blood pressure is 110/70, respiratory rate 14/min, and O_2 saturation 98%. ECG is shown. Carotid massage and Valsalva maneuver do not improve the heart rate. Which of the following is the initial therapy of choice?

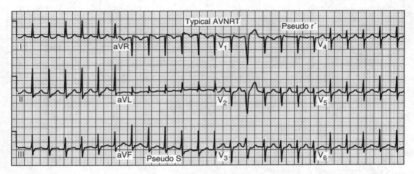

Reproduced, with permission, from Fuster V, Walsh RA, Harrington RA. *Hurst's the Heart*. 13th ed. New York: McGraw-Hill Education, 2011. Figure 41-3.

a. Adenosine 6-mg rapid IV bolus
b. Verapamil 2.5 to 5 mg IV over 1 to 2 minutes
c. Diltiazem 0.25-mg/kg IV over 2 minutes
d. Digoxin 0.5 mg IV slowly
e. Electrical cardioversion at 50 J

166. A patient has been in the coronary care unit for the past 24 hours with an acute anterior myocardial infarction. He develops the abnormal rhythm shown in the following figure, although blood pressure remains stable at 110/68. Which of the following is the best next step in therapy?

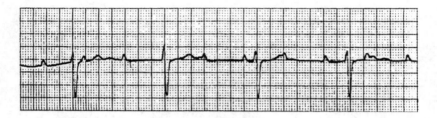

a. Perform cardioversion
b. Arrange for pacemaker placement
c. Give digoxin
d. Give propranolol
e. Give lidocaine

167. A 70-year-old man with a history of coronary artery disease presents to the emergency department with 2 hours of substernal chest pressure, diaphoresis, and nausea. He reports difficulty "catching his breath." An electrocardiogram shows septal T-wave inversion. The patient is given 325 mg aspirin and sublingual nitroglycerin while awaiting the results of his blood work. His troponin I is 0.65 ng/mL (normal <0.04 ng/mL). The physician in the emergency department starts the patient on low-molecular-weight heparin. His pain is 3/10. Blood pressure is currently 154/78 and heart rate is 72. You are asked to assume care of this patient. What is the best next step in management?

a. Arrange for emergent cardiac catheterization
b. Begin intravenous thrombolytic therapy
c. Admit the patient to a monitored cardiac bed and repeat cardiac enzymes and ECG in 6 hours
d. Begin intravenous beta-blocker therapy
e. Begin clopidogrel 75 mg po each day

168. A 55-year-old obese woman presents with pressure-like substernal chest pain lasting 1 hour. She works as a housekeeper. In the past few months, exertion at work has precipitated similar pain that goes away after a few minutes of rest. There is a family history of gallstones (mother and sister). On examination, the patient is pale and diaphoretic. Blood pressure is 90/50 and heart rate is 50 beats/min. Lungs are clear, but the jugular column is elevated to 10 cm above the sternal angle. ECG is shown in the following figure. Aspirin 325 mg is given. While you are waiting for the interventional cardiologist to take the patient to the cardiac catheterization laboratory, what treatment should be administered?

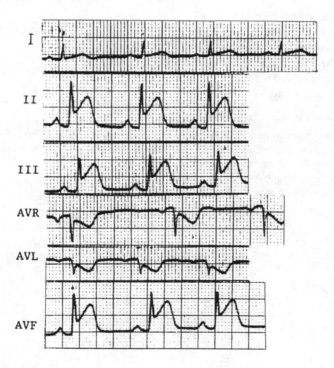

a. IV fluids and atropine
b. Beta-blocker
c. ACE inhibitor
d. Nitroglycerin drip
e. Verapamil

169. A 30-year-old construction worker continues to have elevated blood pressure of 180/100 despite therapeutic doses of hydrochlorothiazide, lisinopril, amlodipine, and metoprolol. He has had persistent hypokalemia despite taking KCl 20 mEq twice daily. He does not use illicit drugs or over-the-counter medications. Pill counts have shown that he is compliant with his antihypertensive regimen. He was found to be hypertensive at age 17 during a routine physical examination; his serum potassium was 3.0 mEq/L at that time. He has a BMI of 23; thyroid examination is normal, and no abdominal bruit is appreciated.

Routine blood chemistry show:

Sodium: 145 mEq/L
Chloride: 110 mEq/L
Potassium: 3.0 mEq/L
HCO_3: 30 mEq/L
Creatinine 0.9 mg/dL
Glucose: 90 mg/dL

Which of the following is the best next step?

a. Add a fifth antihypertensive medication and monitor blood pressure closely
b. Urinary vanillylmandelic acid (VMA), metanephrines, and catecholamines
c. Bilateral renal artery Doppler ultrasound
d. Polysomnography
e. Plasma aldosterone to plasma renin activity ratio

170. A 35-year-old woman was recently diagnosed with systemic lupus erythematosus. She presents with progressive dyspnea and chest pain for 2 weeks. Jugular venous distension is present and heart sounds are muffled. ECG shows electrical alternans. Chest x-ray is shown in the following figure.

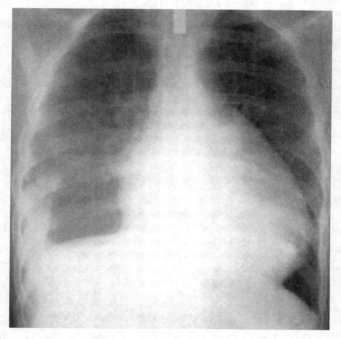

Reproduced, with permission, from Chen MYM, Pope TL, Ott DJ. *Basic Radiology*. 2nd ed. New York, NY: McGraw-Hill Education, 2011. Figure 4-63.

Which of the following is the most likely additional physical finding?
a. Basilar rales halfway up both posterior lung fields
b. S₃ gallop
c. Pulsus paradoxus
d. Strong apical beat
e. Epigastric tenderness

171. A 24-year-old Hispanic woman is found to have rheumatic mitral stenosis and is a candidate for mitral valve replacement. She is in sinus rhythm. You are meeting with her to discuss the option of a mechanical or bioprosthetic (tissue) valve implantation. Which of the following statements is true?

a. Compared with mechanical prosthetic valves, the rate of structural deterioration of bioprosthetic valves is less and the expected valve life is greater
b. In the absence of atrial fibrillation, long-term anticoagulation is not needed in most patients with bioprosthetic valves
c. The hemodynamic demands of pregnancy are better tolerated in patients with bioprosthetic valves
d. Antibiotic prophylaxis for dental procedures that manipulate gingival tissue is recommended for patients with mechanical but not bioprosthetic valves
e. Patients with bioprosthetic valves do not need regular follow-up

172. A 35-year-old woman notices fatigue and exertional dyspnea gradually worsening for the past several months. She denies cough and is a nonsmoker. On physical examination, her pulse rate is 100 and RR is 20. Room air O_2 saturation is 94%. On examination her neck veins are distended 12 cm above the sternal angle with prominent v-waves. Her lungs are clear. On cardiac examination the pulmonic component of the second heart sound (P2) is prominent, and she has a right parasternal heave. An S_4 gallop increases in intensity with inspiration. Chest x-ray shows cardiomegaly but clear lung fields; there is no pulmonary edema or cephalization of flow. Central pulmonary arteries are prominent but the peripheral vessels appear truncated or "pruned." ECG is shown in the following figure.

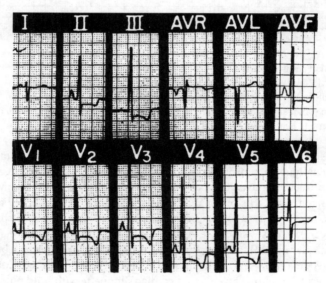

What is the likely pathogenesis of her cardiac problem?

a. Plexiform changes in the small pulmonary arteries, leading to pressure overload on the right ventricle.
b. Constriction of diastolic filling of both ventricles from pericardial fibrosis, leading to equalization of diastolic pressure in all four chambers.
c. Left-to-right shunt across an atrial septal defect, leading to chronic volume overload of the right ventricle.
d. Impaired diastolic relaxation of the left ventricle leading to elevated pulmonary capillary wedge pressure.
e. Impaired oxygen transport across damaged and distended alveoli, leading to reversible pulmonary vasoconstriction.

173. A 62-year-old man with underlying COPD develops a viral upper respiratory infection and begins taking an over-the-counter decongestant. Shortly thereafter he experiences palpitations and presents to the emergency room, where the following rhythm strip is obtained. What is the most likely diagnosis?

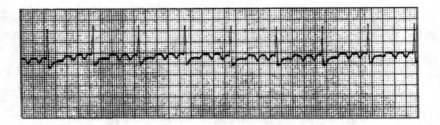

a. Normal sinus rhythm
b. Junctional rhythm
c. Atrial flutter with 4:1 atrioventricular block
d. Paroxysmal supraventricular tachycardia (SVT) with 2:1 atrioventricular block
e. Complete heart block

174. A 32-year-old man presents to your office with concern about progressive fatigue and lower extremity edema. He has experienced decreased exercise tolerance over the past few months, and occasionally awakens coughing at night. His medical history is significant for sickle cell anemia and diabetes mellitus. He has had multiple admissions to the hospital for vaso-occlusive crises since the age of 3. Physical examination reveals a laterally displaced PMI, an S_3 gallop, and scattered basilar rales. 1+ bilateral pitting edema is present. ECG shows a first-degree AV block and low voltage. Chest x-ray shows an enlarged cardiac silhouette with mild pulmonary vascular congestion. Which of the following would be the best initial diagnostic approach?

a. Order serum iron, iron-binding capacity, and ferritin level
b. Order BNP
c. Order CT scan of the chest
d. Arrange for placement of a 24-hour ambulatory cardiac monitor
e. Arrange for cardiac catheterization

175. You are volunteering with a dental colleague in a community indigent clinic. A nurse has prepared a list of patients who are scheduled for a dental procedure and may need antibiotic prophylaxis beforehand. Of the patients listed below, who would be most likely to benefit from antibiotic prophylaxis to prevent infective endocarditis (IE)?

a. A 17-year-old adolescent boy with coarctation of the aorta
b. A 26-year-old woman with a ventricular septal defect (VSD) repaired in childhood
c. A 42-year-old woman with mitral valve prolapse
d. A 65-year-old man with prosthetic aortic valve
e. A 72-year-old woman with aortic stenosis (AS)

176. A 60-year-old woman develops chest pain, respiratory distress, and confusion after right hip replacement surgery. She is minimally responsive and appears in respiratory distress. Blood pressure is 80/50 and heart rate is 155/min. Her extremities are poorly perfused, cold, and mottled. ECG reveals new-onset atrial fibrillation with rapid ventricular response. Which of the following is the best management of this patient's arrhythmia?

a. Immediate defibrillation with 360 J
b. Intravenous amiodarone
c. Intravenous metoprolol
d. Intravenous adenosine
e. Immediate electric cardioversion with 120 J

177. An 18-year-old male military recruit reports several episodes of palpitation and syncope over the past several years. Physical examination is unremarkable. His ECG is shown in the following figure. What is the most likely diagnosis?

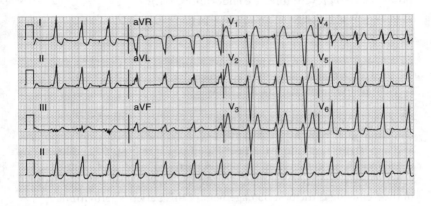

a. Prior myocardial infarction secondary to coronary artery disease
b. Congenital prolonged QT syndrome
c. Hypertrophic cardiomyopathy (HCM)
d. Pre-excitation syndrome (Wolff-Parkinson-White syndrome)
e. Rheumatic mitral stenosis

178. You are seeing for the first time a 45-year-old female patient of your partner. A review of the patient's medical record shows that her systolic blood pressure was greater than 140 mm Hg at both of her last clinic appointments. Her medical history is significant only for diabetes mellitus. She takes metformin 850 mg twice daily but is not on an antihypertensive. Her blood pressure today is 164/92. What is the best next step in her blood pressure management?

a. Ask the patient to keep a written record of her blood pressure and bring with her to a return appointment
b. Advise the patient to begin a heart healthy, low-sodium diet and refer to a nutritionist
c. Prescribe an ACE inhibitor in addition to heart healthy diet
d. Prescribe a dihydropyridine calcium-channel blocker in addition to a heart-healthy diet
e. Arrange for echocardiogram to assess for end-organ damage

179. A 67-year-old man presents to your clinic to establish primary care; he is asymptomatic. He has a history of hypertension for which he takes hydrochlorothiazide. His father had a myocardial infarction at age 62. The patient smoked until 5 years ago, but has been abstinent from tobacco since then. His blood pressure in the office today is 132/78. Aside from being overweight, the remainder of the physical examination is unremarkable. Which of the following preventive health interventions would be most appropriately offered to him today?

a. Carotid ultrasound to evaluate for carotid artery stenosis
b. Abdominal ultrasound to evaluate for aortic aneurysm
c. Lipoprotein(a) assay to evaluate coronary heart disease risk
d. Exercise (treadmill) stress testing to evaluate for coronary artery disease
e. Homocysteine level to evaluate coronary heart disease risk

180. A 68-year-old man complains of pain in his calves while walking. He also notes bilateral foot pain, which awakens him at night. His blood pressure is 117/68. Physical examination reveals diminished bilateral lower extremity pulses. An ankle:brachial index measures 0.6. The patient's current medications include aspirin and hydrochlorothiazide. Which of the following is the best initial management plan for this patient's complaint?

a. Smoking cessation therapy, cilostazol
b. Smoking cessation therapy, graduated exercise regimen, atorvastatin
c. Smoking cessation therapy, outpatient lower-extremity arteriogram
d. Smoking cessation therapy, warfarin, peripherally acting calcium-channel blocker
e. Smoking cessation therapy, consultation with a vascular surgeon

181. A 70-year-old man with a history of mild chronic kidney disease, diabetes mellitus, and CHF is admitted to your inpatient service with decreased urine output, weakness, and shortness of breath. He takes several medications but cannot remember their names. Laboratory tests are pending; his ECG is shown in the following figure. Based on the information available, what is the best initial step in management?

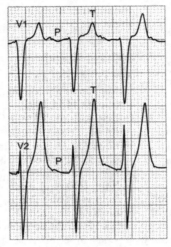

Reproduced, with permission, from Fauci A, et al. *Harrison's Principles of Internal Medicine*. 17th ed. New York, NY: McGraw-Hill Education, 2008.

a. Administration of intravenous insulin
b. Administration of intravenous sodium bicarbonate
c. Administration of intravenous 3% hypertonic saline
d. Administration of oral sodium polystyrene sulfonate
e. Administration of intravenous calcium gluconate

182. A 72-year-old man presents with chest pain. He is found to have ST segment depression in the inferior leads of his ECG and modest troponin I elevation at 2.2 ng/mL (normal <0.04 ng/mL). He is diagnosed with unstable coronary syndrome; left heart catheterization reveals two-vessel CAD with 90% stenosis in the proximal right coronary artery and 80% stenosis in the proximal left anterior descending coronary artery. Both lesions are treated by angioplasty and deployment of drug-eluting stents (DES). The patient does well and is discharged on aspirin, clopidogrel, atorvastatin, metoprolol, and prn sublingual nitroglycerin. Two months later he returns for medical advice. He has had no more chest pain, but he did have one episode of severe abdominal pain classic for biliary colic. He was evaluated in the emergency department where RUQ sonogram revealed several gallstones. Elective laparoscopic cholecystectomy was advised, and he returns to you for advice about his preoperative management. What is your best advice?

a. Proceed with surgery. Continue dual antiplatelet agents until the morning of surgery
b. Proceed with surgery. Discontinue clopidogrel 1 week before the planned operation
c. Obtain exercise stress test for risk stratification
d. Proceed with surgery. Discontinue both antiplatelet agents 1 week before surgery, but bridge the patient with low-molecular-weight heparin until the day before surgery
e. Defer elective surgery for at least 1 year after the percutaneous coronary intervention (PCI)

183. A 48-year-old man with a history of hypercholesterolemia presents to the emergency department with 1 hour of substernal chest pain, nausea, and sweating. His ECG is shown in the following figure. There is no history of hypertension, stroke, or any other serious illness. Which of the following is most appropriate at this time?

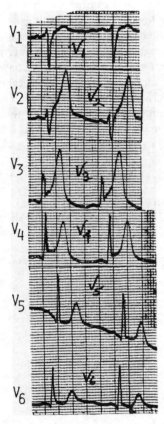

Reproduced, with permission, from Fauci A, et al. *Harrison's Principles of Internal Medicine*. 17th ed. New York, NY: McGraw-Hill, 2008.

a. Aspirin, calcium-channel blocker, morphine, primary percutaneous coronary intervention
b. Aspirin, beta-blocker, morphine
c. Aspirin, beta-blocker, morphine, primary percutaneous coronary intervention
d. Aspirin, morphine, primary percutaneous coronary intervention
e. Aspirin, beta-blocker

Questions 184 to 186

You are working in the university student health clinic, seeing adolescents and young adults for urgent care problems, but you remain attuned to the possibility of more serious underlying disease. For each of the numbered cases below, select the associated valvular or related heart disease. Each lettered option may be used once, more than once, or not at all.

a. Tricuspid stenosis
b. Tricuspid regurgitation
c. Mitral stenosis
d. Mitral regurgitation
e. Aortic regurgitation (insufficiency)
f. Aortic stenosis
g. Hypertrophic cardiomyopathy
h. Pulmonic stenosis
i. Pulmonic regurgitation (insufficiency)

184. This tall, thin 19-year-old white woman with little previous health care complains primarily of decreased vision and occasional diplopia. You note a strong pulse, blood pressure of 180/70, and a high-pitched, blowing, diastolic decrescendo murmur.

185. A 23-year-old graduate student complains of extreme fatigue and a vague sense of feeling ill the past few weeks. He has been under much stress recently and is slightly agitated. On examination, BP is 110/70, pulse is 100, and temperature is 38.0°C (100.5°F). The neck veins are distended with prominent *v* waves. A holosystolic murmur is heard at the left sternal border; the murmur intensifies on inspiration.

186. An asymptomatic 18-year-old man is referred for a pre-participation physical examination before starting a swimming class. He is asymptomatic. Vital signs are normal, but on auscultation you hear a 3/6 systolic ejection murmur at the left upper sternal border. A soft ejection click is present. With inspiration, the murmur becomes louder and the click becomes softer. Jugular venous pressure is 5 cm above the RA with a prominent "a" wave.

Questions 187 to 189

Which of the following diagnostic tests represent the most useful initial study for the patient in each vignette? Each lettered option may be used once, more than once, or not at all.

a. Exercise ECG
b. Vasodilator nuclear perfusion test
c. Dobutamine echocardiography
d. Transthoracic echocardiogram (TTE)
e. Transesophageal echocardiogram (TEE)
f. Cardiac MR imaging
g. Coronary angiography
h. Tilt table test
i. No further testing

187. A 23-year-old woman is referred by her family physician because of a heart murmur. She exercises regularly and is asymptomatic. Her mother died suddenly at age 47, and a brother is on medications for a heart murmur. On examination, her vital signs are normal, her neck veins are flat, and her lungs clear. The apex impulse is forceful, and she has an S_4 gallop. Auscultation reveals a 3/6 systolic ejection murmur at the lower left sternal border (LLSB) without radiation. Valsalva maneuver increases the intensity of the murmur.

188. A 72-year-old man presents for follow-up of chest pain. He was diagnosed with angina pectoris 5 years ago. At that time, coronary arteriography revealed two-vessel CAD with 70% narrowing of the left circumflex and 60% narrowing of the right coronary artery. The patient was started on aspirin, atorvastatin, metoprolol, and prn sublingual nitroglycerine (NTG). He has chest pain about once a month when he overexerts. His pain pattern is stable, and he is able to complete his usual activities without limitation.

189. A 68-year-old woman presents with mild dyspnea. She is able to complete her usual activities, but becomes winded when hiking at 11,500 feet. She has a history of breast cancer, and received adjuvant treatment 5 years ago with a regimen including daunorubicin. On physical examination, she is comfortable, with normal blood pressure and clear lung fields. Her jugular venous column is 4 cm above the sternal angle, and she has a soft S_3 gallop.

Cardiology

Answers

143. The answer is b. This patient presents with acute coronary syndrome (ACS) as indicated by an increase in the frequency and severity of his previously stable angina. The unchanged ECG and normal cardiac biomarkers indicate unstable angina (UA) rather than non-ST segment elevation myocardial infarction (NSTEMI). Patients with ACS should be admitted to a cardiac unit and their medical regimen intensified, in this case with the addition of antithrombotic therapy (IV unfractionated heparin or subcutaneous low-molecular-weight heparin) and additional antiplatelet therapy (such as clopidogrel). Intravenous nitrates, glycoprotein IIb/IIIa inhibitors, and early coronary angiography can be considered. There is no role for digoxin, which would increase myocardial oxygen consumption and exacerbate the situation. Thrombolytic therapy is reserved for the treatment for ST-segment elevation myocardial infarction (STEMI), where occlusive intracoronary thrombosis is demonstrated in 70% of patients. ACS is usually associated with unstable plaque and platelet activation but not major coronary thrombosis. The patient is at high risk for myocardial necrosis and should be admitted to the hospital for stabilization; simple observation and failure to intensify his treatment would be inappropriate.

144. The answer is a. This patient's ECG reveals significant QT prolongation (QTc >460 mm). The syncopal episode was likely related to polymorphic ventricular tachycardia (VT) (torsades de pointes). Both quetiapine and ciprofloxacin can prolong the QT interval; in combination with possible hypokalemia and hypomagnesemia from HCTZ, this could have caused life-threatening polymorphic VT. The patient should be admitted for telemetry, and any electrolyte abnormality promptly treated. If the patient's QT remains prolonged, beta-blockers can be started and the patient can be assessed for ICD placement.

An ICD is indicated in patients with symptomatic sustained (>30 seconds) ventricular tachycardia and in patients at high risk of sudden cardiac death (especially patients who have symptomatic heart failure and LVEF under 35%). ICD implantation would be premature in this patient until reversible abnormalities are corrected. Amiodarone is a class III antiar-rhythmic that blocks cardiac potassium channels. It is used to treat ven-tricular fibrillation and sustained monomorphic VT, but is less effective than IV magnesium and beta-blockers in polymorphic VT. Genetic coun-seling would be considered if the patient is found to have hypertrophic car-diomyopathy or one of the congenital prolonged QT syndromes. Coronary angiography is not indicated unless noninvasive testing suggests underly-ing CAD.

145. The answer is a. The patient has hypertrophic cardiomyopathy, an important cause of exertional syncope in young persons. It is commonly associated with left ventricular hypertrophy and prominent "septal" Q waves on ECG. The typical murmur of hypertrophic cardiomyopathy is a harsh systolic diamond-shaped murmur heard best at the lower sternal border and apex. Factors that increase myocardial contractility (eg, exer-cise or sympathomimetics) or that decrease preload (eg, Valsalva maneu-ver or standing) lead to reduced left ventricular end-diastolic volume. This increases the turbulence of blood flow exiting the ventricle during sys-tole, and hence accentuates the murmur. On the other hand, factors that increase venous return or preload (eg, leg raising), or that expand blood volume (pregnancy) all increase left ventricular volume and decrease inten-sity of the murmur. The diagnosis of hypertrophic cardiomyopathy can be confirmed by echocardiography.

Answer b describes valvular aortic stenosis (AS) due to congenitally bicuspid aortic valve. Although AS can cause syncope; it causes fixed (rather than dynamic) outflow obstruction. The described maneuvers would not change the intensity of an AS murmur. Answer c indicates con-genital pulmonary stenosis (PS). The murmur of PS would increase with inspiration, as decreased intrathoracic pressure would pull blood back to the right side of the heart and increase flow across the valve. If severe, PS would cause right (not left) ventricular hypertrophy. Answer d describes the pathogenesis of mitral valve prolapse (MVP) which is characterized by a mid or late (nonejection) systolic click. The click may be followed by a high-pitched, late-systolic crescendo-decrescendo murmur heard best at the apex. The click and murmur occur earlier (and sometimes become louder) with maneuvers that decrease left ventricular volume (standing, Valsalva maneuver), just as in hypertrophic cardiomyopathy. Maneuvers that increase left ventricular volume, such as squatting and isometric exer-cise, diminish the degree of prolapse, and the click-murmur is delayed and decreases in intensity. However, mitral valve prolapse would be accompanied by a midsystolic click and would not cause syncope or LVH. Answer e describes the common "innocent" pulmonic flow murmur. A physiologic flow murmur, however, would not change with maneuvers and would not account for this patient's syncope or ECG changes.

146. The answer is e. The patient in question has symptomatic tachycardia-bradycardia syndrome. Sinus node automaticity is suppressed by the tachyarrhythmia and results in a prolonged sinus pause following termination of the tachycardia. The patient in this case is symptomatic, and pacemaker placement is warranted; reassurance would put the patient at risk of further syncopal episodes and bodily harm from fall or accident. Although a pacemaker will prevent bradycardia, it does not prevent tachycardia. The patient may need beta-blockers or calcium-channel blockers to prevent tachycardia if she continues to be symptomatic after pacemaker placement. It is unlikely that any positive findings on a stress test could be correlated with her ECG findings. The tachy-brady syndrome does increase the patient's risk of cardioembolic event, and aspirin or anticoagulation should be considered according to her CHADS2 score. Clopidogrel, however, is not a first-line agent to prevent cardiogenic embolism.

147. The answer is c. The patient has post-cardiac injury syndrome (PCIS), also known as Dressler syndrome, which may occur several weeks post-myocardial infarction. It is thought to be an autoimmune phenomenon. The patient may have fever, leukocytosis, and pericardial or pleural effusion. The chest pain associated with pericarditis tends to be pleuritic and improves with upright posture. Lying back (or leaning too far forward) causes the heart to press against the posterior (or anterior) parietal pericardium, thus increasing the pain. A pericardial friction rub is present in about 85% of patients. Typical ECG changes of pericarditis include diffuse ST-segment elevation and PR-segment depression (the latter due to a concomitant atrial injury current). Both are present in this patient. Acute ST elevation with myocardial infarction is usually regional, depending on the infarcted area (V_1-V_4 in anteroseptal infarction; I, aVL, V_5, V_6 in lateral infarction; and II, III, arteriovenous fistula [aVF] in inferior infarction). This is in distinction to the ST segment elevation in acute pericarditis, which often involves all leads (except for AVR).

Treatment of PCIS is the same as for other forms of pericarditis. A short course of a nonsteroidal anti-inflammatory agent or corticosteroid may help relieve symptoms. Anticoagulation would put the patient at risk for hemorrhagic pericarditis, which can lead to potentially fatal pericardial tamponade. A patient recently discharged from the hospital warrants suspicion of pneumonia, but this patient does not have other signs and symptoms suggesting pneumonia. Likewise the patient's symptoms are not suggestive of anginal pain or panic attack, for which nitrates or anxiolytics might be prescribed.

148. The answer is b. There is very good evidence that ACE inhibitors should be used in patients with heart failure (HF) and a depressed left ventricular ejection fraction. ACE inhibitors stabilize left ventricular remodeling, improve symptoms, reduce hospitalization, and decrease mortality. Beta-blocker therapy represents a major advance in the treatment of patients with HF and depressed systolic function. These drugs interfere with the harmful effects of sustained activation of the adrenergic nervous system by competitively blocking beta-receptors. When given with ACE inhibitors, beta-blockers stabilize left ventricular remodeling, improve patient symptoms, reduce hospitalization, and decrease mortality. An aldosterone antagonist is recommended for patients with NYHA class III or IV symptoms who have a left ventricular ejection fraction of less than 35% and who are still symptomatic despite receiving standard therapy with diuretics, ACE inhibitors, and beta-blockers. Likewise, digoxin may improve symptoms and decrease hospitalization rates in patients with HF but has not been shown to prolong life. Neither of these drugs is indicated in this patient with mild symptoms. Furosemide is used to improve symptoms but does not prolong survival. Since this patient wants to minimize medications, an ACE inhibitor and beta-blocker are better first choices because they confer a survival advantage. An implantable defibrillator is indicated in systolic heart failure with left ventricular ejection fraction less than 35% in order to prevent sudden cardiac death, but is not indicated in this patient whose ejection fraction is 40%.

149. The answer is b. Although peripartum (or postpartum) cardiomyopathy may occur during the last trimester of pregnancy or within 6 months of delivery, it most commonly develops in the month before or after delivery. The most common demographics are multiparity, African-American ethnicity, and age greater than 30. About half of patients will recover completely, with most of the rest improving with treatment, although the mortality rate is still 10% to 20%. These women should avoid future pregnancies because peripartum cardiomyopathy often recurs with subsequent pregnancies. Treatment is the same as for other dilated cardiomyopathies. Beta-blockers, digoxin, and diuretics can be used cautiously during pregnancy; ACE inhibitors should be started after delivery. Diagnosis can typically be made without invasive testing.

150. The answer is d. The choice of initial stress test modality depends on the patient's resting ECG, ability to exercise, and the availability of expertise and technology. Exercise electrocardiographic test should be the initial stress test in patients with an interpretable ECG who are able to exercise. When certain resting ECG abnormalities are present (ST depression > 1 mm, left ventricular hypertrophy, left bundle branch block, paced rhythm, or pre-excitation), either echocardiography or nuclear imaging is the preferred initial stress imaging. For patients with concomitant valve disease, pericardial disease, or aortic disease, echocardiography has the advantage of providing information regarding these issues. The major limitation of echocardiography is in patients in whom satisfactory imaging may be technically difficult. This is often the case in patients with COPD or morbid obesity. Therefore, nuclear imaging would be best in this patient. In this patient an exercise test would be difficult because of his claudication and severe osteoarthritis. Thus he will need a pharmacologic nuclear imaging test. In the setting of COPD, however, adenosine is best avoided because it can aggravate bronchospasm. Therefore, a pharmacologic nuclear perfusion scan using dipyridamole as the vasodilator is the best test for this patient.

151. The answer is a. The classic triad of symptoms in aortic stenosis includes exertional dyspnea, angina pectoris, and syncope. Physical findings include a narrow pulse pressure, delayed aortic upstroke, S_4 gallop, early systolic ejection click, and the described systolic murmur. The murmur of aortic stenosis is diamond-shaped and often radiates to the carotids. The diastolic decrescendo murmur (answer b) indicates aortic insufficiency. The holosystolic murmur (answer c) suggests mitral regurgitation. A midsystolic click is seen with mitral valve prolapse, and the scratchy precordial sounds indicate pericarditis. Of these conditions, only aortic stenosis causes syncope.

152. The answer is c. Coronary artery disease has become the predominant cause of congestive heart failure in industrialized countries, causing 60% to 75% of cases. Coronary artery disease, hypertension, and diabetes mellitus interact to augment the risk of heart failure in many patients, but coronary artery disease is the primary cause in most. In 20% to 30% of patients the exact etiology is not known. These patients are referred to as having nonischemic, dilated, or idiopathic cardiomyopathy. Prior viral infection or toxins (eg, alcohol or chemotherapy) may also lead to a dilated cardiomyopathy, but the echocardiogram would show global (not segmental) hypokinesis. Infiltrative conditions such as amyloidosis or sarcoidosis can cause myocardial infiltration with beta-amyloid or granulomas, but they are rare; amyloidosis often produces a characteristic ground-glass thickening of the myocardium on echocardiogram. Valvular diseases can cause heart failure but would be expected to produce a characteristic murmur. Echocardiography is a very sensitive test for valvular disease.

153. The answer is a. The history and physical examination findings suggest mitral stenosis. Dyspnea may be present secondary to pulmonary edema; palpitations are often related to atrial arrhythmias (PACs, SVT, atrial flutter, or fibrillation); hemoptysis may occur as a consequence of pulmonary hypertension with rupture of bronchial veins. A diastolic rumbling apical murmur is characteristic. If the patient is in sinus rhythm, a late diastolic accentuation of the murmur occurs because of increased flow across the mitral valve with atrial contraction. A loud first heart sound and early diastolic opening snap may also be present. The etiology of mitral stenosis is almost always rheumatic; so it is infrequently encountered in developed nations. Hypertension may cause an S_4 gallop but not a diastolic murmur. Myocardial infarction may cause mitral regurgitation because of papillary muscle dysfunction and anemia may cause a pulmonic flow murmur; both of these are systolic murmurs.

154. The answer is b. This patient likely has experienced a paradoxical embolus causing acute embolic stroke. In paradoxical embolism, a venous thrombus (usually from the leg or pelvic veins) passes into the systemic circulation through an intracardiac defect, typically an atrial septal defect (ASD) or less commonly through a ventricular septal defect (VSD). In ASD, a mid-systolic murmur can often be appreciated due to increased flow across the pulmonic valve. During diastole, a mid-diastolic rumbling murmur may occur at the sternal border due to increased flow across tricuspid valve. A prominent right ventricular impulse and palpable pulmonary artery pulsation may sometime be appreciated. The second heart sound is widely split and fixed in relation to respiration. Ventricular septal defect usually presents as a holosystolic murmur at the mid-left sternal border. Aortic insufficiency causes a diastolic decrescendo murmur at the mid-left sternal border. A patent ductus arteriosus (PDA) results in a continuous "machinery" murmur heard best at the upper left sternal border. Coarctation of aorta usually presents with a midsystolic murmur over the left interscapular space which may become continuous if the lesion in the vessel is narrowed enough to cause high-velocity jet flow. Coarctation of aorta causes arterial hypertension in the upper extremities and normal or low blood pressure, with diminished or delayed pulsations, in the lower extremities. Chest x-ray findings such as sign of "3" (due to indentation of the aorta at the site of coarctation with pre- and post-stenotic dilatation) and rib notching (due to rib erosions by dilated collateral vessels) are classic findings. Aortic insufficiency, PDA, and coarctation of the aorta are not associated with paradoxical embolism.

155. The answer is d. Valvular lesions causing volume overload to the left ventricle (mitral regurgitation and aortic regurgitation) are challenging to manage. If surgical repair is postponed until after overt heart failure (HF) develops, the patient may not improve after surgery and may have persistent LV dysfunction and increased mortality. This is in distinction to aortic stenosis, where LV function will recover after surgery even if the patient presents in florid HF. The criteria for recommending surgery for valvular regurgitation vary; just remember that repair is recommended when the LV begins to dilate EF begins to drop, before symptomatic HF occurs. Medications such as ACE inhibitors, beta-blockers, and digoxin have not been shown to alter the natural history of mitral regurgitation.

Most patients with MVP remain stable for years, but a few develop progressive mitral regurgitation. Indeed, MVP is a more common cause of progressive MR in the United States than is rheumatic heart disease. So-called "functional" mitral regurgitation, where dilation of the LV for other reason causes the papillary muscles to pull the MV apparatus open during systole, has not been proven to respond to valve replacement. IE prophylaxis is not recommended for patients with valvular heart disease who have not had mechanical valve replacement. AICD implantation is recommended for patients with HF who remain in NYHA functional class II or III despite maximal medical treatment and who have LV ejection fraction less than 35%.

156. The answer is e. Minimally symptomatic premature atrial and premature ventricular contractions in the absence of structural heart disease are benign and do not require treatment. Antiarrhythmic therapy in this setting has not been shown to reduce sudden cardiac death or overall mortality. A beta-blocker would be the best choice if symptoms begin to interfere with daily activities. Anxiolytics are unnecessary and would put the patient at risk of habituation. Digoxin is not useful in this setting. Type 1 antiarrhythmics (such as quinidine) carry significant risks, including an increased incidence of ventricular tachycardia.

157. The answer is e. Anticoagulation is important in patients with atrial fibrillation who have risk factors for stroke. Risk factors can be calculated from the CHADS2 score, an easy to remember mnemonic (C—CHF, H—hypertension, D—diabetes mellitus, A—age ≥75 and S—previous stroke or transient ischemic attack). Each risk factor is equivalent to 1 point except for stroke or transient ischemic attack (TIA), which counts for 2 points. Patients with scores of 2 or more benefit from anticoagulation such as warfarin with target INR of 2 to 3. Rheumatic mitral valve stenosis, marked left atrial enlargement (>5.0 cm), and left atrial thrombus seen on echocardiography may be additional risk factors. Other scoring systems are also available. Immediate direct current cardioversion is appropriate for hemodynamically unstable patients with atrial fibrillation but would not be indicated in this patient. Antiplatelet agents might be considered in patients with a CHADS2 score less than 2 or if anticoagulation is contraindicated. An implantable defibrillator is not indicated for atrial fibrillation unless left ventricular ejection fraction is less than 35% or there is a history of sudden cardiac death. Pacemakers are usually reserved for cases refractory to standard therapy and who have received AV nodal ablation.

158. The answer is d. This patient's CHADS2 score is 2, which is the threshold for full anticoagulation (for details of the CHADS2 calculation, see question 157). Aspirin alone is used for CHADS2 of 0. CHADS2 of 1 is a borderline value, since the risk of stroke is approximately the same as the risk of serious bleeding from anticoagulation. Classically, anticoagulation for CHADS2 of 2 or higher is accomplished with adjusted-dose warfarin, but this patient's binge drinking increases his risk of over- or under-anticoagulation. Novel anticoagulants such as dabigatran, rivaroxaban, and apixaban are as effective as warfarin and are less dependent on close follow-up and laboratory testing. The chief drawback of all novel anticoagulants is lack of prompt antidote to reverse the anticoagulant effect.

Aspirin is recommended for patients with CHADS2 score of 0 or those with a score of 1 and increased risk of full anticoagulation. Clopidogrel has not been studied for prevention of emboli in atrial fibrillation. Interestingly, patients who are cardioverted into NSR require continued anticoagulation, as brief episodes of atrial fibrillation can still occur. In addition, chemical (as well as electrical) cardioversion carries a major risk of embolic event. So, amiodarone is not administered to a patient with chronic atrial fibrillation without anticoagulation or proof of absence of thrombus in the atrial appendage via transesophageal echocardiography.

159. The answer is c. Abdominal aortic aneurysms (AAAs) occur in 1% to 2% of men older than 50 years and to a lesser extent in women. Smoking and hypertension are major risk factors for the development of AAA. Abdominal aneurysms are commonly asymptomatic, but acute rupture may occur without warning. Some will expand and become painful, with pain as a harbinger of rupture. The risk of rupture increases with the size of the aneurysm. The 5-year risk of rupture is 1% to 2% if the aneurysm is less than 5 cm, but 20% to 40% if the size is greater than 5 cm. Other studies indicate that, in patients with AAAs less than 5.5 cm, there is no difference in mortality rate between those followed with ultrasound and those who undergo elective aneurysmal repair. Therefore, operative repair is typically recommended in asymptomatic individuals when the AAA diameter is greater than 5.5 cm; other indications for surgery are rapid expansion or onset of symptoms. With careful preoperative evaluation and postoperative care, the surgical mortality rate should be less than 1% to 2%. Renal artery involvement increases the complexity of surgical repair but does not increase the risk of rupture. Endovascular stent grafts for infrarenal AAAs are successful and have largely replaced open surgical repair in many centers.

160. The answer is e. AV conduction block is classified as first, second, or third degree. First-degree AV block is defined simply as a prolongation of the PR interval (>0.20 second). Second-degree AV block is divided into two types, also known as Mobitz types. Mobitz type 1 (usually termed Wenckebach phenomenon) is characterized by progressive PR interval prolongation prior to the nonconducted P wave and a "dropped" QRS complex. Mobitz type 2 refers to intermittent nonconducted P wave without prior PR prolongation. In Mobitz type 2, the ECG shows complexes of normal AV conduction with an intermittent "dropped" QRS complex. Third-degree AV block refers to a complete dissociation between atrial conduction (the P wave) and ventricular conduction (the QRS complex). This ECG shows Wenckebach second-degree AV block (ie, progressive PR interval prolongation before the blocked atrial impulse). This rhythm generally does not require therapy. It may be seen in normal individuals, especially with increased vagal tone due to pain or nausea. Other causes of Wenckebach phenomenon include inferior MI and drug intoxications from digoxin, beta-blockers, or calcium-channel blockers. Even in the post-MI setting, Wenckebach second-degree AV block is usually stable; it rarely progresses to higher-degree AV block with consequent need for pacemaker.

161. The answer is e. This patient meets the Duke criteria for infective endocarditis (IE). He has both major criteria: (1) multiple positive blood cultures for an IE-causing organism (*S aureus*, viridans streptococci, *Enterococcus*, HACEK, and certain other organisms) and (2) evidence of endocardial involvement (new regurgitant murmur, vegetation visualized on echocardiogram). Minor criteria include predisposing condition (such as IV drug use), fever, embolic phenomena, immunological event (including immune-mediated glomerular involvement), and positive blood cultures for organisms other than the classic IE group. Indications for surgery in IE have expanded, now that it is apparent that patients in these categories treated surgically have improved outcomes; almost 50% of patients with IE now undergo surgery. The list of surgical indications is long, but the major factors are the (1) development of significant HF (remember, these are patients with regurgitant valvular lesions, leading to volume overload—the kind of valvular physiology that requires early surgery); (2) persistent bacteremia despite appropriate treatment; and (3) presence or high risk of embolization while on medical therapy. This patient's acute pulmonary edema indicates wide-open mitral regurgitation and is an indication for surgery.

A large vegetation (>1–1.5 cm), especially if caused by a difficult-to-treat organism, is a criterion for surgery, but an 8-mm vegetation will often resolve with antibiotics alone. It is certainly important to treat IE with bactericidal antibiotics, traditionally beta-lactams (if the organism is susceptible), but we now have several highly active antibiotics (eg, daptomycin) that are effective in the penicillin-allergic patient. Immunological phenomena are important indicators of IE but will improve with infection control, whether with antibiotics alone or antibiotics combined with surgery. Patients with substance abuse are treated in the same manner as other patients; they are more likely to have *S aureus* (rather than the less destructive streptococcal species) but decision for surgery is still based on clinical features of the illness.

162. The answer is d. This patient's presentation strongly suggests aortic dissection. Aortic insufficiency is common with proximal dissection, as are hypertension and evidence of myocardial ischemia due to dissection of the coronary arteries. Hypotension may be present in severe cases. Distal dissection can lead to obstruction of other major arteries with neurological symptoms, bowel ischemia, or renal compromise. In aortic dissection, the first line of defense is emergent therapy with parenteral beta-blockers. After beta-blockade is confirmed with HR around 60, nitroprusside is commonly used to titrate systolic blood pressure to less than 120. The diagnosis is established with transesophageal echo, MR, or CT angiography. Urgent surgery is usually required in proximal (type A) dissections. Type B dissections, where the aortic arch is spared, are managed medically unless complications occur.

Although endocarditis may cause aortic insufficiency, this patient's sudden onset of symptoms as well as widened mediastinum would be unusual in endocarditis. Myocardial ischemia can cause mitral (but not aortic) insufficiency. Furosemide might help the pulmonary edema but would not address the primary problem; digoxin increases shear force on the aortic wall and could worsen the dissection. Anticoagulation is contraindicated if aortic dissection is suspected, as it may increase the risk of fatal rupture and exsanguinating hemorrhage.

163. The answer is b. A hypertensive emergency occurs when diastolic blood pressure above 130 is associated with acute (or ongoing) target-organ damage. The blood pressure number itself does not define hypertensive emergency. This patient shows evidence of damage, namely hypertensive encephalopathy (headache, visual disturbance, and altered mental status). Other indications for treatment with intravenous antihypertensives include pulmonary edema, acute ischemic chest pain, acute kidney injury (especially if associated with RBC fragmentation), and aortic dissection. Immediate therapy with continuous-infusion nicardipine in the ICU setting is indicated. Other options include intravenous nitroprusside, or enalapril. Intravenous labetalol is often used in hypertensive emergencies but, as a nonselective beta-blocker, is relatively contraindicated in moderate-to-severe asthma. An oral medication such as clonidine would be slow-acting and difficult to administer in a lethargic patient. Sublingual nifedipine is no longer advised because of increased potential for overshoot hypotension with adverse cardiovascular events such as MI, stroke, or ischemic optic neuropathy. Loop diuretics do not lower blood pressure rapidly. If target organ function is normal in the setting of severe hypertension, the condition is termed hypertensive "urgency." Rapidly acting intravenous antihypertensives are not necessary in hypertensive urgency and carry the risk of overshoot hypotension.

164. The answer is c. The most likely explanation for this patient's presentation is heart failure with preserved ejection fraction (HFPEF), also known as diastolic dysfunction. As many as 50% of patients presenting with definite HF will have an ejection fraction above 50%. HFPEF is more common in the elderly, in women, and those with conditions (especially hypertension) that lead to LV hypertrophy. Often the echocardiogram will show evidence of impaired relaxation or increased stiffness of the LV (the latter often suggested by decreased flow across the MV during atrial systole, giving the so-called reversed e/a flow ratio). Tachycardia, by decreasing diastolic filling time, will often worsen HF symptoms in diastolic dysfunction. As opposed to systolic HF, beta-blockers and ACE inhibitors have not demonstrated long-term survival benefit. Management focuses on controlling BP, preventing tachycardia, and treating pulmonary and peripheral fluid overload with diuretics; so many of the modalities used in systolic HF are also employed in HFPEF, just without proof of survival benefit.

High output HF due to an AV fistula, Paget disease, or hyperthyroidism can mimic diastolic HF, but the patient usually has evidence of a hyperdynamic circulation (tachycardia, wide pulse pressure, hyperdynamic precordium). Occult CAD should be considered in patients with exertional dyspnea (which can be an angina equivalent), but this patient's rest symptoms and pulmonary vascular congestion would be unusual. In HF due to coronary artery disease, there is almost always evidence of prior MI or ischemic change on ECG. Nevertheless, a stress test is often obtained in patients with unexplained HF to rule out this possibility. Interstitial lung disease can cause rales and interstitial changes on CXR, but would not explain the cephalization of flow nor the elevated venous pressure. Measuring B-type natriuretic peptide (BNP) will resolve the issue in equivocal cases; BNP will be elevated in HF and normal or minimally elevated in ILD. Anemia can cause fatigue and exertional dyspnea and, rarely, even overt HF, but to cause HF the anemia would have to be very severe (usually Hb 7 g/dL or below) and should be apparent from the physical examination. In addition, severe anemia would usually cause evidence of hyperdynamic circulation as seen in high-output HF.

165. The answer is a. Adenosine, with its excellent safety profile and extremely short half-life, is the drug of choice for supraventricular tachycardia (SVT). The initial dose is 6 mg. A dose of 12 mg can be given a few minutes later if necessary. Verapamil is the next alternative; if the initial dose of 2.5 to 5 mg does not yield conversion, one or two additional boluses 10 minutes apart can be used as long as systolic BP stays above 100. Diltiazem and digoxin may be useful in rate control and conversion, but have a slower onset of action. Electrical cardioversion is reserved for hemodynamically unstable patients. Lidocaine is occasionally used in ventricular (not supraventricular) arrhythmias.

166. The answer is b. The ECG shows complete heart block. Although at first glance the P waves and QRS complexes may appear related, on closer inspection they are completely independent of each other (ie, dissociated). Complete heart block in the setting of acute myocardial infarction requires temporary (and often permanent) transvenous pacemaker placement. Atropine may be used as a temporizing measure. You would certainly want to avoid digoxin, beta-blockers, or any other medication that promotes bradycardia. There is no indication on this strip for cardioversion such as for atrial fibrillation/flutter or ventricular tachycardia/fibrillation. Lidocaine is contraindicated because it might suppress the ventricular pacemaker, leading to asystole.

167. The answer is d. The patient's history suggests acute coronary syndrome (ACS). The combination of elevated troponin and lack of ST segment elevation on ECG is most consistent with non–ST elevation myocardial infarction (NSTEMI). Initial therapy for acute coronary syndrome includes aspirin, nitroglycerin, anticoagulation, and morphine. An intravenous beta-blocker, such as metoprolol, is frequently given in the immediate management of ACS to decrease myocardial oxygen demand, limit infarct size, reduce pain, and decrease the risk of ventricular arrhythmias. Elevated blood pressure also increases myocardial oxygen demand. Given this patient's increased blood pressure and continued pain, administration of a beta-blocker is the appropriate next step in his management. Administration of intravenous morphine would also be appropriate.

Cardiac catheterization may well be necessary at some point during his evaluation, but there is no mortality benefit for emergent catheterization in NSTEMI. There is no role for thrombolytic therapy in patients with ACS without ST segment elevation. All patients with ACS should be admitted to a monitored cardiac unit with serial cardiac biomarkers to estimate the extent of cardiac damage, but the patient's continued pain demands urgent treatment, not just further observation. Clopidogrel therapy is indicated for patients with ACS who will not be undergoing immediate coronary artery bypass grafting (CABG). Clopidogrel therapy, however, will not improve this patient's elevated blood pressure nor promptly decrease myocardial oxygen demand. The correct dose of clopidogrel is a loading dose of 300 to 600 mg, then 75 mg po daily.

168. The answer is a. This patient has typical ECG abnormalities of an acute myocardial infarction of the inferior wall (ST segment elevation in II, III, and aVF) with reciprocal ST depression in aVL. The right coronary artery supplies blood to the right ventricle, the SA node, the inferior portions of the left ventricle, and usually to the posterior portion of the left ventricle and the AV node. Infarctions involving the SA node may produce sinus dysrhythmias, including bradycardia and sinus arrest; atropine is the first choice for the inappropriate bradycardia. Inferior infarction may cause the syndrome of right ventricular infarction, which is characterized by hypotension and elevated right-sided filling pressures. Obtaining right-sided precordial ECG tracings will confirm the diagnosis. Even though right-sided pressures are elevated, hypotension in RV infarction often responds to saline bolus. Then, since this patient is having an acute ST-elevation MI, she should receive prompt percutaneous intervention or thrombolytics, with the goal of opening the culprit artery within 90 minutes of arrival. The use of verapamil or beta-blockers can further worsen the sinus node dysfunction and result in hypotension or shock. The use of nitroglycerin drip also can precipitate profound hypotension, as these patients are preload dependent. The use of ACE inhibitor at this time is not appropriate since patient is hemodynamically unstable.

169. The answer is e. This patient likely has secondary hypertension caused by hyperaldosteronism. Resistant hypertension and hypokalemia especially in the young should raise this suspicion.

In a hypertensive patient with unprovoked hypokalemia (ie, unrelated to diuretics, vomiting, or diarrhea), the prevalence of primary aldosteronism approaches 40% to 50%. Other metabolic derangements such as mild hypernatremia and metabolic alkalosis are also seen. The ratio of plasma aldosterone to plasma renin activity (PA/PRA) is a useful screening test. These measurements are preferably obtained in an ambulatory setting. A ratio greater than 30:1 in conjunction with a plasma aldosterone concentration of greater than 555 pmol/L (20 ng/dL) has a sensitivity of 90% and a specificity of 91%.

Urinary VMA, metanephrines, and catecholamines are tests for pheo-chromocytoma. Patients with pheochromocytoma often present with episodes of palpitations, headaches, and sweating. Bilateral renal artery Doppler is used to diagnose bilateral renal stenosis (RAS). Hypertension due to obstruction of a renal artery is a potentially curable form of hyper-tension. The mechanism of hypertension is generally related to activation of the renin-angiotensin system. Two groups of patients are at risk for this disorder: older arteriosclerotic patients who have a plaque obstructing the renal artery and younger patients, usually female, with fibromuscular dys-plasia. This patient, however, does not have a renal bruit; his normal serum creatinine while on ACE inhibitors also speaks against RAS. Hyperten-sion due to obstructive sleep apnea is increasing in frequency. The sever-ity of hypertension correlates with the severity of sleep apnea. Obesity is an important risk factor. Hypertension related to obstructive sleep apnea should also be considered in patients with drug-resistant hypertension and in patients with a history of snoring. The diagnosis can be confirmed by polysomnography.

170. The answer is c. This patient has the typical water bottle heart seen on the chest x-ray of patients with pericardial effusion, which may occur in patients with lupus. Patients with pericardial effusion may develop cardiac tamponade, a condition in which pericardial fluid impedes diastolic fill-ing, resulting in reduced cardiac output and hypotension. In these patients, the ECG may show pulsus alternans due to the heart sloshing around in the pericardial sac. Typical physical examination findings in cardiac tam-ponade include elevation of jugular venous pressure and pulsus paradoxus (paradoxical pulse). Pulsus paradoxus is defined as more than 10-mm Hg decline in systolic arterial pressure during inspiration. Normally during inspiration the intrathoracic pressure drops, facilitating increased venous return and increased blood volume in the right ventricle. This causes bulg-ing of the interventricular septum into the left ventricular cavity, which impedes left ventricular filling slightly and causes a drop in systolic blood pressure. In normal patients, the inspiratory BP drop is less than 10 mm Hg. That is to say, pulsus paradoxus is not really paradoxical—it is instead an exaggeration of the normal slight drop of systolic blood pressure with inspi-ration. In contrast to pulmonary edema, the lungs of patients with cardiac tamponade are usually clear. Instead of a strong apical beat, one would expect a weak apical pulse and absent or muffled heart sound due to the fluid accumulation in the pericardial sac. An S_3 or third heart sound signifies systolic heart failure in adults. An S_3 is not found in cardiac tamponade. Epigastric and right upper quadrant tenderness can be seen in either acute right-sided heart failure or cardiac tamponade due to passive congestion of the liver, but this finding is not specific. Cardiac tamponade is often fatal unless promptly relieved by pericardiocentesis.

171. The answer is b. Patients contemplating heart valve replacement may choose either a mechanical or a bioprosthetic (tissue) valve. Bioprosthetic valves are most commonly xenografts (usually porcine); homografts (from cadavers) and autografts (from the pulmonary position) are less commonly implanted. Thromboembolic complications are common after implantation of a mechanical heart valve. This increased risk of thromboembolic phenomena is not seen beyond 3 months after implantation of a bioprosthetic valve. Thus, in the absence of atrial fibrillation, long-term anticoagulation is not necessary for most patients who receive a bioprosthetic valve. For many patients this confers significant advantage, as it eliminates the risk of hemorrhagic complications related to long-term anticoagulant therapy. The major disadvantage of bioprosthetic valves is that the rate of structural deterioration is faster and the expected valve life is shorter. Most mechanical valves have an expected life of 20 to 30 years. In contrast, one-third of patients with porcine bioprosthetic valves will require repeat valve replacement in 10 years, and half will need a new valve in 15 years.

Tolerance of the increased cardiac output associated with pregnancy is the same irrespective of implanted valve type. Most experts favor a bioprosthetic valve for women who are contemplating pregnancy. Mechanical valves require long-term anticoagulation with warfarin, which is teratogenic. Women with mechanical valves who are planning pregnancy should switch to an injectable heparin (which is inconvenient and more costly) before conception and continue this during most of pregnancy.

Patients with a prosthetic heart valve are at increased risk of infective endocarditis. For prosthetic heart valve patients, prophylactic antibiotics are recommended before and after certain high-risk procedures. Though official recommendations have recently eliminated many procedures for which antibiotic prophylaxis was traditionally recommended, antibiotic prophylaxis is still recommended for patients undergoing dental procedures that manipulate gingival tissue. This is recommended for all patients with a prosthetic heart valve irrespective of valve type or location. All patients with a prosthetic heart valve need regular follow-up. Many experts recommend yearly echocardiography beginning 5 years after valve implantation.

172. The answer is a. This patient has a disease process that causes pure right-sided heart failure (HF). The ECG shows right ventricular hypertrophy. Think about RVH whenever the R wave in larger than the S wave in lead V1. Secondary changes include right axis deviation (axis greater than +90), right atrial enlargement (large, wide P waves in II, III, and aVF), and ST-T changes in the precordial leads. Causes of pure right-sided HF include chronic pulmonary disease (such as COPD), primary pulmonary hypertension, right-sided valvular lesions (which are rare), and pericardial disease. This woman's gender, her age, the absence of evidence of lung disease on the CXR, and the cardiomegaly all point to primary pulmonary hypertension (PPH) as the most likely cause of her symptoms. In PPH, the fundamental problem lies in the small pulmonary arteries; plexiform changes lead to failure of pulmonary vasoconstriction. This raises pressure in the normally low-resistance pulmonary circuit. The right ventricle does not compensate well in response to increased afterload.

Answer b describes the physiological changes in constrictive pericarditis. This woman's predominant right-sided findings would be consistent with pericardial constriction, but cardiomegaly and right ventricular hypertrophy would not occur. In addition, constrictive pericarditis usually causes the jugular pressure to rise with inspiration (so-called Kussmaul sign) and would not cause prominent v waves (which indicate tricuspid regurgitation). Answer c describes the physiological changes of atrial septal defect (ASD). Rather than causing decreased peripheral lung markings, ASD usually causes prominent pulmonary vasculature (due to increased blood flow through the pulmonary circuit). Fixed splitting of the second heart sound would also be expected in ASD. Answer d describes the pathophysiology of HFPEF. Diastolic heart failure, however, causes left-sided failure initially, leading to orthopnea and pulmonary edema. LVH (rather than RVH) would be anticipated. This patient has no evidence of left ventricular dysfunction. Answer e describes the changes of cor pulmonale. Chronic hypoxia leads to reactive vasoconstriction of the pulmonary arteries. Cor pulmonale associated with COPD usually improves with oxygen administration, which relieves the hypoxic stimulus to vasoconstriction. The absence of pulmonary disease on CXR and the lack of hypoxia provide strong evidence against cor pulmonale.

173. The answer is c. The rhythm strip reveals atrial flutter with 4:1 atrioventricular (AV) block. Atrial flutter is characterized by an atrial rate of 250 to 350/min; the electrocardiogram typically reveals a sawtooth baseline configuration characteristic of flutter waves. In this strip, every fourth atrial depolarization is conducted through the AV node, resulting in a ventricular rate of 75/min (although 2:1 conduction is more commonly seen). The rapid atrial rate excludes sinus rhythm (where the atrial and ventricular rates are the same) and junctional rhythm. In SVT the atrial rate is around 150, and inverted P waves usually follow the QRS complexes because of retrograde atrial conduction from the AV node. Regular atrial depolarizations at a rate of 300/min (as in this case) would exclude SVT.

174. The answer is a. The patient's history of sickle cell disease should raise the suspicion of iatrogenic iron overload. Multiple transfusions in a patient whose anemia is not attributed to blood loss can lead to tissue iron accumulation and end-organ damage just like genetic hemochromatosis. Measures to assess body iron status (transferrin saturation, serum ferritin level) are the initial diagnostic studies. This patient's diabetic status may also be related to iron accumulation. Evidence of cardiomegaly (from physical examination and chest x-ray) together with a low voltage on ECG suggests an infiltrative process affecting the heart. BNP is released from the cardiac myocytes in response to ventricular stretch and can be a useful tool in determining whether someone is suffering from heart failure. BNP will not, however, help determine the cause of the heart failure. Holter monitoring and cardiac catheterization is not necessary in patients without evidence of intermittent arrhythmias or coronary ischemia, respectively. CT of the chest is used to assess lung nodules or parenchymal abnormalities (such as interstitial lung disease) but would not be useful in this patient with only vascular congestion on CXR.

175. The answer is d. Recommendations for prophylaxis of infective endocarditis (IE) from transient bacteremia associated with dental, genitourinary, or gastrointestinal procedures have recently undergone major revision. Only patients with history of prior infective endocarditis (IE), patients with prosthetic heart valves, patients with unrepaired congenital cyanotic heart disease, and patients with prosthetic graft material which has not yet endothelialized (typically 6 months from placement of the graft material) are given prophylactic antibiotics. Therefore, the patients with coarctation of the aorta, repaired VSD, mitral valve prolapse, and aortic stenosis do not require pretreatment. A typical adult prophylactic regimen is a single dose of amoxicillin 2 g orally 30 to 60 minutes prior to the procedure. Any dental procedure that causes bleeding can cause transient bacteremia.

Sterile procedures (ie, cardiac catheterization) and procedures with a very low risk of bacteremia (ie, endoscopy without biopsy) do not need pre-procedure antibiotics.

176. The answer is e. This woman has hemodynamically unstable atrial fibrillation which requires immediate electrical cardioversion. Rate control with metoprolol or adenosine is not appropriate because these drugs may further worsen her hypotension. Though embolic stroke is a concern during cardioversion, the benefit of promptly stabilizing the patient's hemodynamic compromise outweighs this risk. Additionally, atrial fibrillation must be present for 24 to 48 hours before clots have time to form in the left atrial appendage. With atrial fibrillation, synchronized cardioversion (which delivers an electric shock timed to the R wave of QRS complex on the ECG) is preferred. Defibrillation using an unsynchronized electric shock of 360 J is used in ventricular fibrillation and pulseless ventricular tachycardia. In the absence of hemodynamic compromise, the initial goals in the management of atrial fibrillation are (1) ventricular rate control, and (2) prevention of embolic stroke by anticoagulation. Ventricular rate control is best established with beta-blockers and/or calcium-channel blocking agents (such as verapamil or diltiazem). These can be given by oral or intravenous route depending on the ventricular rate and clinical status of the patient. Digoxin may be added for rate control. An antiarrhythmic such as amiodarone can be started once sinus rhythm has been established or in anticipation of cardioversion in an attempt to maintain sinus rhythm. In the long-term management of atrial fibrillation, clinical trials have demonstrated no advantage for rhythm control over rate control.

177. The answer is d. The ECG reveals shortened PR interval and a delta wave causing widening of the QRS. The delta wave is a "slurring" of the upstroke of the R wave caused by the early depolarization of ventricular myocardium. This is consistent with an accessory conduction pathway or WPW. The aberrant conduction tissue bypasses the normal AV node (hence the PR interval of <0.12 seconds); it leads the electrical impulse directly to the ventricle (bypassing the His-Purkinje fibers and widening the QRS complex). Q waves are not infrequent and can be mistaken for evidence of prior MI. Myocardial infarction, however, does not cause shortened PR interval or delta wave. This patient's QT interval is normal (<0.46 second). Patients with HCM usually have voltage criteria for left ventricular hypertrophy, prominent ST/T-wave changes, and may even have large Q waves owing to hypertrophy of the septum. Rheumatic mitral stenosis would cause left atrial enlargement and perhaps atrial fibrillation, not the changes seen on this ECG.

178. The answer is c. Hypertension is defined as elevated blood pressure on two or more separate readings. In a patient with stage 1 HTN and no other cardiac risk factors, consideration may be given to a therapeutic trial of diet and lifestyle modification. This patient, however, has diabetes mellitus. JNC-8 recommends a target blood pressure of 140/90 or lower in patients below 60 years of age, including those with diabetes. It is unlikely that the patient will be able to reach target blood pressure with diet and lifestyle modification alone, although these interventions will be important adjunct therapies. The JNC-8 recommends thiazide diuretic, calcium-channel blocker, ACE inhibitor or angiotensin-receptor blocker (ARB) as initial therapy for most patients with hypertension. Patients with diabetes and hypertension, however, benefit more from an ACE inhibitor or ARB, especially if they have signs of renal damage (elevated creatinine or micro-albuminuria). There is no contraindication to the use of calcium-channel blockers, but their increased expense without increased benefit would prevent answer d from being correct. Evidence of end-organ damage, such as left ventricular hypertrophy on an echocardiogram, is unlikely to change your initial management.

179. The answer is b. The U.S. Preventive Services Task Force recommends that all men between the ages of 65 and 75 with any history of smoking undergo one-time screening for abdominal aortic aneurysm (AAA). There is no evidence that screening carotid ultrasonography (ie, in the patient without cerebrovascular symptoms or carotid bruits) or treadmill testing are beneficial screening tests. Although lipoprotein(a) and homocysteine levels have some predictive value in assessing CAD risk, their measurement is not recommended by the USPS Task Force. The USPSTF instead recommends that standard lipids (cholesterol, HDL cholesterol, triglycerides) be measured every 5 years, beginning at age 35 in men and at age 40 in women.

180. The answer is b. This patient has symptomatic peripheral arterial disease (PAD). Initial intervention should focus on symptom improvement and cardiovascular disease prevention. Lifestyle modification, most notably smoking cessation, would help with both issues. The most effective way to improve his symptoms is a graduated exercise regimen. Cilostazol, a phosphodiesterase inhibitor, improves exercise tolerance but is less effective than exercise. Patients with PAD usually have underlying coronary disease. Aggressive risk factor modification (smoking cessation, lipid and blood pressure control) will decrease their main risk of death, which is coronary artery disease. It would be wrong, therefore, to start cilostazol without managing his cardiac risk with a statin. Calcium-channel blockers have not been shown to improve exercise tolerance, and there is no role for systemic anticoagulation in patients with PAD. Invasive interventions (angioplasty, surgery) are typically reserved for patients who have failed medical therapy or have limb-threatening ischemia. Arteriography would likely be needed before invasive intervention is attempted.

181. The answer is e. The patient's ECG findings (peaked T waves, AV dissociation) strongly suggest hyperkalemia. Additional ECG findings may include prolongation of the PR and QRS intervals. Further electrical deterioration may lead to QRS widening and development of a sine wave. Ventricular fibrillation and asystole are potential terminal consequences. The patient's diabetes mellitus and kidney disease are predisposing factors; ACE inhibitors, beta-blockers, and spironolactone can increase the serum potassium.

Hyperkalemia less than 7.5 mEq/L usually does not result in fatal arrhythmias, but evidence of hyperkalemia on an ECG should prompt rapid intervention. Calcium gluconate is commonly administered to decrease membrane excitability. Its effects begin within 5 to 10 minutes and last up to 1 hour. There are no contraindications to calcium in this patient. Insulin causes K+ to shift into the intracellular space and decreases serum potassium concentration. In euglycemic patients, a combination of insulin and glucose is typically administered concomitantly to decrease the risk of hypoglycemia. In hyperglycemic patients insulin alone should be given. In our patient, however, laboratory tests are still pending. It would be prudent to check a blood sugar before administering insulin. Sodium bicarbonate therapy also will shift K+ into the cells but is less effective than insulin administration. Patients with severe kidney disease or hypervolemic states, such as CHF, may not tolerate alkalinization or the associated sodium load. Ideally, the serum bicarbonate and creatinine should be checked before intravenous sodium bicarbonate is administered. Inhaled albuterol is also an effective intervention in hyperkalemia, since beta-receptor activation will shift potassium into cells.

Each of the above therapies only shifts K+ into the cells. Attention must then be given to removing excess K+ from the body. Sodium polystyrene sulfonate (Kayexalate) is a cation exchange resin that binds K^+ in the GI tract and decreases serum K^+. The delayed onset of action of this drug prevents this from being the best initial intervention. Diuretic therapy (eg, furosemide) or hemodialysis can also decrease total body K^+. Depending on the patient's kidney function and volume status, these may be considered, but they too take hours to work and should not take the place of immediate therapy. There is no role for hypertonic saline in the management of hyperkalemia.

182. The answer is e. Stents are used to prevent artery closure after angioplasty. Bare metal stents are complicated by in-stent stenosis in 20% to 30% of cases. In-stent stenosis is associated with intimal thickening and gradual constriction of the lumen, leading to recurrence of angina. Drug-eluting stents combat this problem by using antiproliferative agents (sirolimus, paclitaxel) to decrease ingrowth of intimal cells. A consequence, however, is that the drug-eluting stent (DES) is slow to re-endothelialize. Whereas bare metal stents remain thrombogenic for just 4 to 6 weeks, it takes the DES at least a year to re-endothelialize. If the patient is not maintained on dual antiplatelet therapy, there is a significant risk of stent thrombosis, a potentially catastrophic event. Whereas in-stent stenosis is a gradual process, stent thrombosis usually causes sudden occlusion of the stent and an acute myocardial infarction. The mortality of stent thrombosis is 40%. Therefore, premature discontinuation of dual antiplatelet therapy early after DES placement should be avoided if possible. Elective surgery should be deferred at least a year. If the patient requires emergency surgery in the meantime, the cardiology service should be informed and aware.

Although minor surgery (eg, cataract extraction) could be carried out in this patient, dual-antiplatelet therapy leads to significantly increased risk of bleeding with major surgery. Few surgeons will schedule elective surgery unless the clopidogrel has been stopped. This patient has no symptoms of active CAD; a stress test will not predict his susceptibility to stent thrombosis. LMW heparin can be used to bridge patients who are on warfarin but has not been studied for prevention of stent thrombosis. A major risk of thrombosis occurs in the immediate postoperative period when tissue thromboplastin has been activated. LMW heparin would be on hold for the procedure at this time in any circumstance.

183. The answer is c. The ECG shows acute ST-segment elevation in the anterior precordial leads. The symptoms have persisted for only 1 hour, so the patient is a candidate for primary percutaneous intervention (angioplasty and/or stenting) or thrombolytic therapy, depending on the setting. Aspirin 325 mg should be given on arrival. Nitroglycerin and morphine are indicated for pain control. Beta-blockers reduce pain, limit infarct size, and decrease ventricular arrhythmias. There is no role for calcium-channel blockers in this acute setting (in fact, short-acting dihydropyridines may increase mortality). ACE inhibitors are given to decrease post-infarct remodeling and to improve LV function, but they are usually started orally within 24 hours of the initial infarct if systolic BP remains >100 mm.

184 to 186. The answers are 184-e, 185-b, 186-h. The first patient displays the classic triad of Marfan syndrome: (1) long, thin extremities, possibly with arachnodactyly or other skeletal changes; (2) reduced vision as a result of lens dislocations; and (3) aortic root dilatation or aneurysm. The diastolic murmur described is characteristic of aortic regurgitation (insufficiency), accompanied by the peripheral signs of water-hammer pulse and widened pulse pressure. Findings in the second patient suggest tricuspid regurgitation. Recall that inspiration increases right heart volume and therefore augments right-sided murmurs. The symptoms and low-grade fever raise the suspicion of infective endocarditis; the vegetations of IE usually cause regurgitant murmurs. Further history and physical signs of IV drug abuse should be sought. The final vignette suggests congenital pulmonary valve stenosis. Patients are often asymptomatic and may be diagnosed in adulthood. "Innocent" pulmonic flow murmurs are common, but pulmonic stenosis causes a loud murmur, often associated with an ejection click. Prominent increase in the murmur with inspiration (Carvallo sign) is characteristic. The prominent "a" wave in the jugular pulse is due to vigorous contraction of the right atrium as it squeezes blood into the stiff right ventricle. Right ventricular hypertrophy on ECG would be anticipated. Symptomatic pulmonary valve stenosis responds well to balloon valvuloplasty.

187 to 189. The answers are 187-d, 188-i, 189-d. The patient in question 187 has features suggestive of hypertrophic cardiomyopathy (HCM). The positive family history (including, worrisomely, family history of sudden death), the S4 gallop (usually indicating abnormal LV stiffness due to hypertrophy), and the dynamic murmur are all indicative of this diagnosis. Transthoracic echocardiography will always show the LV thickening (sometimes primarily involving the septum, occasionally involving the LV symmetrically) of HCM. The murmur of HCM is related either to LV outflow obstruction from the thickened septum or to mitral regurgitation from systolic anterior motion (SAM) of the mitral valve apparatus. The patient in question 188 has stable angina pectoris. Controlled studies have shown no advantage of invasive management (PCI or CABG) over medical treatment in stable angina; so this patient would not benefit from further testing. The patient in question 189 is at risk for dilated cardiomyopathy due to her anthracycline treatment; even those with low-dose exposure (<550 mg/M^2) are at some risk. Either radionuclide ventriculogram or echocardiogram would be indicated. Although radionuclide ventriculogram is a more sensitive test for systolic dysfunction, many cardiologists prefer echocardiography because it can pick up diastolic dysfunction, the earliest stage in chemotherapy-induced cardiomyopathy.

Exercise ECG should be the first test for most patients with intermediate-probability chest pain. Pharmacologic stress is used in those patients who cannot exercise, and more sophisticated tests for ischemic changes (radionuclide perfusion deficits, echocardiographic wall-motion abnormalities) are used in those whose ECGs are difficult to interpret for ischemia (LBBB etc). TTE is the first test for most patients with suspected ventricular or valvular abnormalities. Transesophageal echocardiography is better for subtle valvular disease (ie, infective endocarditis) or aortic disease (dissection). Cardiac MRI scanning may be helpful in patients with obscure cardiomyopathy. Coronary angiography is expensive and invasive; it is reserved for patients in whom revascularization is likely to be of benefit. Tilt-table testing is performed in patients with recurrent, unexplained, high-risk syncope.

Suggested Readings

1. Kasper DL, Fauci AS, Hauser SL, Longo DL, Jameson LJ, Loscalzo J. *Harrison's Principles of Internal Medicine*, 19th ed. New York: McGraw-Hill; 2015. Chapters 19, 52, 264, 279, 280, 283, 284, 288, 293, 300.

2. Fusler V, Walsh RA, Harrington RA. *Hurst's The Heart*. 13th ed. New York: McGraw-Hill; 2011.

3. American College of Cardiology/American Heart Association, available at: http://www.my.americanheart.org/professional/StatementsGuidelines/

4. Link MS. Clinical Practice. Evaluation and initial treatment of supraventricular tachycardia. *JAMA*. 2012;367:1438-1448.

5. Vongpatanasin W. Resistant hypertension: A review of diagnosis and management. *JAMA*. 2014;311:2216-2224.

6. Wilson JF. In the clinic. Stable ischemic heart disease. *Annals Int Med*. 2014;160:ITC 1-16.

Endocrinology and Metabolic Disease

Questions

190. A 50-year-old obese woman has long-standing type 2 diabetes mellitus inadequately controlled on metformin and pioglitazone. Insulin glargine (15 units subcutaneously at bedtime) has recently been started because of a hemoglobin A1C level of 8.4. Over the weekend, she develops nausea, vomiting, and diarrhea after exposure to family members with a similar illness. Afraid of hypoglycemia, the patient omits the insulin for 3 nights. Over the next 24 hours, she develops lethargy and is brought to the emergency room. On examination, she is afebrile and unresponsive to verbal command. Blood pressure is 84/52. Skin turgor is poor and mucous membranes dry. Neurological examination is nonfocal; she does not have neck rigidity. Laboratory results are as follows:

Na: 126 mEq/L
K: 4.0 mEq/L
Cl: 95 mEq/L
HCO_3: 22 mEq/L
Glucose: 1100 mg/dL
BUN: 84 mg/dL
Creatinine: 3.0 mg/dL

Which of the following is the most likely cause of this patient's coma?

a. Diabetic ketoacidosis
b. Hyperosmolar nonketotic state
c. Syndrome of inappropriate antidiuretic hormone (ADH) secretion
d. Drug-induced hyponatremia
e. Bacterial meningitis

191. A 24-year-old white man presents with a persistent headache for the past few months. The headache has been gradually worsening and is unresponsive to over-the-counter medicines. He notices diminished peripheral vision while driving. He takes no medications. He denies illicit drug use but has smoked one pack of cigarettes per day since the age of 18. His medical history is significant for passage of a kidney stone last year. At that time, he was told to increase his fluid intake.

Family history is positive for diabetes in his mother. His brother (age 20) has had kidney stones from too much calcium and a "low-sugar problem." His father died of some type of tumor at age 40. Physical examination reveals a deficit in temporal fields of vision and a few subcutaneous lipomas. Laboratory results are as follows:

Calcium: 11.8 mg/dL (normal 8.5-10.5)
Cr: 1.1 mg/dL
BUN: 17 mg/dL
Glucose: 70 mg/dL
Prolactin: 220 µg/L (normal 0-20)
Intact parathormone: 90 pg/mL (normal 8-51)

You suspect a pituitary tumor and order an MRI which reveals a 0.7 cm pituitary mass. Based on this patient's presentation, which of the following is the most probable diagnosis?

a. Tension headache
b. Multiple endocrine neoplasia type 1 (MEN1)
c. Primary hyperparathyroidism
d. Multiple endocrine neoplasia type 2A (MEN2A)
e. Prolactinoma

192. A 50-year-old woman is 5 ft 7 in tall and weighs 185 lb. There is a family history of diabetes mellitus. Fasting blood glucose (FBG) is 160 mg/dL and 155 mg/dL on two occasions. HgA1c is 7.9%. You educate the patient on medical nutrition therapy. She returns for reevaluation in 8 weeks. She states she has followed diet and exercise recommendations, but her FBG remains between 140 and 150 and HgA1C is 7.7%. She is asymptomatic, and physical examination shows no abnormalities. Which of the following is the treatment of choice?

a. A thiazolidinedione such as pioglitazone
b. A dipeptidyl peptidase-4 (DPP-4) inhibitor such as sitagliptin.
c. Insulin glargine at bedtime
d. Metformin
e. A glucagon-like-peptide-1 receptor agonist such as liraglutide

193. A 24-year-old woman presents 6 months after the delivery of her first child, a healthy girl, for evaluation of fatigue. She suspects that the fatigue is related to getting up at night to breastfeed her baby, but she has also noticed cold intolerance and mild constipation. She recalls having a tremor and mild palpitations for a few weeks, beginning 3 months after delivery. On examination, her BP is 126/84 and her pulse rate is 56. The thyroid gland is two times normal in size and nontender. The rest of the physical examination is normal. Laboratory studies reveal a free T_4 level of 0.7 ng/mL (normal 0.9-2.4) and an elevated thyroid-stimulating hormone (TSH) at 22 microU/mL (normal 0.4-4). What is the likely course of her illness?

a. Permanent hypothyroidism requiring lifelong replacement therapy
b. Eventual hyperthyroidism requiring methimazole therapy
c. Recovery with euthyroidism
d. Infertility
e. Increased risk of thyroid cancer

194. A 65-year-old white woman presents for an annual examination. She feels well except for occasional nocturnal leg cramp and mild abdominal bloating. She takes a multivitamin and a supplement containing 600 mg calcium carbonate and 200 international units of vitamin D twice daily. She takes no prescription medications. Physical examination is unremarkable for her age. In completing the appropriate screening tests, you order a dual-x-ray absorptiometry (DXA) to evaluate whether the patient has osteoporosis. DXA results reveal a T-score of −3.0 at the total hip and −2.7 at the femoral neck (osteoporosis: less than −2.5). Since her Z-score is −2.0, you proceed with an evaluation of secondary osteoporosis. Laboratory evaluation reveals

Calcium: 8.2 mg/dL
Cr: 1.0 mg/dL
BUN: 19 mg/dL
Glucose: 98 mg/dL
25,OH vitamin D: 12 ng/mL (optimal >30)

Liver enzymes including alkaline phosphatase: normal

WBC: 7700/µL
Hg: 10.3 g/dL
HCT: 32 g/dL
MCV 68
PLT: 255,000/µL

What is the likely cause of her osteoporosis?

a. Hypoparathyroidism
b. Estrogen deficiency
c. Renal leak hypercalciuria
d. Primary biliary cirrhosis
e. Celiac disease

195. A 27-year-old woman presents with palpitations, fatigue, heat intolerance, and insomnia. She has an otherwise unremarkable medical history. She is on no medications and does not use illicit drugs, weight loss products, or caffeine. On physical examination, her extremities are warm and she is tachycardic. Her neck shows diffuse, nontender thyroid enlargement. She has mild proptosis, as well as thickening of the skin in the pretibial area. Her laboratory values show a free T_4 value of 3.2 ng/dL (normal 0.9-2.4), and increased radioiodine uptake at 24 hours. Which of the following statements about the pathogenesis of her disease process is most accurate?

a. Immune globulins produced in the thyroid, lymph nodes, and bone marrow stimulate the thyroid directly to produce high levels of T_4.
b. Antibodies against TSH cause its level to appear low when in reality it is being overproduced, leading to high levels of T_4.
c. Microscopic thyroid lesions present in the enlarged thyroid gland produce T_4 in an autonomous and unregulated fashion.
d. Multiple nodules that will be evident on a thyroid ultrasound secrete a TSH analog which leads to hyperthyroidism.
e. A pituitary tumor which is actively secreting TSH is the usual mechanism of this process.

196. A 50-year-old woman is evaluated for hypertension. Her blood pressure is 130/98. She complains of polyuria and mild muscle weakness. She is on no blood pressure medication. On physical examination, the PMI is displaced to the sixth intercostal space. There is no sign of congestive heart failure and no edema. Laboratory values are as follows:

Na^+: 147 mEq/dL
K^+: 2.6 mEq/dL
Cl^-: 112 mEq/dL
HCO_3: 27 mEq/dL

The patient denies the use of diuretics or over-the-counter agents to decrease fluid retention or promote weight loss. She does not eat licorice. Which of the following is the most useful initial diagnostic test?

a. 24-hour urine for cortisol
b. Urinary metanephrine
c. Plasma renin activity
d. Renal angiogram
e. Ratio of plasma aldosterone to plasma renin activity

197. A 36-year-old woman presents with delirium and congestive heart failure. Her husband indicates that she has been losing weight and becoming more anxious and irritable over the past 3 months. Over the past several weeks she has developed dyspnea and peripheral edema. She has previously been healthy and takes no medications. Her husband says that she drinks alcohol moderately and has never used illicit drugs. On physical examination, she is awake, anxious, and confused. Her temperature is 38°C (100°F) and her heart rate is 142 and regular. She has jugular venous distension to 16 cm above the sternal angle as well as bibasilar rales. In addition, she has a diffuse goiter with a soft bruit over each lobe, as well as a stare expression and exophthalmos. Chest x-ray (CXR) shows pulmonary edema and cardiomegaly. Her ECG reveals sinus tachycardia but is otherwise unremarkable. What is the best approach to management of this patient?

a. Admit to the general medicine ward, obtain serum-free T_4 and TSH, order a radioiodine uptake and scan, and begin furosemide 40 mg IV daily.
b. Order free T_4 and TSH, start the patient on propranolol 20 mg po tid and Lasix 40 mg po bid, obtain a radioiodine uptake and scan, and follow closely as an outpatient.
c. Obtain free T_4, TSH, and thyroid-stimulating immunoglobulin levels, begin methimazole 10 mg po tid, and follow closely as an outpatient.
d. Admit to the general medicine ward, obtain blood and urine cultures and an echocardiogram, and begin treatment with broad-spectrum antibiotics and furosemide.
e. Admit the patient to the intensive care unit (ICU), order free T_4 and TSH, and begin high-dose propranolol, propylthiouracil, potassium iodide, corticosteroids, furosemide, and acetaminophen.

198. A 58-year-old man is referred to your office after evaluation in the emergency room for abdominal pain. The patient was diagnosed with gastritis, but a CT scan with contrast performed during the work-up of his pain revealed a 2-cm adrenal mass. The patient has no history of malignancy and denies erectile dysfunction (ED). Physical examination reveals a BP of 122/78 with no gynecomastia or evidence of Cushing syndrome. His serum potassium is normal. What is the next step in determining whether this patient's adrenal mass should be resected?

a. Plasma aldosterone/renin ratio
b. Estradiol level
c. Plasma metanephrines and dexamethasone-suppressed cortisol level
d. Testosterone level
e. Repeat CT scan in 6 months

199. On routine physical examination, a 28-year-old woman is found to have a thyroid nodule. She denies pain, hoarseness, hemoptysis, or local symptoms. Thyroid examination shows a 1.5-cm nodule in the right lobe of the thyroid; it moves normally with deglutition (ie, it is not fixed). No cervical lymphadenopathy is found. Serum TSH is normal. Which of the following is the best next step in evaluation?

a. Thyroid ultrasonography
b. Thyroid scan
c. Surgical resection
d. Suppression of the nodule with exogenous thyroxine
e. No further evaluation

200. An 80-year-old woman is admitted to the intensive care unit with sepsis due to a urinary tract infection. While in the ICU she develops atrial fibrillation with rapid ventricular response and is treated with a loading dose of amiodarone. She converts to sinus rhythm and is sent home on amiodarone to prevent recurrences of atrial fibrillation. In the following weeks she develops increasing fatigue, dry skin, and constipation and her internist finds her TSH to be 25. She is in sinus rhythm. What is the best approach in this situation?

a. Stop the amiodarone and follow the TSH and the clinical response.
b. Start low dose levothyroxine and repeat TSH in 6 weeks.
c. Start a beta-blocker and begin weaning off the amiodarone.
d. Check for anti-TPO antibodies to help guide your decision.
e. Start prednisone.

201. A 55-year-old man presents to the office with erectile dysfunction. He has mild diabetes and is on an angiotensin converting enzyme (ACE) inhibitor for hypertension. He and his wife enjoy a good relationship, and there is little external stress. He has, however, noted a lessening of sexual desire; they have not had intercourse in the past 6 months. The general physical examination is normal. In particular, his peripheral sensation to monofilament is intact, and vascular examination of the lower extremities is normal. Testicular size is mildly decreased bilaterally. Which of the following is the most appropriate first step in evaluation?

a. Serum-free testosterone and gonadotropin levels
b. Hemoglobin A1C and ankle-brachial index
c. Psychological evaluation
d. Therapeutic trial of sildenafil
e. Morning total testosterone level

202. A 65-year-old diabetic patient is hospitalized because of acute chole-cystitis. His diabetes is normally controlled with metformin 850 mg twice daily; a recent hemoglobin A1C level was 6.4. Cholecystectomy is per-formed, but is complicated by postoperative pneumonia and septic shock. The patient requires endotracheal intubation and ICU care. Blood cul-tures grow gram-negative rods, and vasopressors are required to maintain peripheral perfusion. What is the best method of controlling blood sugars in this patient?

a. Continue metformin via nasogastric tube.
b. IV insulin infusion to maintain blood glucose 140 to 180 mg/dL.
c. Sliding scale regular insulin to maintain blood glucose 80 to 120 mg/dL.
d. IV insulin infusion to maintain blood glucose below 100 mg/dL.
e. Contact endocrinology for subcutaneous insulin pump and continuous glucose monitoring.

203. A 58-year-old postmenopausal woman presents to your office on suggestion from an urologist. She has passed three kidney stones in the past 3 years. She is taking no medications. Her basic laboratory work shows the following:

Na: 139 mEq/L
K: 4.2 mEq/L
HCO_3: 25 mEq/L
Cl: 101 mEq/L
BUN: 19 mg/dL
Creatinine: 1.1 mg/dL
Ca: 11.2 mg/dL

A repeat calcium level is 11.4 mg/dL; Po_4 is 2.3 mmol/L (normal above 2.5). Which of the following tests will confirm the most likely diagnosis?

a. Serum ionized calcium
b. Thyroid function profile
c. Intact parathormone (iPTH) level
d. Liver function tests
e. 24-hour urine calcium

204. A patient comes to your office for a new-patient visit. He has moved recently to your city due to a job promotion. His last annual examination was 1 month prior to his move. He received a letter from his primary physician stating that laboratory work-up had revealed an elevated alkaline phosphatase and that he needed to have this evaluated by a physician in his new location. On questioning, his only complaint is pain below the right knee that has not improved with over-the-counter medications. The pain increases with standing. He denies trauma to the area. On examination you note slight warmth just below the knee, no deformity or effusion of the knee joint, and full ROM of the knee without pain. You order an x-ray, which shows cortical thickening of the superior fibula and sclerotic changes. Laboratory evaluation shows an elevated alkaline phosphatase of 297 mg/dL with an otherwise normal metabolic panel. In particular, the liver transaminases and gamma glutamyl transpeptidase (GGT) levels are normal. Which of the following is the treatment of choice for this patient?

a. Observation
b. Nonsteroidal anti-inflammatory drugs
c. High-dose bisphosphonate
d. Melphalan and prednisone
e. Ursodeoxycholic acid (UDCA)

205. Your patient is a 48-year-old Hispanic man with a 4-year history of type 2 diabetes mellitus. He is currently utilizing a combination NPH/regular 70/30 insulin product, injecting 60 units prior to breakfast and 30 units prior to supper. His supper time has become variable due to a new job and ranges from 5 to 8 PM. In reviewing his glucose diary you note some very low readings (40-60 mg/dL) during the past few weeks at 3 AM. When he awakens to urinate, he feels sweaty or jittery so has been checking fingerstick blood glucose. Morning glucose levels following these episodes are always higher (200-250) than his average fasting glucose level (120-150). Which change in his insulin regimen is the best and most likely to resolve this patient's early morning hypoglycemic episodes?

a. Increase morning dose of NPH/regular 70/30 and decrease evening dose.
b. Decrease morning dose of NPH/regular 70/30 and decrease evening dose.
c. Change regimen to glargine or detemir at bedtime and institute morning and evening use of regular insulin.
d. Discontinue NPH/regular 70/30 insulin and institute lispro insulin using a sliding scale before each meal.
e. Change regimen to glargine at bedtime combined with lispro insulin adjusted according to blood glucose prior to each meal.

206. A 40-year-old alcoholic man is being treated for tuberculosis, but he has been only intermittently compliant with his medications despite the health department's best efforts at directly observed therapy. He complains of increasing weakness, fatigue, weight loss, and nausea over the preceding 3 weeks. He appears thin, and his blood pressure is 80/50 mm Hg. There is increased pigmentation over the elbows and in the palmar creases. Cardiac examination is normal. Which of the following is the best next step in evaluation?

a. CBC with iron and iron-binding capacity
b. Erythrocyte sedimentation rate (ESR)
c. Early morning serum cortisol and cosyntropin stimulation
d. Blood cultures
e. Esophagogastroduodenoscopy (EGD)

207. A 37-year-old woman presents with difficult-to-control diabetes. The diabetes developed 3 years prior to this visit, when the patient began to notice fatigue, nocturia, and visual blurriness. She has been placed on metformin, glyburide, and finally pioglitazone at maximal doses, and yet her hemoglobin A1C is still above target at 8.2. She has been compliant with her medical regimen and is concerned about her health status. There is no family history of diabetes. On examination, her BP is 126/80, BMI is 23.7, and general physical examination is normal. She has no evidence or retinopathy or peripheral neuropathy. Anti-islet cell autoantibodies, including anti-glutamic acid decarboxylase (GAD) antibodies, are positive. What is the likely diagnosis?

a. Cushing syndrome
b. Glucagonoma
c. Type 2 diabetes mellitus
d. Late-onset autoimmune diabetes of adulthood (LADA)
e. Maturity-onset diabetes of the young (MODY)

208. A 45-year-old G2P2 woman presents for annual examination. She reports regular menstrual cycles lasting 3 to 5 days. She exercises five times per week and reports no difficulty sleeping. Her weight is stable at 140 lb and she is 5 ft 8 in tall. Physical examination is unremarkable. Laboratory studies are normal with the exception of a TSH value of 6.6 mU/L (normal 0.4-4.0 mU/L). Free T_4 is normal. Which of the following represents the best option for management of this patient's elevated TSH?

a. Repeat TSH in 3 to 6 months and reassess for symptoms of hypothyroidism.
b. Begin low-dose levothyroxine (25-50 µg/d).
c. Recommend dietary iodide supplementation.
d. Order thyroid uptake scan.
e. Measure thyroid peroxidase antibodies (TPO Ab).

209. A family brings their 82-year-old grandmother to the emergency room stating that they cannot care for her anymore. They tell you, "She has just been getting sicker and sicker." Now she stays in bed and won't eat because of abdominal pain. She is too weak to go to the bathroom on her own. Her symptoms have been worsening over the past year, but she has refused to see a doctor. The patient denies symptoms of depression. Blood pressure is 90/54 with the patient supine; it drops to 76/40 when she stands. Heart and lungs are normal. Skin examination reveals a bronze coloring to the elbows and palmar creases. What laboratory abnormality would you expect to find in this patient?

a. Low serum Ca^+
b. Low serum K^+
c. Low serum Na^+
d. Normal serum K^+
e. Microcytic anemia

210. A 60-year-old woman comes to the emergency room in a coma. The patient's temperature is 32.2°C (90°F). She is bradycardic. Her thyroid gland is enlarged. There is diffuse hyporeflexia. BP is 100/60. Which of the following is the best next step in management?

a. Await results of T_4 and TSH.
b. Obtain T_4 and TSH; begin intravenous thyroid hormone and glucocorticoid.
c. Begin rapid rewarming.
d. Obtain CT scan of the head.
e. Begin intravenous fluid resuscitation.

211. A 56-year-old woman with diabetes, hypertension, and hyperlipidemia is found to have an A1C of 11 despite her best attempts at diet and faithfully taking her metformin and glyburide. The patient mentions that she has been unable to exercise much, partially due to severe fatigue and sleepiness in the daytime. On examination she is obese, has a full appearing posterior pharynx, clear lungs, a normal heart examination, and trace bilateral edema. Reflexes and skin are normal. Her TSH is 2.0 µ/L (normal). The patient asks if there is anything else that can be done before adding another oral agent or switching to insulin. What is the best next step?

a. Educate the patient on sleep hygiene to ensure better rest and more energy.
b. Prescribe zolpidem as a sleep aid to help her sleep and increase her energy to exercise during the day.
c. Explore for possible depression as a contributor to the fatigue which is keeping her from exercising.
d. Arrange for a sleep study to check the patient for obstructive sleep apnea.
e. Check vitamin D level.

212. A 25-year-old woman is admitted for hypertensive crisis. The patient's urine drug screen is negative. In the hospital, blood pressure is labile and responds poorly to antihypertensive therapy. The patient complains of palpitations and apprehension. Her medical history shows that she developed hypertension during an operation for appendicitis at age 23.

Hct: 49% (normal range 37%-48%)
WBC: 11,000/mm^3 (4.3-10.8)
Plasma glucose: 160 mg/dL (75-115)
Plasma calcium: 11 mg/dL (9-10.5)

Which of the following is the most likely diagnosis?

a. Panic attack
b. Renal artery stenosis
c. Essential hypertension
d. Type 1 diabetes mellitus
e. Pheochromocytoma

213. A 23-year-old man complains of persistent headache. He has noticed gradual increase in his ring size and his shoe size over the years. On physical examination, he has a peculiar deep, hollow-sounding voice and a prognathic jaw. Bedside visual field testing suggests bitemporal hemianopsia. What initial studies are indicated?

a. Serum insulin-like growth factor 1(IGF-1) and prolactin levels
b. Morning growth hormone levels
c. Overnight dexamethasone-suppressed cortisol level
d. Lateral skull film to assess sella turcica size
e. GHRH-stimulated growth hormone level

214. A patient with small cell carcinoma of the lung develops increasing fatigue but is otherwise alert and oriented. Serum electrolytes show serum sodium of 118 mEq/L. There is no evidence of edema, orthostatic hypotension, or dehydration. Urine is concentrated with an osmolality of 550 mmol/L. Serum BUN, creatinine, and glucose are within normal range. Which of the following is the next appropriate step?

a. Normal saline infusion
b. Diuresis
c. Fluid restriction
d. Demeclocycline
e. Hypertonic saline infusion

215. The 40-year-old woman shown in the following figure complains of weakness, amenorrhea, and easy bruisability. She has hypertension and diabetes mellitus. She denies use of any medications other than hydrochlorothiazide and metformin. What is the most likely explanation for her clinical findings?

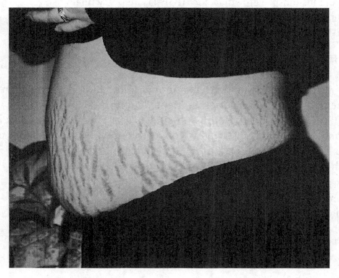

Reproduced, with permission, from Fauci A, et al. *Harrison's Principles of Internal Medicine*. 17th ed. New York, NY: McGraw-Hill Education, 2008.

a. Pituitary tumor
b. Adrenal tumor
c. Ectopic adrenocorticotropic hormone (ACTH) production
d. Hypothalamic tumor
e. Partner abuse (domestic violence)

216. A 24-year-old man presents with gynecomastia and infertility. On examination, he has small, firm testes and eunuchoid features. He has scant axillary and pubic hair. Which of the following is correct?

a. The patient has Turner syndrome.
b. The patient will have a normal testosterone level.
c. His most likely karyotype is 47 XXY.
d. The patient will have normal sperm count.
e. The patient is likely to have low levels of gonadotropins.

217. A 52-year-old man complains of impotence. On physical examination, he has an elevated jugular venous pressure, S$_3$ gallop, and hepatomegaly. He also appears tanned, with pigmentation along skin folds. He has joint pain and bony overgrowth primarily affecting the second and third metacarpophalangeal joints bilaterally. The plasma glucose is 250 mg/dL, and liver enzymes are elevated. Which of the following studies will help establish the diagnosis?

a. Detection of nocturnal penile tumescence
b. Determination of iron saturation
c. Determination of serum copper
d. Detection of hepatitis B surface antigen
e. Echocardiography

218. A 30-year-old man is evaluated for a thyroid nodule. The patient reports that his father died from thyroid cancer and that a brother had a history of recurrent renal stones. Blood calcitonin concentration is 2000 pg/mL (normal is <100); serum calcium and phosphate levels are normal. The patient is referred to a thyroid surgeon. Which of the following studies should also be obtained?

a. Obtain a liver scan.
b. Measure parathormone level.
c. Measure urinary metanephrines.
d. Administer suppressive doses of thyroxine and measure levels of thyroid-stimulating hormone.
e. Treat the patient with radioactive iodine.

219. A 32-year-old woman has a 3-year history of oligomenorrhea that has progressed to amenorrhea during the past year. She has observed loss of breast fullness, reduced hip measurements, acne, increased body hair, and deepening of her voice. Physical examination reveals frontal balding, clitoral hypertrophy, and a male escutcheon. Urinary free cortisol and dehydroepiandrosterone sulfate (DHEAS) are normal. Her plasma testosterone level is 6 ng/mL (normal is 0.2-0.8). Which of the following is the most likely diagnosis?

a. Cushing syndrome
b. Arrhenoblastoma
c. Polycystic ovary syndrome
d. Granulosa-theca cell tumor
e. Ovarian teratoma

220. A 36-year-old woman presents with amenorrhea. She has two children aged 8 and 6 years. She took oral contraceptives until her husband had a vasectomy 18 months ago. Since then she has not had a menstrual period. Otherwise she feels well. She takes no medications and exercises regularly but not to excess. She denies headache or galactorrhea. Her physical examination is normal. In particular, visual fields to confrontation are normal. Initial laboratory testing reveals negative pregnancy testing and normal CBC, creatinine, and TSH. Her prolactin level is 225 ng/mL (normal < 20). MRI of the pituitary is shown in the figure below. What is the best treatment for this patient's condition?

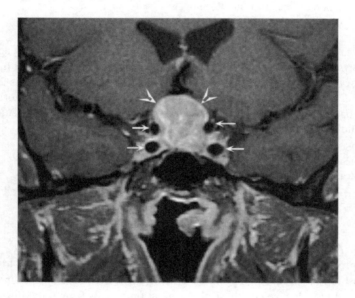

a. Transsphenoidal hypophysectomy
b. Resume oral contraceptives to reestablish menstrual cycles
c. Somatostatin analogue
d. Dopamine agonist such as cabergoline
e. Observation with yearly prolactin levels and MRI scanning

221. A 73-year-old man with a history of Parkinson disease, hypertension, and benign prostatic hypertrophy is noted by his wife to have abnormal mental status which progresses rapidly to lethargy. On arrival to the hospital he is febrile, tachycardic, and has a blood pressure of 80/50 mm Hg. His bladder is distended. Rapid laboratory assessment shows a WBC of 21,000, 8 bands, 85 segmented cells and 7 lymphocytes, Hgb 11 g/dL, BUN 70 mg/dL, and Cr 4.3 mg/dL. A Foley catheter is placed and 1050cc of turbid urine is obtained. Urinalysis reveals too numerous to count WBCs and bacteria present on microscopic examination. Blood cultures are drawn and broad-spectrum antibiotics administered along with aggressive IV fluids. He remains hypotensive. An echocardiogram shows no wall motion abnormalities and an ejection fraction of 60%. Norepinephrine drip is started. What is the next best step in his management?

a. Request emergent dialysis given the patient's uremic state.
b. Add a dobutamine drip and titrate upward until blood pressure is adequate.
c. Request the patient be sedated and intubated to reduce overall workload.
d. Add an antifungal antimicrobial IV stat.
e. Start hydrocortisone 60 mg IV q6h for 5 to 7 days and taper per clinical response.

222. A 48-year-old woman with a history of hypertension, hypertriglyceridemia, hypothyroidism, and obesity presents at her 6-monthly clinic visit complaining of pain in her feet. The pain is bilateral, symmetrical, and characterized as burning although the pain feels sharp when the feet are constricted in any way. She does not even like the bedsheets to lie firmly on her feet at night when the pain is the worst. There is no family history of neurologic problems; her personal social history is positive for one alcoholic drink nightly and for smoking 1 pack of cigarettes per day. On examination her BMI is 36, her blood pressure is 165/95, lungs are clear, heart is regular, abdomen normal, and extremities have no edema with distal pulses present. Careful neurologic examination reveals decreased pin prick sensation bilaterally up to the mid foot. Strength, vibration, and position sense are preserved. What is the most likely cause of her foot pain?

a. Alcoholic neuropathy.
b. Diabetic polyneuropathy.
c. Peripheral neuropathy due to peripheral arterial disease.
d. Peripheral neuropathy due to B12 deficiency.
e. Chronic use of restrictive footwear.

223. A 50-year-old woman presents with complaints of more than 10 severe hot flashes per day. Her last menstrual period was 13 months ago. She denies fatigue, constipation, or weight gain. Current medical issues include osteopenia diagnosed by central DXA. Family history is positive for hypertension in her father and osteoporosis in her mother. The patient uses no medications other than calcium 600 mg and vitamin D 400 IU twice daily.

Physical examination reveals weight 145 lb, height 5 ft 6 in, BMI 24, BP 126/64, and HR 68. Otherwise the examination is normal.

Screening laboratory studies:

Fasting glucose: 98
Cholesterol: 200 mg/dL
LDL: 100 mg/dL
Triglycerides: 150 mg/dL
HDL: 50 mg/dL
TSH: 1.0 mU/L

The patient requests hormone therapy to decrease hot flashes. Which of the following statements is true regarding hormone replacement therapy?

a. Progesterone therapy alone can alleviate hot flashes.
b. Hormone therapy does not affect bone density.
c. Her symptoms do not warrant systemic HT.
d. Oral estrogen therapy does not affect lipid levels.
e. The risk of breast cancer is directly related to duration of estrogen use.

Questions 224 to 226

Select the most likely disease process for the clinical syndromes described. Each lettered option may be used once, more than once, or not at all.

a. Acromegaly
b. Exogenous human growth hormone (HGH) use
c. Empty sella syndrome
d. Cushing disease
e. TSH-secreting adenoma
f. Chronic oral glucocorticoid use
g. Prolactin-secreting adenoma

224. A 30-year-old woman has prominent cervical and dorsal fat pads, hirsutism, acne, purple abdominal striae, unexplained hypokalemia, and diabetes mellitus.

225. A 28-year-old nursing student complains of joint pains and malaise. She is treated by a local alternative health practitioner. She has prominent central fat pads, striae, abnormal bruising, and hyperglycemia. Her serum potassium is normal.

226. An obese hypertensive woman has chronic headaches, normal visual fields, and normal pituitary function.

Questions 227 to 229

Match each symptom or sign with the appropriate disease. Each lettered option may be used once, more than once, or not at all.

a. Subacute thyroiditis
b. Graves disease
c. Factitious hyperthyroidism
d. Struma ovarii
e. Multinodular goiter
f. Thyroid nodule
g. Iodide deficiency
h. TSH-secreting pituitary adenoma

227. A 35-year-old woman is referred to for evaluation of elevated free T_4 and goiter. She complains of weight loss despite a voracious appetite, tremor, and rapid heartbeat. Thyroid examination shows mild diffuse enlargement without nodularity. She does not have exophthalmos or pretibial myxedema. Free T_4 is again elevated. TSH level is 2.8 (normal 0.4-4).

228. A 63-year-old woman who recently arrived as a refugee from Somalia complains of difficulty swallowing. She denies weight loss and chronic reflux symptoms. On examination her vital signs are normal. She has palpable enlargement and nodular lobularity of her thyroid, with the remainder of her examination being normal. Her T_3, T_4, and TSH are all normal.

229. A 20-year-old woman presents after recent upper respiratory infection. She complains of neck pain and heat intolerance. The thyroid is tender. Erythrocyte sedimentation rate is elevated; free thyroxine value is modestly elevated.

Endocrinology and Metabolic Disease

Answers

190. The answer is b. This woman with poorly controlled diabetes has developed hyperglycemia and lethargy during an episode suggestive of viral gastroenteritis. Her presentation is most consistent with hyperosmolar nonketotic state. This condition typically occurs in type 2 diabetics who become volume depleted and develop renal insufficiency. Glucose is no longer able to spill out into the urine, the blood glucose skyrockets, and severe hypertonicity leads to brain dysfunction and coma. Serum osmolarity is calculated by the formula:

$$\frac{\text{Plasma glucose}}{18} + 2(\text{Na}^+ + \text{K}^+) + \frac{\text{blood urea nitrogen}}{2.8}$$

This patient's serum osmolarity is as follows:

$$\frac{1100}{18} + 2(126 + 4) + \frac{84}{2.8} = 61 + 260 + 30 = 351$$

Thus, the serum osmolarity is greater than 350 mOsm/L. Although the serum sodium is usually the main determinant of osmolarity, extreme hyperglycemia contributes significantly to this patient's hypertonicity. Osmotically active particles in the extracellular fluid space pull water out of the intracellular space. This causes cellular dehydration in the brain and consequently the patient's CNS changes.

Diabetic ketoacidosis would be associated with a much lower serum bicarbonate level and with an elevated anion gap. This patient's anion gap is 9 mEq/L (126 − [95 + 22]), which is well within the normal range. This patient's hyponatremia is minimal and is related to the osmotic effects of hyperglycemia. Patients with SIADH have an inappropriate production of ADH, leading to water retention and consequent hypotonicity (not hypertonicity, as in this case). The diagnosis of SIADH or drug-induced hyponatremia cannot be made in the setting of severe hypovolemia. Although the oral hypoglycemic chlorpropamide can cause drug-induced hyponatremia, this patient was not taking a sulfonylurea. Although meningitis can be associated with hyponatremia, this patient's hypertonicity and lack of meningeal signs point toward hyperosmolar nonketotic state as the cause of her illness.

191. The answer is b. This young man presents with two obvious serum abnormalities—hypercalcemia and hyperprolactinemia (most likely secondary to the pituitary tumor). This, along with his positive family history of a younger sibling with high calcium and low blood sugar and a father who died from an unknown tumor, indicates this family has one of the multiple endocrine neoplasia syndromes. MEN1 is associated with hyperparathyroidism, pituitary tumors (usually prolactinomas), and islet cell tumors (most commonly gastrinomas, occasionally insulinomas). This patient's personal and family history, therefore, suggests MEN1. The MEN2 syndromes include medullary carcinoma of the thyroid and pheochromocytoma. MEN2A is associated with hyperparathyroidism; MEN2B with mucosal and GI tract neuromas. There is no pituitary abnormality with the MEN2 syndromes. It would not be prudent to treat the patient's issues as two separate abnormalities (primary hyperparathyroidism and prolactinoma). Tension headache is untenable in the face of a pituitary tumor and visual field deficit.

192. The answer is d. The classification of diabetes mellitus has changed to emphasize the process that leads to hyperglycemia. Type 2 DM is a group of heterogeneous disorders characterized by insulin resistance, impaired secretion of insulin, and increased glucose production. In this type 2 patient, the first intervention, medical nutrition therapy, failed to achieve the goal HgA1c of less than 7.0%. *Medical nutrition therapy* (MNT) is a term now used to describe the best possible coordination of calorie intake, weight loss, and exercise. It emphasizes modification of risk factors for hypertension and hyperlipidemia, not just weight loss and calorie restriction. This was appropriately instituted in the question. Blood glucose control should be evaluated after 4 to 6 weeks and additional therapy should be added if the goal has not been reached. Metformin is considered first-line therapy in that it promotes mild weight loss, has known efficacy and side-effect profile, and is available as a generic with very low cost. Thiazolidinediones ("glitazones"), DPP-4 inhibitors, GLP-1 agonists, sulfonylureas, and insulin are all considered second-line or add-on therapy for most patients with type 2 DM.

193. The answer is c. This patient has postpartum thyroiditis, a condition that follows 5% to 8% of all pregnancies. Like other forms of destructive thyroiditis (including subacute or de Quervain thyroiditis), this illness is triphasic. Initially there is hyperthyroidism due to inflammation and release of preformed thyroid hormone from the inflamed follicles; this phase usually lasts 2 to 4 weeks. In subacute thyroiditis, the initial phase is usually noticed because of pain and tenderness over the thyroid gland, but in postpartum thyroiditis the thyroid is usually painless, and the hyperthyroid phase may be overlooked. This phase is then followed by transient hypothyroidism, usually lasting 1 to 3 months. The third phase is resolution and euthyroidism. Whereas Hashimoto thyroiditis usually leads to permanent autoimmune hypothyroidism, most patients with destructive thyroiditis have a full recovery. Some will be symptomatic enough to require thyroid supplementation for 1 to 3 months until the process resolves.

Although the initial hyperthyroid phase can suggest Graves disease, in thyroiditis the absence of infiltrative ophthalmopathy and a suppressed radioiodine uptake will make the distinction. Antithyroid drug treatment of thyroiditis is ineffective and puts the patient at unnecessary risk of toxicity such as agranulocytosis. Although hypothyroidism can cause amenorrhea and hence impair fertility, the hypothyroid phase of postpartum thyroiditis is transient. Low-level radiation exposure, but not thyroiditis, increases the risk of subsequent development of thyroid cancer. Interestingly, therapeutic radioactive iodine, such as is given for Graves disease, does *not* increase the long-term risk of cancer, probably because the thyroid cells are destroyed.

194. The answer is e. Screening for osteoporosis in women is recommended at age 65 for most women and at age 60 for those with risk factors, including hyperparathyroidism, corticosteroid use greater than 3 months, cigarette smoking, low body weight, or documented fragility fracture. Although most women with osteoporosis will have primary osteoporosis, this woman's hypocalcemia and low vitamin D levels suggest that her osteoporosis is due to a secondary cause. The GI symptoms and the iron deficiency anemia suggest that her hypovitaminosis D is due to intestinal malabsorption. Celiac disease is relatively common (as high as 1% of the Caucasian population) and often presents with mild symptoms. A tissue transglutaminase or antiendomysial antibody test will provide important diagnostic information.

Hypoparathyroidism causes hypocalcemia but is not associated with vitamin D deficiency or osteoporosis. Estrogen deficiency is an important contributing factor to the skeletal loss of calcium that occurs in women at the time of menopause, but is associated with normal calcium and vitamin D levels and would not account for the iron deficiency. Hypercalciuria of any cause will lead to kidney stones but does not cause hypocalcemia or hypovitaminosis D. Although primary biliary cirrhosis may present with mild symptoms (usually pruritus) and vitamin D deficiency, the alkaline phosphatase is always elevated (often three to five times upper normal) in this disease. Again, recent studies show that sprue (celiac disease) is much commoner than PBC.

195. The answer is a. Immune globulins produced in the thyroid, lymph nodes, and bone marrow stimulate the thyroid directly to produce high levels of T_4. These thyroid stimulating immunoglobulins (TSIs) directly stimulate the TSH receptor and can be readily measured. Anti-TPO (thyroid peroxidase) antibodies are also present in over 80% of the patients. Cytokines such as tumor necrosis factor, interleukin-1, and others activate fibroblasts, leading to production of glycosaminoglycans which then trap water in muscles and lead to swelling of ocular muscles and hence the ophthalmopathy. The other choices are not pathogenetic mechanisms of Graves disease, although answer e describes a rare condition where a pituitary microadenoma can produce TSH and cause a hyperthyroid state. Pituitary-tumor induced hyperthyroidism does not cause infiltrative ophthalmopathy or pretibial myxedema.

196. The answer is e. The patient has diastolic hypertension with unprovoked hypokalemia. She is not taking diuretics. There is no edema on physical examination. Inappropriate aldosterone overproduction is a prime consideration in hypertension with hypokalemia. Hypersecretion of aldosterone increases distal tubular exchange of sodium for potassium with progressive depletion of body potassium. The hypertension is caused by increased sodium absorption. Interestingly, peripheral edema does not occur despite the sodium retention.

Elevated aldosterone level and low plasma renin activity suggest the diagnosis of primary hyperaldosteronism. The plasma aldosterone to renin ratio is a useful screening test. A high ratio of greater than 30 strongly suggests aldosterone oversecretion. Lack of suppression of aldosterone (ie, autonomous overproduction), however, is necessary to definitively diagnose primary hyperaldosteronism. High aldosterone levels that are not suppressed by a 2-L saline load prove the diagnosis. CT scan of the adrenal glands is then ordered to distinguish an aldosterone-producing tumor from bilateral adrenal hyperplasia. Renin levels alone lack specificity. Suppressed renin activity occurs in about 25% of hypertensive patients with essential hypertension. Twenty-four-hour urine for free cortisol would be used in the work-up of a patient with Cushing syndrome. Urinary metanephrine is a screening test for pheochromocytoma. Renal angiography is a test for renal artery stenosis. None of these diagnoses are as likely as hyperaldosteronism, given this clinical presentation.

197. The answer is e. This patient has thyroid storm, a medical emergency. The presence of fever, severe tachycardia, congestive heart failure, and CNS changes (delirium, psychosis, seizure, or coma) help separate thyroid storm from uncomplicated hyperthyroidism. Other factors that point toward storm or impending storm include atrial fibrillation, abdominal symptoms, jaundice, and the absence of a precipitating event. Even with treatment, the mortality of thyroid storm can be 10% to 20%, so admission to an intensive care unit for close monitoring is mandatory. Propranolol, generally contraindicated in decompensated congestive heart failure, improves the high-output CHF and, in high doses, helps block conversion of T_4 to the active hormone T_3. Propylthiouracil blocks the uptake and organification of iodide by the thyroid gland, and oral iodides prevent the release of preformed T_4 and T_3 from the thyroid gland. Relative adrenal insufficiency is often present, so corticosteroids are administered routinely in thyroid storm.

Patients with mild to moderate hyperthyroidism are usually evaluated and treated as an outpatient. Impending or threatened thyroid storm can be managed on the general medicine ward or in the ICU as clinically indicated, but overt thyroid storm (as in this patient) requires ICU care. If an outpatient has a diffuse goiter and if the cause of hyperthyroidism is unclear, radioiodine uptake can be measured to distinguish Graves disease (normal or increased RAI uptake) from painless thyroiditis (low RAI uptake). In thyroid storm, however, immediate treatment takes precedence over measuring the 24-hour radioiodide uptake. Furthermore, thyroiditis rarely, if ever, causes thyroid storm. Thyroid-stimulating immunoglobulin assays are rarely needed to diagnose Graves disease. Methimazole is often used in mild to moderate hyperthyroidism because of ease of dosing, but propylthiouracil blocks T_4 to T_3 conversion and should be used in thyroid storm. Although the febrile, tachycardic patient with hyperthyroidism can appear septic, other features of this case strongly suggest that thyroid storm, not infection, is the cause of her illness. Antibiotics without proper management of her hyperthyroidism would probably prove fatal.

198. The answer is c. This patient has what is commonly referred to as an adrenal incidentaloma. If the mass is greater than 1 cm, the first step is to determine whether it is a functioning or nonfunctioning tumor via measurement of serum metanephrines (pheochromocytoma) and dexamethasone-suppressed cortisol (Cushing syndrome) levels. As the patient has no history of malignancy, a CT-guided fine-needle aspiration is not required. The patient has normal BP and potassium; therefore, plasma aldosterone/plasma renin ratio to evaluate primary hyperaldosteronism is not required. There are no signs of feminization or erectile dysfunction, so sex-steroid measurement is not indicated. Contrast-enhanced CT after appropriate serum work-up determines true size and characteristics (Hounsfield units [HU]). Malignant indicators include large-size (>4-6 cm), irregular margins, soft tissue calcifications, tumor inhomogeneity, high CT attenuation (values greater than 10 HU), or delayed washout of contrast. CT scan should be repeated in 6 months and again in 1 year to ensure stability of the adrenal mass, but only after a functioning tumor has been excluded.

199. The answer is a. Palpable thyroid nodules are common, occurring in about 5% of all adults. The first test is serum TSH. Low TSH suggests an autonomously functioning ("hot") nodule, which is almost always benign. The diagnosis is confirmed by RAI uptake and scan. If the patient is biochemically euthyroid (as in this case), thyroid ultrasound is obtained to characterize the nodule and to stratify the patient for fine-needle aspiration (FNA). Pure thyroid cysts are aspirated and followed. Nodules with benign characteristics (less than 1 cm, hyperechogenicity, "comet tail" on ultrasound, among others) in a patient with no clinical features worrisome for cancer (ie, no previous radiation to neck, no family history) may be followed sonographically. For other nodules, FNA is generally recommended. About 15% of thyroid nodules will be found to harbor malignancy. False-negative rate for FNA is 4%; so some patients with benign pathology will still require surgery. If malignancy is confirmed, total thyroidectomy is necessary to eradicate thyroid cancer. Attempting to "shrink" the nodule with exogenous thyroxine is not a reliable way to distinguish benign from malignant nodules and is no longer recommended. Thyroid cancer can present even in a young, asymptomatic patient like this, so answer e would not be appropriate.

200. The answer is b. Amiodarone is a widely used antiarrhythmic drug. It is related structurally to thyroid hormone and is stored in adipose tissue. The drug has a high iodine content as well. Taking amiodarone on an ongoing basis can lead to hypothyroidism by inhibiting deiodinase activity and by acting as a direct antagonist to T_4. In some cases, amiodarone-induced hypothyroidism resolves within a few months; however, in many, especially when accompanying anti-TPO antibodies are present, treatment with levothyroxine is needed. This can be easily monitored and adjusted. While answer a is a consideration, the patient likely needs the amiodarone given her tendency toward paroxysms of atrial fibrillation and the attendant risk of stroke. While starting a beta-blocker may prevent episodes of rapid ventricular response, this decision would be made with the help of her cardiologist, which is not mentioned. Anti-TPO antibodies increase the risk of hypothyroidism but are not necessary to guide therapy in this patient. Although prednisone may be used for treatment of amiodarone-induced hyperthyroidism, this patient has hypothyroidism, and prednisone is not indicated.

201. The answer is e. Although the commonest causes of erectile dysfunction are vascular (including small vessel disease), neurological, and psychological, endocrine causes should not be overlooked. Most patients with vascular or neurological causes retain libido, which is driven by testosterone. This patient's diminished libido, as well as his small testicular size, suggests hypogonadism as a potential cause. The first step in evaluation for endocrine causes of ED is a morning testosterone level. Free testosterone is more specific but much more expensive. A testosterone level above 350 effectively excludes hypogonadism. Levels between 200 and 350 are equivocal and should either be repeated or be followed by a free testosterone. If the testosterone level is low, gonadotrophin levels will help determine if the cause is central (low LH) or peripheral (ie, testicular failure with high gonadotrophin level). If central (pituitary or hypothalamic) hypogonadism is demonstrated, a prolactin level is necessary to exclude a hormonally active pituitary tumor.

Although peripheral neuropathy and peripheral arterial disease can cause erectile dysfunction, this patient has a normal neurological and vascular examination. Diabetic autonomic neuropathy is usually associated with a distal sensory neuropathy that would be detected on physical examination. In a diabetic with ED and loss of libido, you should not assume that neuropathy is the cause of the ED, as a sight-threatening pituitary tumor may be missed. Psychological factors were once felt to be the leading cause of ED; now organic causes are felt to be more common, although in few areas of life are psychological factors more important than in sexual function. Psychogenic impotence is usually associated with preservation of spontaneous morning erections and is often partner-specific. This patient's loss of libido should not be ascribed to psychological causes until hypogonadism has been ruled out. Although phosphodiesterase-5 inhibitors are effective treatments for ED, organic causes should be considered first, or important medical diseases might be overlooked.

202. The answer is b. The best way to maintain glucose control in the critically ill patient is to use continuous glucose infusion with frequent fingerstick blood glucose measurements and dosage adjustments. Although initial studies suggested benefit from "tight" glucose control (especially in septic or postoperative patients), subsequent trials showed that a more modest target (140-180) leads to better outcomes and prevents complications (especially adverse cardiac events and severe hypoglycemia). Once stabilized and taking enteral nutrition, the patient can often be easily transitioned to a basal-bolus regimen (ie, a long-acting insulin supplemented by pre-meal boluses of a short-acting insulin).

Although metformin is usually the initial oral agent chosen for the outpatient management of type 2 diabetes, it should not be used in the setting of critical illness, where fluctuations in renal perfusion and glomerular filtration rate (GFR) increase the risk of lactic acidosis. Metformin should be withheld around the time of surgery and radiographic procedures involving the use of IV contrast agents for the same reason. "Sliding scale" insulin has fallen out of favor in this setting as well; it is reactive rather than proactive and often leads to wide fluctuations and inadequate glucose control. Although continuous insulin infusion using a subcutaneous pump may be employed as an outpatient for tight glucose control, its use in the critical care setting has not been well studied and is probably inferior to IV insulin.

203. The answer is c. Hypercalcemia must first be confirmed since misleading laboratory values can be caused by hemoconcentration of the serum sample. Ninety percent of hypercalcemia is attributed either to hyperparathyroidism or to malignancy. Almost all patients with malignancy-associated hypercalcemia have previously diagnosed cancer or symptoms (weight loss, anorexia, cough, and hemoptysis) to suggest this diagnosis. In this otherwise healthy patient, confirmed hypercalcemia should lead to measurement of intact parathyroid hormone (iPTH). Other causes of hypercalcemia include familial hypocalciuric hypercalcemia, vitamin D intoxication, sarcoidosis and other granulomatous diseases, hyperthyroidism, prolonged immobilization, and milk-alkali syndrome. Thyroid studies and liver enzymes (to evaluate for granulomatous hepatitis) might be ordered if the iPTH level is suppressed. Urine calcium excretion is assessed before parathyroidectomy to rule out familial hypocalciuric hypercalcemia, which can mimic hyperparathyroidism but is associated with very low 24 hour urine calcium levels. Urine calcium determination, however, would not be the first test obtained in the assessment of hypercalcemia. Osteoporosis should be considered in this postmenopausal woman with hyperparathyroidism and appropriate screening for osteoporosis performed with central dual-x-ray absorptiometry (DXA).

204. The answer is c. The radiographs and elevated alkaline phosphatase suggest Paget disease of the bone. Most patients with Paget disease do not require treatment, as they are asymptomatic. Bone pain, hearing loss, bony deformity, congestive heart failure, hypercalcemia, and repeated fractures are all indications for specific therapy beyond just symptomatic treatment for pain. Bisphosphonates bind to hydroxyapatite crystals to decrease bone turnover; they are now recommended as the treatment of choice for symptomatic Paget disease. Bisphosphonates such as alendronate, risedronate, pamidronate, and zoledronic acid have replaced etidronate because they are more potent and do not produce mineralization defects. The recommended dose in Paget disease is higher than the bisphosphonate dose used to treat osteoporosis. Subcutaneous injectable calcitonin is still used in patients who cannot tolerate the GI side effects of bisphosphonates. Melphalan and prednisone can be used to treat multiple myeloma, but myeloma causes osteolytic (rather than sclerotic) changes and does not cause elevation of the serum alkaline phosphatase. Ursodeoxycholic acid (UDCA) is utilized in the treatment of primary biliary cirrhosis (which can also present with elevated alkaline phosphatase) but has no effect on bone mineralization.

205. The answer is e. To recognize the best insulin regimen, you must first understand the pharmacokinetics of different insulin preparation—namely the peak time of onset of action and effective duration. The following describes the insulin preparations from shortest to longest duration. Lispro (as well as the newer aspart and glulisine) has a peak onset of 0.5 to 1.5 hours and effective duration of 3 to 4 hours. Regular insulin has a peak onset of 2 to 3 hours and effective duration of 4 to 6 hours. NPH has a peak onset of 6 to 10 hours and effective duration of 10 to 16 hours. Glargine or detemir provides basal insulin with an effective duration of 24 hours and no peak effect. This patient is experiencing early morning hypoglycemia resulting from his erratic supper time; in addition his fasting blood glucose levels (120-150 mg/dL) are not adequately controlled. The most appropriate insulin regimen for this patient is a long-acting insulin such as glargine at bedtime along with a short-acting insulin such as lispro, aspart, or glulisine before each meal. This will allow better regulation of basal glucose levels while providing coverage at mealtime and will address the issue of variable mealtimes. Twice-daily regimens with NPH and regular insulin rarely provide sufficient coverage for either basal or meal-associated glucose production. Although the 70/30 combination is less expensive, the use of a basal plus rapid-acting insulin will more closely match the meal-associated glucose surge and will provide better overall control.

206. The answer is c. This patient's symptoms of weakness, fatigue, and weight loss in combination with hypotension and extensor hyperpigmentation are all consistent with adrenal insufficiency (Addison disease). Tuberculosis can involve the adrenal glands and result in adrenal insufficiency. Measurement of serum cortisol baseline and then stimulation with cosyntropin (a synthetic ACTH analogue) will confirm the clinical suspicion. The cosyntropin stimulation test is used to determine the adrenal reserve capacity for steroid production. Cortisol response is measured 30 and 60 minutes after cosyntropin is given intramuscularly or intravenously; a value of 18 µg/dL or above effectively excludes adrenal insufficiency. ACTH level (drawn before cosyntropin administration) will demonstrate whether the problem is based in the adrenal gland (primary) or hypothalamus/pituitary axis (secondary). Hemochromatosis can cause hyperpigmentation but not the weight loss and hypotension. Bacteremia would not cause the gradually increasing symptoms or the hyperpigmentation. In some patients with weight loss and nausea, an esophagogastroduodenoscopy (EGD) may be warranted; however, the clinical features of adrenal insufficiency in conjunction with poorly treated tuberculosis would first direct attention toward adrenal status.

207. The answer is d. Classically, the pathophysiology of type 1 diabetes is considered to be immune-mediated destruction of beta cells leading to insulin-dependent disease in children or adolescents, and type 2 diabetes to be insulin resistance in obese adults with a positive family history of the disease—but reality is more complex. Late-onset autoimmune diabetes of adults (LADA) typically occurs in nonobese adults, often without a family history of diabetes. It is slower in onset and less ketosis-prone than classic type 1 diabetes, but responds poorly to agents such as metformin that improve insulin sensitivity. Autoantibodies (anti-GAD antibodies being the most sensitive and specific) characterize LADA as well as type 1 DM. An important aspect of LADA is that early use of insulin is necessary to adequately control the blood glucose levels.

Maturity-onset diabetes of young (MODY) is the opposite of LADA; it is a condition resembling type 2 diabetes (ie, often associated with obesity and a positive family history) yet occurring before the age of 20. This patient's autoantibodies, thin body habitus, and unresponsiveness to oral hypoglycemic would not go with MODY. Cushing syndrome is often associated with hyperglycemia due to the insulin counter-regulatory effect of cortisol, but this patient does not have the other clinical features that almost always accompany cortisol excess. Glucagonomas are rare islet cell tumors that produce weight loss, malabsorption, and a severe skin rash. The patient in question has none of the features of this rare syndrome.

208. The answer is a. In this patient with a TSH below 10 µU/L and no symptoms of hypothyroidism, the diagnosis is subclinical hypothyroidism. Recommendations include checking a free thyroxine level (it should be normal in subclinical hypothyroidism) and repeating the TSH in 3 to 6 months to monitor for progression toward overt hypothyroidism. The patient should be informed about the symptoms of hypothyroidism. Thyroxine therapy is not currently recommended for most asymptomatic patients with a TSH level below 10 mU/L. One exception is women contemplating pregnancy, whose TSH should be lowered with l-thyroxine to less than 2.5 mU/L before conception.

Although an abnormal TPO Ab increases the risk of progression to overt hypothyroidism, it does not affect your present management. Thyroid uptake scan may be useful in the diagnosis of hyperthyroidism, but not in possible hypothyroidism. Iodide deficiency is not seen in the United States because of dietary iodide supplementation although it could be considered in immigrants or refugees from developing countries.

209. The answer is c. This patient's presentation suggests adrenal insufficiency (Addison disease). Hyponatremia is caused by loss of sodium in the urine (aldosterone deficiency) and free-water retention. Sodium loss causes volume depletion and orthostatic hypotension. Hyperkalemia is caused by aldosterone deficiency, impaired glomerular filtration, and acidosis. Ten to twenty percent of patients with adrenal insufficiency will have mild hypercalcemia; hypocalcemia is not expected. Complete blood count can reveal a normocytic anemia, relative lymphocytosis, and a moderate eosinophilia. Microcytic anemia would suggest an iron disorder or thalassemia if the mean corpuscular volume is quite low. The hyperpigmentation results from the release of pro-opiomelanocortin which has melanocyte-stimulating activity. Hyperpigmentation is not seen if pituitary dysfunction is causing the adrenal insufficiency (ie, in secondary hypoadrenalism).

210. The answer is b. The clinical picture strongly suggests myxedema coma. Unprovoked hypothermia is a particularly important sign. Myxedema coma constitutes a medical emergency; treatment should be started immediately. Should laboratory results fail to support the diagnosis, treatment can be stopped. An intravenous bolus of levothyroxine is given (200-500 µg loading dose), followed by daily intravenous doses (50-100 µg). If high doses are used, the patient should be carefully monitored for cardiac arrhythmias. Impaired adrenal reserve may accompany myxedema coma, so parenteral hydrocortisone is given concomitantly. Intravenous fluids are also needed but are less important than thyroxine and glucocorticoids; rewarming should be accomplished slowly, so as not to precipitate cardiac arrhythmias. If alveolar ventilation is compromised, then intubation may also be necessary. Hyponatremia and an elevated Pco_2 are laboratory markers of severe myxedema. CT of the head would not be the first choice, since a structural brain lesion would not explain the hypothermia, diffuse goiter, or hyporeflexia seen in this case.

211. The answer is d. Obstructive sleep apnea (OSA) that has gone untreated contributes to increased insulin resistance. This appears to have an additional effect even beyond the common co-occurrence of obesity as in this patient. Treatment of OSA can lead to improvement in glucose control. This patient is obese, has a crowded oropharynx on examination, and has daytime somnolence. Although overnight oxygen saturation monitor may be performed at home as screening, this patient is at high risk of complications of OSA should proceed directly to formal overnight polysomnography. Sleep hygiene is important for patients with sleep disturbance but is not likely to help in this patient with probable severe OSA. Similarly, sedative hypnotic agents such as zolpidem are widely prescribed for sleep but could exacerbate the OSA. Depression should always be explored but there are no clues beyond fatigue to suggest this diagnosis. Low vitamin D levels are generally asymptomatic unless the condition is severe and prolonged and would not affect sleep apnea or glucose control specifically.

212. The answer is e. Hypertensive crisis in this young woman suggests a secondary cause of hypertension. In the setting of palpitations, apprehension, and hyperglycemia, pheochromocytoma should be considered. Pheochromocytomas are derived from the adrenal medulla. They are capable of producing and secreting catecholamines. Unexplained hypertension associated with surgery or trauma may also suggest the disease. Clinical symptoms are the result of catecholamine secretion. For example, the patient's hyperglycemia is a result of a catecholamine effect of insulin suppression and stimulation of hepatic glucose output. Hypercalcemia has been attributed to decreased plasma volume or to ectopic secretion of parathormone-related protein. Renal artery stenosis can cause severe hypertension but would not explain the systemic symptoms or laboratory abnormalities in this case. An anxiety attack can produce palpitations, apprehension, and mild to moderate elevation in blood pressure but would not produce hypercalcemia nor elevated blood pressure poorly responsive to treatment. Essential hypertension can occur in a 25-year-old but again would not account for the laboratory changes. Diabetes mellitus does not cause hypertension unless renal insufficiency has already developed; her hyperglycemia will likely resolve when the pheochromocytoma is removed. Once pheochromocytoma is suspected, a urine or plasma specimen for metanephrines or fractionated catecholamines is the commonly used diagnostic study. If a plasma sample is used, it is drawn from an indwelling IV catheter so that the pain of phlebotomy does not raise the catecholamine levels. After biochemical evidence of catecholamine overproduction is found, imaging studies (CT scan, radionuclide imaging) will localize the problem for curative surgery.

213. The answer is a. The patient has excessive growth of soft tissue that has resulted in coarsening of facial features, prognathism, and frontal bossing—all characteristic of acromegaly. This growth hormone–secreting pituitary tumor will result in bitemporal hemianopsia when the tumor impinges on the optic chiasm, which lies just above the sella turcica. Growth hormone–secreting tumors are the second commonest functioning pituitary tumors (second to prolactinomas). Serum insulin-like growth factor-1 (IGF-1) level will be elevated and is usually the first diagnostic test. Since 40% of GH-producing tumors also produce prolactin, a prolactin level should be obtained as well. Growth hormone secretion is pulsatile and a single GH level is often equivocal; the GH level must be suppressed (usually with glucose) to diagnose autonomous overproduction.

Dexamethasone suppression is used in the evaluation of Cushing syndrome, with partial suppressibility suggesting a pituitary cause, but this patient's presentation strongly suggests acromegaly, not Cushing syndrome. Once GH overproduction is documented, MRI scan of the pituitary will show the size and extent of the tumor (most are macroadenomas >1 cm). The lateral skull film is insufficiently sensitive for this purpose. Growth hormone stimulation tests (insulin-induced hypoglycemia, arginine plus GHRH) may be used to diagnose growth hormone deficiency, but would not be useful to diagnose GH overproduction, where a suppression test should be used.

214. The answer is c. The patient described has hyponatremia, euvolemia, and concentrated urine. These features are sufficient to make a diagnosis of inappropriate antidiuretic hormone secretion. If ADH were responding normally to the patient's hypotonic state, the urine would be dilute and the excess water load would be excreted. Treatment necessitates restriction of fluid (free-water) intake. Insensible and urinary water loss results in a rise in serum Na^+ and serum osmolality and symptom improvement. If the patient has CNS symptoms such as confusion, obtundation, or seizures, hypertonic saline is cautiously administered to raise the serum sodium out of the danger zone (usually a rise of 4-6 mEq/L). Normal saline would treat volume depletion, but this patient is euvolemic. Isotonic saline would not address the free-water excess. Loop diuretics lead to modest free-water loss in the urine but would be less effective than fluid restriction. The tetracycline derivative demeclocycline decreases renal response to ADH and can be used in cases where the hyponatremia does not respond to fluid restriction. SIADH can occur as a side effect of many drugs or from carcinoma (especially small cell carcinoma of the lung), CNS disorders (head trauma, CNS infection), or benign lung diseases (especially lung abscesses or other chronic infections).

215. The answer is a. The clinical findings all suggest an excess production of cortisol by the adrenal gland. Hypertension, truncal obesity, and dark abdominal striae are common physical findings; patients often have ecchymoses at points of trauma (especially legs and forearms) because of increased capillary fragility. The process responsible for hypercortisolism is most often an ACTH-producing pituitary microadenoma. An adrenal adenoma that directly produces cortisol is the next most likely option. Most ectopic ACTH-producing neoplasms (usually small cell carcinoma of the lung) progress too rapidly for the full Cushing syndrome to develop. These patients usually present with muscle weakness due to profound hypokalemia. The initial test to diagnose endogenous cortisol overproduction is either 24 hour urine collection for free cortisol or overnight dexamethasone suppression test (in normal patients, the AM cortisol should suppress to <2 µg/dL after a midnight dose of 1 mg dexamethasone). More extensive testing is then required to determine the source. Hypothalamic tumors can affect ADH production and eating behavior but do not produce cortisol or ACTH. Unexpected bruising should prompt questions about domestic violence, but partner abuse would not account for the constellation of this patient's findings.

216. The answer is c. The picture of infertility, gynecomastia, and tall stature (arms and legs longer than expected for truncal size) is consistent with Klinefelter syndrome and an XXY karyotype. The patient has abnormal gonadal development with hyalinized testes that result in low testosterone levels. Pituitary function in Klinefelter syndrome is normal, so gonadotropin levels are elevated in response to underproduction of testosterone. Although Klinefelter patients may have sexual function, they do not produce sperm and are infertile. Turner syndrome refers to the 45 XO karyotype that results in abnormal sexual development in a female.

217. The answer is b. Iron overload should be considered among patients who present with any one or a combination of the following: hepatomegaly, weakness, hyperpigmentation, atypical arthritis, diabetes, erectile dysfunction, unexplained chronic abdominal pain, or cardiomyopathy. Diagnostic suspicion should be particularly high when the family history is positive for similar clinical findings. The most frequent cause of iron overload is the common genetic disorder, idiopathic hemochromatosis. Secondary iron storage problems can occur after multiple transfusions in a variety of anemias. The most practical screening test is the determination of serum iron, transferrin saturation, and ferritin. Transferrin saturation greater than 50% in males or 45% in females suggests increased iron stores. Substantially elevated serum ferritin levels confirm total body iron overload. Genetic screening is now used to assess which patients are at risk for severe fibrosis of the liver. Definitive diagnosis can be established by liver biopsy. Determination of serum copper is needed when Wilson disease is the probable cause of hepatic abnormalities. Wilson disease does not cause hypogonadism, heart failure, diabetes, or arthropathy. Chronic liver disease caused by hepatitis B would not account for the heart failure, hyperpigmentation, or diabetes. Nocturnal penile tumescence and echocardiogram can confirm clinical findings but will not establish the underlying diagnosis.

218. The answer is c. For the patient described, the markedly increased calcitonin level indicates the diagnosis of medullary carcinoma of the thyroid. In view of the family history, the patient most likely has multiple endocrine neoplasia (MEN) type 2A, which includes medullary carcinoma of the thyroid gland, pheochromocytoma, and parathyroid hyperplasia. Pheochromocytoma may exist without sustained hypertension, as indicated by excessive urinary catecholamine metabolites. Before thyroid surgery is performed on this patient, a pheochromocytoma must be ruled out through urinary metanephrine determinations; the presence of such a tumor might expose him to a hypertensive crisis during surgery. The serum calcium serves as a screening test for hyperparathyroidism. At surgery, the entire thyroid gland must be removed because foci of parafollicular cell hyperplasia, a premalignant lesion, may be scattered throughout the gland. Successful removal of the medullary carcinoma can be monitored with serum calcitonin levels. Medullary carcinoma of the thyroid rarely metastases to the liver, so a liver scan would be unnecessary if liver enzymes are normal. Thyroxine will be needed after surgery, but MEN type 2 is not associated with hypothyroidism. Radioactive iodine can be used to treat malignancies that arise from the follicular cells of the thyroid; parafollicular cells, however, do not take up iodine and do not respond to radioactive iodine. Hyperparathyroidism, while unlikely in this eucalcemic patient, is probably present in his brother.

219. The answer is b. The symptoms of masculinization (eg, alopecia, deepening of voice, clitoral hypertrophy) in this patient are characteristic of an active androgen-producing tumor. Such extreme virilization is very rarely observed in polycystic ovary syndrome or in Cushing syndrome; moreover, the presence of normal cortisol and adrenal androgens (DHEA-S) plus markedly elevated plasma testosterone levels indicates an ovarian rather than adrenal cause of the findings. Arrhenoblastomas are the most common androgen-producing ovarian tumors. Their incidence is highest during the reproductive years. Composed of varying proportions of Leydig and Sertoli cells, they are generally benign. In contrast to arrhenoblastomas, granulosa-theca cell tumors produce feminization, not virilization. Dermoid cysts (benign teratomas) do not produce androgens but cause symptoms by enlargement, ovarian torsion (pain), or rupture with contents spilling into the peritoneal cavity. Ovarian teratomas can also contain autonomously functioning thyroid tissue, causing hyperthyroidism (so-called struma ovarii).

220. The answer is d. This woman's amenorrhea is due to her elevated prolactin level. Although certain medications (especially dopamine blockers), hypothyroidism, renal failure, and pregnancy can cause hyperprolactinemia, there is no evidence of these conditions in this patient's case. Nonpituitary causes rarely elevate the prolactin level above 150. In addition, the MRI shows a macroadenoma (tumor >1 cm). Prolactin-producing pituitary tumors, even macroadenomas, remain under control of dopamine, which is the physiological prolactin inhibitory factor. In most patients, with dopamine agonist therapy, the prolactin level will normalize, menses will return, and tumor shrinkage will occur. While previously bromocriptine was used, now the longer-acting cabergoline is usually prescribed.

Pituitary surgery can usually be avoided, even if visual symptoms are present, with the use of dopamine agonist therapy. Transsphenoidal hypophysectomy is therefore not the best choice. Although some minimally symptomatic patients with microadenomas are treated with hormone replacement therapy, macroadenomas should be shrunken with dopamine agonist therapy. Somatostatin analogues are used to treat certain growth hormone producing tumors, but are not first-line treatment for prolactinomas. Watchful waiting would expose this woman to the risk of osteoporosis from estrogen deficiency as well as tumor growth with possible visual compromise, and would not be the best choice for this young woman.

221. The answer is e. This elderly patient with multiple comorbidities is profoundly ill with sepsis due to his urinary tract infection following urinary obstruction. All appropriate initial management steps have been instituted and yet the patient remains profoundly hypotensive. This suggests the possibility of "relative" adrenal insufficiency, which is common in the setting of sepsis, trauma, surgery, and shock from any cause. Prompt administration of stress doses of hydrocortisone has been shown to shorten the length of need for pressors and to reduce mortality if the patient has severe septic shock. It is no longer recommended that a random cortisol level or cosyntropin stimulation test be obtained in an attempt to determine who should receive the corticosteroid treatment. While the patient does have significant renal dysfunction, it appears to be prerenal and there is no indication for emergent dialysis (refractory fluid overload, hyperkalemia, refractory metabolic acidosis, certain intoxications, or uremic symptoms such as pericarditis or neuropathy). Norepinephrine has just been initiated to raise systemic vascular resistance in this patient with septic shock. While dobutamine is not contraindicated, it is not the drug of choice given his apparently normal heart function with ejection fraction of 60%. It is not recommended to intubate the patient unless he is in respiratory distress, unable to maintain his oxygen saturation or ventilation, or unable to protect his airway. Adding an antifungal agent would not be indicated this early in the patient's course.

222. The answer is b. This patient has the metabolic syndrome given her hypertension, hypertriglyceridemia, and obesity. In some patients, peripheral neuropathy can precede the diagnosis of diabetes. Fasting blood glucose or hemoglobin A1C levels are likely to establish the diagnosis. Neuropathy occurs in more than 50% of diabetic patients, particularly those with poor glucose control, obesity, smoking, and alcohol use, most of which are mentioned in this patient's history. While alcohol may be contributing to the condition, it is unlikely that one drink per day is the main cause of the pain. Peripheral vascular disease is unlikely in view of normal pulses and no description of poor capillary refill, lack of hair on the feet, or of resting erythema. B_{12} deficiency can cause peripheral neuropathy but usually affects proprioception and vibratory sensation first. Restrictive footwear could contribute to foot pain but not the peripheral neuropathy.

223. The answer is e. Estrogen is the most effective medication for decreasing vasomotor symptoms related to menopause. Hormone therapy (HT) favorably affects the lipid panel by decreasing LDL and increasing HDL, but HT also increases triglyceride levels and has pro-thrombotic effect. HT has an antiresorptive effect on bone, thus stabilizing or increasing bone density. In the Women's Health Initiative Study, HT was shown to decrease the incidence of hip fractures. Hormone therapy should be implemented in women with moderate to severe hot flashes who lack contraindications to use (endometrial cancer, history of venous thromboembolism, breast cancer, or gallbladder disease). This patient has a low risk for cardiovascular disease and has no direct contraindications for HT. The risk of breast cancer with HT use is directly related to the length of use. Five or more years is considered long-term use and is the cutoff where most research studies and meta-analyses found increasing risk of breast cancer. Progestational agents alone do not improve vasomotor symptoms.

224 to 226. The answers are 224-d, 225-f, 226-c. Cushing disease produces hypercortisolism secondary to excessive secretion of pituitary ACTH. It often affects women in their childbearing years. Prominent cervical fat pads, purple striae, hirsutism, and glucose intolerance are characteristic features, as well as muscle wasting, easy bruising, amenorrhea, and psychiatric disturbances. Diabetes mellitus can result from chronic hypercortisolism. Exogenous glucocorticoid use will produce cervical fat pads, purple striae, muscle wasting, easy bruising, and secondary diabetes mellitus. Since, however, most oral glucocorticoids (eg, prednisone, dexamethasone) have little mineralocorticoid and no androgenic effect, hypokalemia and hirsutism are rare. Empty sella syndrome is enlargement of the sella turcica from CSF pressure compressing the pituitary gland. It is most common in obese, hypertensive women. There are no focal findings. Some patients have chronic headaches; others are asymptomatic. MRI will distinguish this syndrome from a pituitary tumor. These patients have normal pituitary function, the rim of pituitary tissue being fully functional. Acromegaly is usually due to a pituitary macroadenoma; the characteristic physical changes develop so slowly as to be imperceptible to the patient. Interestingly, exogenous growth hormone administration (as a performance enhancing drug, for instance) rarely causes acromegaloid changes. TSH-producing pituitary tumors are rare causes of hyperthyroidism. Prolactinomas cause amenorrhea and galactorrhea in women and hypogonadism in men.

227 to 229. The answers are 227-h, 228-e, 229-a. This woman has clinical and chemical hyperthyroidism, but her TSH is not suppressed. A TSH-producing pituitary tumor should be suspected, and imaging of the pituitary with MRI scan ordered. Although the rarest of functional pituitary tumors, a TSH-producing adenoma can mimic Graves disease by causing hyperthyroidism with a diffuse goiter. A TSH-producing tumor does not cause infiltrative ophthalmopathy or pretibial myxedema, but these findings, helpful when present, are absent in over 50% of patients with Graves disease as well. Nontoxic multinodular goiter is very common, affecting up to 12% of adults. It is more common in women than men and is more common in areas of iodine insufficiency. Laboratory studies are typically normal, and the main effects are seen on physical examination and on follow-up imaging studies of the thyroid. The risk of malignancy in multinodular goiter is similar to that of solitary nodules, and suspicious nodules should be biopsied. A tender thyroid gland and elevated ESR make subacute thyroiditis a likely diagnosis. Hyperthyroid symptoms are common early in the illness. The condition is self-limited (usually lasting 6-8 weeks), so antithyroid drugs are not used. Beta-blockers can alleviate symptoms until the inflammation resolves.

Ectopic thyroid tissue in an ovarian teratoma causes struma ovarii. This syndrome leads to hyperthyroidism without thyroid enlargement, and can be detected by whole-body radioiodide scanning. Factitious hyperthyroidism is caused by ingestion of exogenous thyroid preparations, often to promote weight loss. The thyroid gland will not be palpable. A functioning thyroid adenoma can cause hyperthyroidism, usually associated with a single palpable nodule. Radioiodide scanning shows the "hot" nodule and suppression of iodide uptake in the remainder of the thyroid. Iodide deficiency is no longer seen in the United States. Still found in parts of South America, it causes a large goiter and tendency toward hypothyroidism.

Suggested Readings

1. Kasper DL, Fauci AS, Hauser SL, Longo DL, Jameson LJ, Loscalzo J. *Harrison's Principles of Internal Medicine.* 19th ed. New York: McGraw-Hill; 2015. Chapters 399, 402, 403, 405, 406, 407, 408, 417, 418, 419, 424, 428.

2. Gardner DG, Shoback D. *Greenspan's Basic & Clinical Endocrinology.* 9th ed. New York: McGraw-Hill; 2011. Chapters 3, 7, 20, 24.

3. Stern S, Cifu, AS, Altkorn D. *Symptom to Diagnosis: An Evidence-Based Guide.* 2nd ed. McGraw-Hill Education; 2010. Chapters 4, 11, 21. ISBN 978-0-07-149613-1.

4. Clinical practice guidelines from American Association of Clinical Endocrinology, available at: https://www.aace.com/publications/guidelines

5. Diabetes management guidelines available at: http://www.ndei.org?ADA-2014-guidelines-diabetes-diagnosis-A1C-testing.aspx

6. DeSantis L. Update in endocrinology. *Ann Intern Med.* 2011;154:684-689.

7. Ismail-Beigi F. Clinical practice. Glycemic management of type 2 diabetes mellitus. *N Engl J Med.* 2012;366:1319-1327.

8. Vaidya B, Pearce SH. Diagnosis and management of thyrotoxicosis. *British Medical Journal.* Aug 21, 2014;349:g5128.

Gastroenterology

Questions

230. A 65-year-old woman is admitted with rectal bleeding. She noticed a significant amount of blood in the toilet after going to the bathroom this morning and experienced severe abdominal pain which has persisted for several hours. Her medical history is positive for coronary artery disease (recent drug-eluting stent managed with aspirin and clopidogrel) and osteoarthritis (for which she has been taking ibuprofen). She denies weight loss and has no history of bleeding. On examination she is slightly diaphoretic. Vital signs are BP 124/72 and pulse 88 with the patient supine, BP 94/52 and pulse 110 with the patient standing. Abdomen is nontender and nondistended. NG aspirate is negative for occult blood. After establishing two large-bore intravenous lines, administering an IV fluid bolus and otherwise stabilizing the patient, what will be the most important study to perform?

a. Upper endoscopy
b. Air-contrast barium enema
c. Colonoscopy
d. X-ray of the abdomen—flat and upright
e. CT scan of the abdomen

231. A 60-year-old woman with depression and poorly controlled type 2 diabetes mellitus complains of episodic vomiting over the past 3 months. She has constant nausea and early satiety. She vomits once or twice almost every day. In addition, she reports several months of mild abdominal discomfort localized to the upper abdomen. The pain sometimes awakens her at night. She has lost 5 lb of weight. Her diabetes has been poorly controlled (glycosylated hemoglobin recently was 9.5). Current medications are glyburide, metformin, and amitriptyline.

Her physical examination is normal except for mild abdominal distention and evidence of a peripheral sensory neuropathy. Complete blood count, serum electrolytes, BUN, creatinine, and liver enzymes are all normal. Gallbladder sonogram is negative for gallstones. Upper endoscopy and CT scan of the abdomen are normal.

What is the best next step in the evaluation of this patient's symptoms?

a. Barium esophagram
b. Scintigraphic gastric emptying study
c. Colonoscopy
d. MR cholangiography
e. Small bowel biopsy

232. A 56-year-old woman becomes the chief financial officer of a large company and, several months thereafter, develops upper abdominal pain that she ascribes to stress. She takes an over-the-counter antacid with temporary benefit. She uses no other medications. One night she awakens with nausea and vomits a large volume of coffee grounds-like material; she becomes weak and diaphoretic. Upon hospitalization, she is found to have an actively bleeding duodenal ulcer. Which of the following statements is true?

a. The most likely etiology is adenocarcinoma of the duodenum.
b. The etiology of duodenal ulcer is different in women than in men.
c. The likelihood that she harbors *Helicobacter pylori* is greater than 50%.
d. Lifetime residence in the United States makes *H pylori* unlikely as an etiologic agent.
e. Organisms consistent with *H pylori* are rarely seen on biopsy in patients with duodenal ulcer.

233. A 39-year-old man presents with a 2-month history of constipation, blood-streaked stools, and decreasing stool caliber. Barium enema reveals a lesion in the descending colon (see figure below). Which aspect of the patient's history is most likely to be helpful in understanding the cause of this patient's illness?

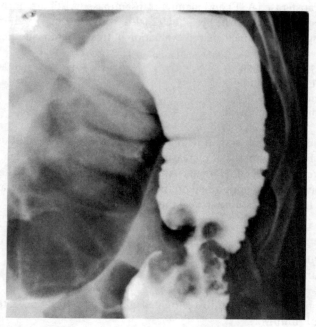

Reproduced, with permission, from Way LW. *Current Surgical Diagnosis & Treatment.* 10th ed. Stamford, CT: Appleton & Lange, 1994:658.

a. Travel history
b. Dietary history
c. Family history
d. Sexual history
e. History of psychiatric disease

234. A 70-year-old man presents with a complaint of fatigue. There is no history of alcohol abuse or liver disease; the patient is taking no medications. Scleral icterus is noted on physical examination; the liver and spleen are nonpalpable. The patient has a normocytic, normochromic anemia. Urinalysis shows bilirubinuria with absent urine urobilinogen. Serum bilirubin is 12 mg/dL, with 9.8 mg/dL direct-reacting fraction. Aspartate aminotransferase (AST) and alanine transaminase (ALT) are normal, and alkaline phosphatase (ALP) is 300 U/L (three times normal). Which of the following is the best next step in evaluation of this patient's jaundice?

a. Ultrasound or CT scan of the abdomen
b. Viral hepatitis profile
c. Reticulocyte count
d. Serum ferritin
e. Antimitochondrial antibody

235. A 52-year-old woman with a long history of daily alcohol use complains of several months of increasing abdominal girth and edema. Examination reveals spider angiomata, palmar erythema, abdominal distention, a fluid wave, shifting abdominal dullness to percussion, and bilateral pitting edema. Laboratory studies reveal the following:

AST = 90 U/L
ALT = 40 U/L
Bilirubin = 3.0 mg/dL
Albumin = 2.9 g/dL
INR = 2.0
Creatinine = 0.9 mg/dL (estimated glomerular filtration rate [GFR] 45 mL/min/M2)

Despite administration of furosemide 40 mg daily, the patient's weight and edema remain unchanged. What is the most likely reason that this patient has not had effective diuresis?

a. Poor intestinal absorption of furosemide.
b. Furosemide is protein bound, and the low albumin results in lower levels of free furosemide.
c. Furosemide is ineffective in persons with a low glomerular filtration rate.
d. High levels of aldosterone result in avid distal tubular reabsorption of sodium.
e. Lymphedema is not responsive to diuretic therapy.

236. A 66-year-old man sees you in clinic with a 3-month history of episodes when he will develop redness of the face and neck associated with a feeling of warmth. These episodes generally last less than 5 minutes and are often associated with watery diarrhea. He believes that some of the episodes may be precipitated by stress, but usually they occur for no particular reason. Over the same period of time he has had episodic cramping abdominal pain and fatigue. His examination is remarkable for a systolic murmur heard at the left base; the murmur increases with inspiration. Which of the following test is most likely to result in the correct diagnosis?

a. Stool for ova and parasites
b. Urinary *5-HIAA*
c. Stool culture
d. Serum-free T_4 level
e. PHQ9 Quick Depression Assessment

237. A 60-year-old woman complains of fever and constant left lower quadrant (LLQ) pain of 2-day duration. She has not had vomiting or rectal bleeding. She has a history of hypertension but is otherwise healthy. She has never had similar abdominal pain, and has had no previous surgeries. Her only regular medication is lisinopril. On examination, blood pressure is 150/80, pulse 110, and temperature 38.9°C (102°F). She has normal bowel sounds and left lower quadrant abdominal tenderness with rebound. A complete blood count reveals WBC = 28,000/μL. Serum electrolytes, BUN, creatinine, and liver enzymes are normal. What is the best next step in evaluating this patient's problem?

a. Colonoscopy
b. Barium enema
c. Exploratory laparotomy
d. Ultrasound of the abdomen
e. CT scan of the abdomen and pelvis

238. A 58-year-old man with cirrhosis and ascites caused by chronic hepatitis C is hospitalized because of subtle personality change that progresses to drowsiness and confusion. The patient's wife reports that his stools have been darker than usual and that he has been unsteady upon arising the past few days. She also reports that he has been reluctant to take several of his medications recently as he has been reading about natural remedies. On physical examination, the patient is lethargic, disoriented, and uncooperative. He is afebrile, has clear lungs, normal heart, distended abdomen with shifting dullness, and no meningeal or focal neurologic findings. There is mild hyperreflexia and a nonrhythmic flapping tremor of the wrists. Stool is positive for occult blood. CT scan of the head is normal. What is the best initial therapy to address this patient's mental status changes?

a. Quetiapine 25 mg orally tid
b. Lorazepam 1 mg orally tid
c. Haloperidol 2 mg intramuscularly q 4 hours prn agitation
d. Omeprazole 20 mg orally bid
e. Lactulose 30 cc orally, titrated to three to four stools daily

239. A 65-year-old woman with diabetes, hypertension, coronary artery disease, gastroesophageal reflux disease, and ongoing use of alcohol and tobacco, presents with several months of increasing midsternal chest discomfort predominantly when swallowing solid food. Recently, even liquids are becoming problematic. She has not noted blood in her stool or melena, weight loss, or change in her energy level. Laboratory studies are normal. What is the most likely cause of her dysphagia?

a. Esophageal cancer
b. Peptic esophageal stricture
c. Achalasia
d. Zenker diverticulum
e. Polymyositis

240. A 34-year-old man presents with substernal discomfort. The symptoms are worse after meals, particularly a heavy evening meal, and are sometimes associated with hot/sour fluid in the back of the throat and nocturnal awakening. The patient denies difficulty swallowing, pain on swallowing, or weight loss. The symptoms have been present for 6 weeks; the patient has gained 20 lb in the past 2 years. Which of the following is the most appropriate initial approach?

a. Therapeutic trial of ranitidine or omeprazole
b. Exercise test with thallium imaging
c. Esophagogastroduodenoscopy
d. CT scan of the chest
e. Coronary angiography

241. A 48-year-old woman presents with a 2-month history of change in bowel habit and 10 lb weight loss despite preservation of appetite. She notices increased abdominal gas, particularly after fatty meals. The stools are malodorous and occur two to three times per day; no rectal bleeding is noticed. The symptoms are less prominent when she follows a clear liquid diet. Which of the following is the most likely histological abnormality associated with this patient's symptoms?

a. Signet ring cells on gastric biopsy
b. Mucosal inflammation and crypt abscesses on sigmoidoscopy
c. Villous atrophy and increased lymphocytes in the lamina propria on small bowel biopsy
d. Small, curved gram-negative bacteria in areas of intestinal metaplasia on gastric biopsy
e. Periportal inflammation on liver biopsy

242. An otherwise healthy 40-year-old woman sees you because of recurrent abdominal pain. In the past month she has had four episodes of colicky epigastric pain. Each of these episodes has lasted about 30 minutes and has occurred within an hour of eating. Two of the episodes have been associated with sweating and vomiting. None of the episodes have been associated with fever or shortness of breath. She has not lost weight. She does not drink alcohol or take any prescription or over-the-counter medications. Other than three previous uneventful vaginal deliveries, she has never been hospitalized.

Her examination is negative except for mild obesity (BMI = 32). Complete blood count and multichannel chemistry profile that includes liver function tests are normal. Gallbladder sonogram reveals multiple gallstones.

What is the best next step in the treatment of this patient?

a. Omeprazole, 20 mg daily for 8 weeks
b. Ursodeoxycholic acid 300 mg po tid
c. Observation without specific therapy
d. Laparoscopic cholecystectomy
e. Weight reduction

243. A 56-year-old chronic alcoholic has a 1-year history of ascites. He is admitted with a 2-day history of diffuse abdominal pain and fever. Examination reveals scleral icterus, spider angiomas, a distended abdomen with shifting dullness, and diffuse abdominal tenderness. Paracentesis reveals slightly cloudy ascitic fluid with an ascitic fluid PMN cell count of $1000/\mu L$. Which of the following statements about treatment is true?

a. Antibiotic therapy is unnecessary if the ascitic fluid culture is negative for bacteria.
b. The addition of albumin to antibiotic therapy improves survival.
c. Repeated paracenteses are required to assess the response to antibiotic treatment.
d. After treatment of this acute episode, a second episode of spontaneous bacterial peritonitis would be unlikely.
e. Treatment with multiple antibiotics is required because polymicrobial infection is common.

244. A 72-year-old woman comes to the emergency department with abdominal pain. She has chronic constipation. Last night she developed nausea and lower abdominal pain that has been intermittent and cramping. She vomited twice this morning. On examination there is distention of the abdomen, high-pitched bowel sounds, and mild diffuse abdominal tenderness. An x-ray of the abdomen is shown (see figure below). What is the most likely diagnosis?

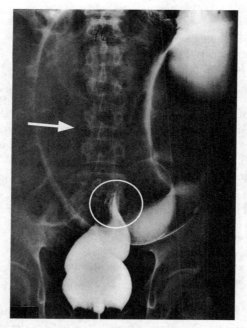

Reproduced, with permission, from Doherty GM. *Current Diagnosis & Treatment*: Surgery. 13th ed. New York, NY: McGraw-Hill Education, 2010. Figure 30-16.

a. Small bowel ileus
b. Small bowel obstruction
c. Large bowel obstruction
d. Pseudo-obstruction of the colon
e. Fecal impaction

245. A 40-year-old white man complains of slowly progressive generalized weakness, weight loss, abdominal pain, and wrist and knee pain over the past several months. He was told at an urgent care visit that his blood sugar was a little higher than normal. There is a family history of liver disease on his father's side. On examination, the patient has diffuse hyperpigmentation and a palpable liver edge. Mild polyarthritis of the wrists and metacarpophalangeal joints is also noted. What is the best test or combination of tests to help you diagnose this patient's problem?

a. Complete blood count with differential and a comprehensive metabolic panel
b. Hemoglobin A1C
c. Iron, total iron-binding capacity, and ferritin
d. Alpha-1-antitrypsin level
e. Liver-spleen scan

246. A 32-year-old white woman complains of abdominal pain off and on since the age of 17. She notices abdominal bloating relieved by defecation as well as alternating diarrhea and constipation. She has no weight loss, GI bleeding, or nocturnal diarrhea. On examination, she has slight LLQ tenderness and gaseous abdominal distension. Laboratory studies, including CBC, are normal. Which of the following is the most appropriate initial approach?

a. Recommend increased dietary fiber, antispasmodics as needed, and follow-up examination in 2 months.
b. Refer to gastroenterologist for colonoscopy.
c. Two weeks of oral tetracycline.
d. Order UGI series with small bowel follow-through.
e. Order small bowel biopsy.

247. A 55-year-old white woman has had recurrent episodes of alcohol-induced pancreatitis. Despite abstinence, the patient develops postprandial abdominal pain, bloating, weight loss despite good appetite, and bulky, foul-smelling stools. Kidney, ureter, bladder (KUB) x-ray shows pancreatic calcifications. In this patient, you should expect to find which of the following?

a. Diabetes mellitus
b. Malabsorption of fat-soluble vitamins D and K
c. Positive fecal occult blood test
d. Courvoisier sign
e. Markedly elevated amylase

248. A 34-year-old white woman is treated for UTI with amoxicillin. Initially she improves, but 5 days after beginning treatment she develops recurrent fever, abdominal bloating, and diarrhea with six to eight loose stools per day. On examination, she appears hypovolemic and moderately ill. Temperature is 38°C (100°F) and the abdomen is moderately tender without guarding. What is the best diagnostic test to confirm your diagnosis?

a. Identification of *Clostridium difficile* toxin in the stool
b. Isolation of *C difficile* in stool culture
c. Stool for white blood cells (fecal lactoferrin)
d. Detection of IgG antibodies against *C difficile* in the serum
e. Visualization of gram-positive rods on microscopic examination of stool

249. A 27-year-old woman is found to have a positive hepatitis C antibody at the time of plasma donation. Physical examination is normal. Liver enzymes reveal ALT of 62 U/L (normal <40), AST 65 U/L (normal <40), bilirubin 1.2 mg/dL (normal), and alkaline phosphatase normal. Hepatitis C viral RNA is 100,000 copies/mL. Hepatitis B surface antigen and HIV antibody are negative. Which of the following statements is true?

a. Liver biopsy is necessary to confirm the diagnosis of hepatitis C.
b. Most patients with hepatitis C eventually resolve their infection without permanent sequelae.
c. This patient should not receive vaccinations against other viral forms of hepatitis.
d. Serum ALT levels are a good predictor of prognosis.
e. Patients with hepatitis C genotype 3 are more likely to have rapid progression to fibrosis.

250. A 72-year-old woman notices progressive dysphagia to solids and liquids. There is no history of alcohol or tobacco use, and the patient takes no medications. She denies heartburn, but occasionally notices the regurgitation of undigested food from meals eaten several hours before. Her barium swallow is shown in the following figure. Which of the following is the cause of this condition?

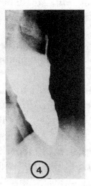

Reproduced, with permission, from Longo DL, Fauci AS. *Harrison's Gastroenterology and Hepatology*. New York, NY: McGraw-Hill, 2010. Figure 13-1.

a. Growth of malignant squamous cells into the muscularis mucosa.
b. Scarring caused by silent gastroesophageal reflux.
c. Spasm of the lower esophageal sphincter.
d. Loss of intramural neurons in the esophagus.
e. Psychiatric disease.

251. A 19-year-old man comes to the student health center because of jaundice. It is finals week and he has been staying up late at night studying for exams. A classmate noted that his eyes looked yellow. He has otherwise felt completely well, and has not had fever, fatigue, nausea, vomiting, or change in the color of his urine. He does not drink alcohol or use any medications. He is not been exposed to any persons with jaundice nor had any foreign travel. He is previously been immunized for hepatitis A and B. On examination he is afebrile and has normal vital signs. There is mild scleral icterus. The liver and spleen are nonpalpable, there is no abdominal tenderness, and the examination is otherwise normal. Laboratory studies disclose the following.

CBC: normal
Total bilirubin: 2.7 mg/dL
Direct bilirubin: 0.9 mg/dL
AST: normal
ALT: normal
Alkaline phosphatase: normal
Urine bilirubin: negative

What is the most likely explanation for this man's jaundice?

a. Glucuronyl transferase deficiency.
d. Warm antibodies directed against red blood cell antigens.
c. Beta-globin gene mutation.
d. Common bile duct obstruction.
e. Hepatocellular injury.

Questions 252 to 254

Match the patient described with the most likely diagnosis. Each lettered option may be used once, more than once, or not at all.

a. Acute diverticulitis
b. Acute pancreatitis
c. Acute cholecystitis
d. Intestinal obstruction
e. Irritable bowel syndrome (IBS)
f. Mesenteric ischemia

252. A 45-year-old diabetic woman presents with 2 days of severe upper abdominal pain that radiates into the back and has been associated with nausea and vomiting. She takes insulin but has been noncompliant for several weeks. She denies alcohol consumption. Her serum is lipemic.

253. A 78-year-old white man with coronary artery disease presents with several months of postprandial generalized abdominal pain that typically lasts 30 to 60 minutes. He has become fearful of eating and has lost 15 lb of weight. On examination the abdomen is nontender. There is no hepato-splenomegaly, but a loud mid-abdominal bruit is detected.

254. A 68-year-old woman who has had a previous hysterectomy presents with an 8-hour history of cramping periumbilical pain. Each episode of pain lasts 3 to 5 minutes and then abates. Over several hours she develops nausea, vomiting, and abdominal distension. She has been unable to pass stool or flatus for the past 4 hours.

Questions 255 and 256

In each scenario below, the patient is diagnosed with cirrhosis of the liver. Match the most likely etiology. Each answer can be used once, more than once, or not at all.

a. Defect in the *HFE* gene.
b. Defect in the *ATP7B* gene.
c. Chronic replication of a DNA virus.
d. Chronic replication of an RNA virus.
e. Immune-mediated destruction of interlobular bile ducts.

255. A 52-year-old man presents with personality change, cognitive impairment and choreoathetosis.

256. A 52-year-old woman with a history of Sjögren syndrome is seen in the clinic with 1 year of fatigue and pruritus.

Questions 257 to 259

Match the clinical description with the most likely disease process. Each lettered option may be used once, more than once, or not at all.

a. Hemolysis secondary to G6PD deficiency
b. Pancreatic carcinoma
c. Acute viral hepatitis
d. Crigler-Najjar syndrome
e. Nonalcoholic fatty liver disease
f. Gilbert syndrome

257. An African-American male patient develops mild jaundice while being treated for a urinary tract infection. Urine bilirubin is negative. Serum bilirubin is 3 mg/dL, mostly unconjugated. Hemoglobin is 7 g/dL.

258. A 55-year-old obese Hispanic man with a history of hypertension, diabetes, and hypertriglyceridemia reports intermittent mild right upper quadrant discomfort. He does not drink alcohol. He has elevated AST and ALT tests two to three times normal. Hepatitis panel is negative. His abdominal ultrasound shows a normal gallbladder without stones and generalized hyperechogenicity of the liver.

259. A young woman complains of 1 week of fatigue, change in skin color, and dark brown urine. She has right upper quadrant tenderness and ALT of 1035 U/L (normal <40) Bilirubin is 15.2 mg/dL (12.1 mg/dL direct-reacting), and the alkaline phosphatase is normal.

Questions 260 to 262

For each case scenario, select the most likely cause of gastrointestinal blood loss. Each lettered option may be used once, more than once, or not at all.

a. Mallory-Weiss tear
b. Aortoenteric fistula
c. Gastric ulcer
d. Esophageal varices
e. Hereditary hemorrhagic telangiectasia (HHT)
f. Dieulafoy lesion

260. An 88-year-old white woman with osteoarthritis has noticed mild epigastric discomfort for several weeks. Naproxen has helped her joint symptoms. She has emesis that resembles coffee grounds on three occasions.

261. A 76-year-old white man presents with painless hematemesis and hypotension. He has no previous GI symptoms but did have resection of an abdominal aortic aneurysm 12 years ago. Emergency esophagogastroduodenoscopy (EGD) shows no bleeding source in the stomach or duodenum.

262. A 56-year-old man with a history of heavy alcohol consumption is admitted with sudden massive hematemesis and hypotension. On examination there is jaundice, spider angiomata, abdominal distension with shifting dullness, and edema.

Questions 263 to 265

For each case scenario, select the most likely cause of lower gastrointestinal bleeding. Each lettered option may be used once, more than once, or not at all.

a. Ulcerative colitis
b. Crohn disease
c. Ischemic colitis
d. Diverticulosis
e. Amebic colitis
f. Tuberculoma of the colon

263. A 35-year-old white man presents with diarrhea, weight loss, and right lower quadrant (RLQ) pain. On examination, a tender mass is noted in the RLQ; the fecal occult blood test is positive. Colonoscopy shows segmental areas of inflammation. Barium small bowel series shows nodular thickening of the terminal ileum.

264. A 75-year-old African-American woman, previously healthy, presents with low-grade fever, diarrhea, and rectal bleeding. Colonoscopy shows continuous erythema from rectum to mid-transverse colon. The cecum is normal.

265. A 70-year-old white woman presents with LLQ abdominal pain, low-grade fever, and mild rectal bleeding. Examination shows LLQ tenderness. Unprepped sigmoidoscopy reveals segmental inflammation beginning in the distal sigmoid colon through the mid-descending colon. The rest of the examination is negative.

Questions 266 to 268

For each of the following case scenarios, select the most likely pathogen. Each lettered option may be used once, more than once, or not at all.

a. *Staphylococcus aureus*
b. *Shigella dysenteriae*
c. *Entamoeba histolytica*
d. *Escherichia coli O157H7*
e. *Salmonella* species
f. *Giardia lamblia*
h. *Clostridium difficile*

266. A 21-year-old man develops bloody diarrhea and fever. He owns and operates an exotic pet store, which specializes in reptile sales.

267. Two hours after ingesting potato salad at a picnic, a 50-year-old white woman develops severe nausea and vomiting. She has no diarrhea, fever, or chills. On examination, she appears hypovolemic, but the abdomen is benign.

268. Last week a 30-year-old woman received treatment with trimethoprim-sulfamethoxazole for bloody diarrhea. She now presents with a creatinine of 6.0 mg/dL (normal 0.5-1.0) and a hemoglobin of 7.2 g/dL (normal 12.5-14.0). Examination of the peripheral blood smear shows fragmented RBCs and schistocytes.

Gastroenterology

Answers

230. The answer is c. This patient has ischemic colitis, which typically occurs in people older than 50. Risk factors include atherosclerotic disease, including peripheral vascular disease and coronary artery disease. Episodes of bleeding are often accompanied by abdominal pain and watery diarrhea. The bleeding in diverticulosis (another common cause of acute rectal bleeding) is usually painless. Colonoscopy in ischemic colitis will reveal inflammatory changes (sometimes patchy) from the splenic flexure to the sigmoid colon with sparing of the rectum. Nonsteroidal-induced colitis is also a possibility and could be evaluated by colonoscopy. Given the history of red blood per rectum, upper endoscopy would not be the first choice of examination. An air-contrast barium enema could be obtained if colonoscopy were unavailable, in order to evaluate for colitis and to rule out a carcinoma. Plain x-rays of the abdomen occasionally show thumbprinting from edematous mucosal folds but are less sensitive than colonoscopy. CT of the abdomen is not a sensitive or specific test for mucosal disease of the colon.

231. The answer is b. Delayed gastric emptying (gastroparesis) is a common cause of recurrent vomiting, nausea, early satiety, and weight loss in poorly controlled diabetics. Abdominal discomfort is often nonspecific, but may be localized to the upper abdomen and often awakens the patient at night. Drugs with anticholinergic properties (such as amitriptyline) may aggravate the problem. The best diagnostic test is a scintigraphic gastric emptying study, which will show delay in gastric emptying. Treatment includes withdrawal of aggravating drugs such as opiates and anticholinergics, good diabetes control, and drug therapy with metoclopramide or erythromycin. The patient's symptoms are not those of esophageal disease (dysphagia, odynophagia), so a barium esophagram would not be useful. Her symptoms also do not suggest colonic pathology; in the absence of iron deficiency, colonoscopy would not be indicated. In the absence of elevated alkaline phosphatase or sonographic evidence of common bile duct dilation, MR cholangiography would not be indicated. Small bowel biopsy would be indicated if her symptoms suggested intestinal malabsorption.

232. The answer is c. Duodenal ulcer is more common in men than women, but *H pylori* is present in 70% of patients (men and women) who have a duodenal ulcer not associated with NSAID ingestion. In gastric ulcer disease, the incidence of *H pylori* is 30% to 60%. *Helicobacter pylori* is more common in developing countries but is often seen in the United States. It is more common in patients with low socioeconomic status, in particular those with unsanitary living conditions, which suggests that *H pylori* is transmitted by fecal-oral or oral-oral routes. In patients with duodenal ulcer, organisms consistent with *H pylori* are frequently seen on biopsy. Before the discovery of *H pylori,* most duodenal ulcers would reoccur. Adenocarcinoma of the duodenum is a rare cause of upper gastrointestinal bleeding.

233. The answer is c. The lesion seen on the barium enema is a classic "apple core" filling defect characteristic of colorectal cancer. The risk of colon cancer increases with age, with peak incidence between 70 and 80. Colon cancer is rare in persons under 50, unless they have predisposing risk factors. The strongest risk factor for the development of colon cancer is one of the hereditary polyposis syndromes (familial adenomatous polyposis, or hereditary non-polyposis colorectal cancer). In patients with familial adenomatous polyposis, the risk for colon cancer is nearly 100% by age 40. Thus, inquiry about family history of premature colon cancer or familial polyposis would be the most helpful historical information in understanding why this young man has colon cancer, a disease usually seen at a much older age. Patients on a high-fat, low fiber diet are also at increased risk for colon cancer, but the excess risk is small. Foreign travel might put him at risk for parasitic diseases of the colon such as amebiasis, but this does not increase the risk of colon cancer. Persons who practice anal sex are at risk for infectious diseases of the colon such as gonorrhea and for anal carcinoma related to human papilloma virus, but these illnesses do not cause apple-core lesions of the colon. Certain types of psychiatric illness can be associated with foreign body insertion into the rectum, but x-ray pattern would reveal the foreign object.

234. The answer is a. Patients with jaundice should be characterized as having unconjugated (indirect reacting) or conjugated (direct) hyperbilirubinemia. Causes of unconjugated hyperbilirubinemia include hemolysis, ineffective erythropoiesis, or enzyme deficiencies (the commonest in adults being Gilbert syndrome). Water-insoluble unconjugated bilirubin circulates bound to serum albumin; because albumin is too large to be filtered at the glomerulus, unconjugated bilirubin does not show up in the urine. This patient, however, has bilirubin in the urine and conjugated hyperbilirubinemia, which almost always indicates significant liver dysfunction, either hepatocellular or cholestatic (obstructive); the predominant elevation of alkaline phosphatase suggests a cholestatic pattern. Normal transaminases rule out hepatocellular damage (such as viral or alcoholic hepatitis). Instead, a disease of bile ducts or a cause of impaired bile excretion should be considered. Ultrasound or CT scan will evaluate the patient for an obstructing cancer or stone disease versus intrahepatic cholestasis. Reticulocyte count would be indicated if the patient had indirect hyperbilirubinemia. Ferritin values would evaluate for hemochromatosis, but this disease typically causes transaminase elevation and hepatomegaly. Primary biliary cirrhosis (PBC, evaluated by the antimitochondrial antibody test) might be considered if imaging studies show normal intra- and extrahepatic bile ducts (suggesting intrahepatic cholestasis), but PBC is usually seen in middle-aged women.

235. The answer is d. This patient presents with classic signs of cirrhosis, which include spider angiomata, palmar erythema, and (in the male) gynecomastia and testicular atrophy. Additionally she has physical examination findings of ascites, which is due to portal hypertension. For reasons that are still not completely understood, patients with portal hypertension have high levels of circulating aldosterone. Furosemide, a loop diuretic, results in increased sodium delivery to the distal nephron, but under the influence of aldosterone the sodium is reabsorbed. Patients with ascites and edema commonly require aldosterone-blocking agents (such as spironolactone) to achieve an effective diuresis. Patients with severe hypoalbuminemia sometimes have bowel wall edema which can inhibit the absorption of certain drugs, but this is much more commonly seen in nephrotic syndrome and in patients with albumin less than 1.0 g/dL. Furosemide is not protein bound. Though furosemide is less effective as glomerular filtration rate (GFR) falls, it is often effective in patients with GFR of less than 30 mL/min/M2. This patient's GFR is only slightly low. Lymphedema is not responsive to diuretic therapy, but this patient does not have lymphedema, which is characterized by non-pitting edema and is often unilateral.

236. The answer is b. This patient has symptoms of carcinoid syndrome, which is characterized by cutaneous flushing, diarrhea, abdominal cramps, and occasional wheezing. A significant proportion of patients with carcinoid syndrome develop right-sided cardiac lesions due to endocardial fibrosis, thickening of the tricuspid valve, and tricuspid regurgitation. Carcinoid tumors most commonly arise in the small bowel and produce a number of active gastrointestinal compounds, most commonly serotonin. A serotonin metabolite, 5-HIAA, is excreted in the urine, and measurement of this metabolite is a common diagnostic test. The active peptides of intestinal carcinoids are frequently metabolized in the liver, and therefore the development of systemic symptoms often suggest metastatic disease at a location that drains into systemic veins rather than the portal circulation. Carcinoids may also arise from the bronchus or ovary, and carcinoids at these sites are more likely to be associated with the carcinoid syndrome. Parasitic and bacterial infections of the gastrointestinal tract are commonly associated with diarrhea, but do not cause flushing and valvular abnormalities. Hyperthyroidism is often associated with loose stools, but not the carcinoid syndrome. Depression is more likely to be associated with constipation than diarrhea.

237. The answer is e. The most likely diagnosis in this patient is acute diverticulitis. Diverticulitis results from obstruction of a preexisting colon diverticulum. Colonic diverticulosis is very common in Western societies, and over half of Americans older than 60 have diverticula. Diverticulosis is asymptomatic. However, obstruction of a diverticulum can result in a microscopic perforation contained by the mesentery, or frank perforation and development of a diverticular abscess. Diverticulitis is classically associated with abdominal pain and fever. The pain is typically located in the left lower quadrant because the sigmoid is the most common region of the colon to be affected by diverticulosis. The marked leukocytosis in this patient combined with rebound tenderness suggests the possibility of a diverticular abscess. Diverticulitis can usually be diagnosed by CT scan of the abdomen and pelvis, which can also detect an associated diverticular abscess. Abdominal ultrasound is rarely useful in assessing colon pathology. Diverticulitis should be treated with antibiotics that are effective against coliforms and anaerobes. A typical choice is ciprofloxacin and metronidazole. Diverticular abscesses over 4 cm in size frequently require drainage, which can often be done percutaneously. Surgery is reserved for cases refractory to antibiotics and percutaneous drainage. Because of the increased risk of colon perforation, colonoscopy and barium enema are usually deferred for 4 to 6 weeks in patients with acute diverticulitis.

238. The answer is e. This patient has hepatic encephalopathy. Precipitating factors include azotemia, acute liver decompensation, use of sedatives or opioids, GI hemorrhage, hypokalemia, constipation, infection, a high-protein diet, and recent placement of a portosystemic shunt (TIPS). The most effective medical treatment is lactulose, a nonabsorbable disaccharide. Antibiotics such as neomycin, metronidazole, and rifaximin can also reduce symptoms. Rifaximin, which has fewer gastrointestinal side effects but is more expensive, has been shown to be as effective as lactulose in treating patients with hepatic encephalopathy. Quetiapine is used for psychosis and depression, lorazepam is useful in alcohol withdrawal and anxiety, and haloperidol in psychosis, but none of these agents would help hepatic encephalopathy. Benzodiazepines often worsen this condition. Omeprazole is useful in peptic ulcer disease but would not improve this patient's encephalopathy.

239. The answer is b. Peptic strictures due to chronic, persistent acid reflux cause 80% of esophageal strictures. Diagnostic esophagogastroduodenoscopy followed by dilation is necessary to relieve the dysphagia; the procedure may need to be repeated from time to time as symptoms recur. A patient with esophageal cancer is likely to have anemia and weight loss. Patients with achalasia often regurgitate undigested food; achalasia is less common than peptic stricture. A Zenker diverticulum is an outpouching in the posterior wall of the hypopharynx, which allows food retention, causing halitosis, recurrent aspiration, and pneumonia. While patients with polymyositis often have dysphagia, they would typically display weakness of the proximal muscles in addition to dysphagia.

240. The answer is a. In the absence of alarm symptoms (such as dysphagia, odynophagia, weight loss, or gastrointestinal bleeding), a therapeutic trial of acid reduction therapy is reasonable. Mild to moderate gastrointestinal reflux disease (GERD) symptoms often respond to H_2 blockers. More severe disease, including erosive esophagitis, usually requires proton-pump inhibitor therapy for 8 weeks to ensure healing. If the patient has recurrent symptoms or symptomatic GERD for over 5 years, endoscopy is indicated to rule out Barrett esophagus (intestinal metaplasia of the lower esophagus). Barrett esophagus is a premalignant condition, and most patients receive surveillance EGD every 2 to 3 years, although evidence of mortality benefit from this approach is not available. In the absence of alarm symptoms, a therapeutic trial is generally favored over more expensive diagnostic studies (endoscopy, CT scan). Classic symptoms of GERD do not mandate an evaluation for coronary artery disease unless other features suggest this diagnosis.

241. The answer is c. The patient's history suggests malabsorption. Weight loss despite increased appetite goes with either a hypermetabolic state (such as hyperthyroidism) or nutrient malabsorption. The gastrointestinal symptoms support the diagnosis of malabsorption. Patients may notice greasy malodorous stools, increase in stool frequency, stools that are tenacious and difficult to flush, as well as changes in bowel habit according to the fat content of the diet. In the United States, celiac disease (gluten-sensitive enteropathy) and chronic pancreatic insufficiency are the commonest causes of malabsorption. Celiac disease is associated histologically with villous atrophy and increased lymphocytes in the lamina propria of the small bowel. IgA antiendomysial antibodies and antibodies against tissue transglutaminase provide supporting evidence. Signet ring cells are seen with gastric cancer. This lesion causes weight loss through anorexia or early satiety but would not cause malabsorption. Colonic mucosal inflammation and crypt abscesses are associated with ulcerative colitis; since this disease affects only the colon, small bowel absorption is not affected. *Helicobacter pylori* (which appears as curved gram-negative rods on gastric biopsy) is not associated with malabsorption. Periportal inflammation is seen in chronic hepatitis but not in malabsorption.

242. The answer is d. Cholelithiasis (gallstone disease) is very common. Risk factors for the development of gallstones include advancing age, female gender, obesity, prior pregnancies, Native American or Hispanic ancestry, and rapid weight loss. Many patients are asymptomatic, but some develop biliary colic. About half of symptomatic patients will have recurrent episodes, and 1% to 2% will develop complications annually. The treatment of choice is cholecystectomy, which can usually be performed laparoscopically. This woman's symptoms are classic for biliary colic; acid reducers such as omeprazole would not be useful. Although ursodeoxycholic acid can dissolve gallstones, they usually recur, and this drug is no longer considered appropriate therapy unless surgery is contraindicated. Weight reduction does not dissolve gallstones, and rapid weight loss can precipitate symptoms. In order to prevent complications, symptomatic patients with low operative risk are usually managed with surgery rather than with observation. Asymptomatic gallstone disease is followed and treated surgically if symptoms develop.

243. The answer is b. Spontaneous bacterial peritonitis is the occurrence of bacterial infection in preexisting ascitic fluid without bowel wall perforation. It is almost always caused by a single species; isolation of multiple species would suggest a bowel wall perforation. The typical patient has preexisting cirrhosis and ascites, and presents with fever and abdominal pain. Acute deterioration of liver function and hepatic encephalopathy are also common. An ascitic fluid PMN cell count of greater than 250/µL confirms the diagnosis, even if the culture is negative. Standard antibiotic therapy is a third-generation cephalosporin or levofloxacin for 7 to 10 days. Response to therapy can be judged clinically, and repeated paracentesis is not usually necessary. The addition of albumin to antibiotic therapy has been shown to improve survival. Recurrence rates are high, and long-term prophylactic therapy with a fluoroquinolone is recommended.

244. The answer is c. The x-ray reveals a dilated sigmoid colon and the classic "birds beak" finding associated with a sigmoid volvulus causing large bowel obstruction. Common causes of large bowel obstruction include colon cancer, acute diverticulitis, sigmoid volvulus, and fecal impaction. Small bowel obstruction is also associated with abdominal distention and high-pitched bowel sounds, but vomiting is usually more copious, and the x-ray would show multiple air fluid levels in the small intestine and paucity of gas in the large bowel. Small bowel ileus is associated with absent or decreased bowel sounds, with air-filled distended loops of small and large bowel. Pseudo-obstruction of the colon can mimic a large bowel obstruction with dilatation of the colon on x-ray, but is usually associated with decreased bowel sounds, and no abrupt cutoff of the large bowel is seen on x-ray. Occasionally large bowel obstruction can be due to fecal impaction, but the x-ray should disclose large amounts of stool in the colon.

245. The answer is c. Hemochromatosis is an autosomal recessive condition that causes increased intestinal absorption of iron and excessive total body iron stores. The cause is a defect in the *HFE* or related gene; it affects Caucasians most frequently at a rate of about 1 in 250 persons. Clinically, the liver is usually enlarged, and excessive skin pigmentation is present in

90% of symptomatic patients at the time of diagnosis. Diabetes occurs secondary to direct damage to the pancreas by iron deposition. Arthropathy develops in 25% to 50% of cases. Initial screening involves transferrin saturation (iron/total iron binding capacity) and ferritin levels. A transferrin saturation of over 40% in women or 50% in men or a ferritin over 300 would be consistent with the diagnosis and would suggest the need for referral and genetic testing. CBC is normal in hemochromatosis in the absence of cirrhosis; liver enzymes would show transaminase elevation but would not be specific for hemochromatosis Hemoglobin A1C is helpful in diagnosing and monitoring diabetes. Patients with alpha-1-antitrypsin deficiency have liver disease but not diabetes or arthropathy. Liver-spleen scan could detect cirrhosis but would not rule out hemochromatosis as the cause.

246. The answer is a. This patient meets the Rome II criteria for irritable bowel syndrome. The major criterion is abdominal pain relieved with defecation and associated with change in stool frequency or consistency. In addition, these patients often complain of difficult stool passage, a feeling of incomplete evacuation, and mucus in the stool. In this young patient with long-standing symptoms and no evidence of organic disease on physical and laboratory studies, further evaluation (ie, colonoscopy or small bowel studies for malabsorption) is unnecessary. Irritable bowel syndrome is a motility disorder associated with altered sensitivity to abdominal pain and distension. It is the commonest cause of chronic GI symptoms and is three times more common in women than in men. Associated lactose intolerance may cause similar symptoms and should be considered in all cases. Patients older than 40 years with new symptoms, weight loss, or positive family history of colon cancer should have further workup, usually with colonoscopy. Initial treatment consists of a high fiber diet. Antispasmodics may be helpful for abdominal cramps. If dietary changes are not effective, many clinicians add psyllium or polyethylene glycol. Two weeks of rifaximin has been shown to be efficacious in patients with symptoms refractory to dietary modification, but is not recommended as initial therapy.

247. The answer is a. Chronic pancreatitis is caused by pancreatic damage from repeated attacks of acute pancreatitis. The classic triad is abdominal pain, malabsorption, and diabetes mellitus. Pancreatic calcifications are frequently seen on abdominal x-rays. Twenty-five percent of cases are idiopathic. Vitamins D and K are absorbed intact from the intestine without digestion by lipase and are therefore absorbed normally in pancreatic insufficiency. Forty percent of patients, however, develop B_{12} deficiency. Treatment of the malabsorption with pancreatic enzyme replacement will lead to weight gain, but the pain can be difficult to treat. Courvoisier sign is a palpable, nontender gallbladder in a jaundiced patient. This finding suggests the presence of a malignancy, usually pancreatic cancer. Chronic pancreatitis per se does not produce heme-positive stools. Amylase is usually normal in patients with chronic pancreatitis.

248. The answer is a. *Clostridium difficile* is an important cause of diarrhea in patients who receive antibiotic therapy. *Clostridium difficile* proliferates in the gastrointestinal tract when the normal enteric microbiome is altered by antibiotics. Commonly implicated antibiotics include ampicillin, clindamycin, cephalosporins, and trimethoprim-sulfamethoxazole. The diarrhea is usually mild to moderate, but can be profuse. Other clinical findings include fever, abdominal pain, abdominal tenderness, leukocytosis, and serum electrolyte abnormalities. The diagnosis is made by demonstration at sigmoidoscopy of yellowish plaques (pseudomembranes) that adhere to the colonic mucosa or by detection of *C difficile* toxin in the stool. The pseudomembranes consist of a tenacious fibrinopurulent exudate that contains extruded leukocytes, mucin, and sloughed mucosa. Isolation of *C difficile* from stool cultures is nonspecific because of asymptomatic carriage, particularly in infants. Testing for fecal leukocytes is also nonspecific and may be negative in *C difficile* colitis. Serological tests are not clinically useful for diagnosing this infection. Although *Clostridia* are indeed gram-positive bacilli, they cannot be distinguished microscopically from numerous other anaerobic organisms in stool. Pseudomembranous colitis demands discontinuation of the offending antibiotic. Recommended antibiotic therapy is metronidazole, or oral vancomycin for severe disease (which is defined by a leukocyte count >= 15,000 or creatinine >= 1.5 mg/dL). Cholestyramine can be used in mild cases to bind the diarrheogenic toxin.

249. The answer is e. This patient has chronic hepatitis C. A positive test for hepatitis C viral RNA confirms the diagnosis. Liver biopsy is not necessary for confirmation, but may be useful in predicting need for treatment. Chronic hepatitis C rarely resolves spontaneously. Untreated, about 15% of patients with hepatitis C will eventually develop cirrhosis. The levels of ALT and viral RNA correlate poorly with histologic disease and eventual prognosis. Treatment is aimed at achieving virologic cure and preventing progression to cirrhosis. Untreated patients with ongoing alcohol use, genotype 3, or co-infection with HIV or hepatitis B are more likely to progress rapidly to fibrosis. All patients with chronic hepatitis C should receive vaccination against hepatitis A and B, which can cause fulminant hepatic failure in patients with preexisting hepatitis C.

250. The answer is d. The barium swallow shows the dilated baglike proximal esophagus and tapered distal esophageal ring characteristic of achalasia. This is a motor disorder of the esophagus characterized by loss of intramural neurons and classically produces dysphagia to both solids and liquids. In achalasia, manometry shows elevated pressure and poor relaxation of the lower esophageal sphincter. In classic achalasia the contractions of the esophagus are weak, although a variant called *vigorous achalasia* is associated with large-amplitude prolonged contractions. Medications such as nitrates, calcium channel blockers, botox injections into the lower esophageal sphincter (LES) or physical procedures (balloon dilatation or surgical myotomy) that decrease LES pressure are the recommended treatments. Cancer causes dysphagia when malignant cells grow into the muscularis or when the tumor narrows the lumen. This usually causes trouble swallowing solids as the first manifestation. This pattern of early dysphagia to solids is also seen in the scarring associated with gastroesophageal reflux. Squamous cell carcinoma would not cause esophageal dilation and would be associated with ratty rather than smooth tapering of the esophagus. Achalasia is not associated with gastroesophageal reflux disease. Although anxiety can cause dysphagia and a globus-like sensation in the cricoid region, it would not cause the anatomical changes seen on this barium swallow.

251. The answer is a. This patient has isolated hyperbilirubinemia (hepatocellular enzymes and alkaline phosphatase are normal). Furthermore, his hyperbilirubinemia is unconjugated (direct bilirubin is normal and indirect bilirubin is high). Causes of unconjugated isolated hyperbilirubinemia include overproduction of bilirubin from hemolysis or defective conjugation of bilirubin related to deficiencies in glucuronyl transferase. Hemolysis, such as that associated with the beta-globin gene mutation of sickle cell disease or warm antibody production associated with autoimmune hemolysis, is always associated with anemia. Mild deficiency of glucuronyl transferase is seen in Gilbert syndrome. This benign disorder affects up to 7% of the population and is much more common in males. Episodes of mild jaundice are often precipitated by stress or fasting, and resolve spontaneously. More severe deficiency or absence of glucuronyl transferase is seen in Crigler-Najjar syndrome. In patients with this disorder, the bilirubin is greater than 5. Common bile duct obstruction can cause jaundice, but would be associated with an elevated alkaline phosphatase. Hepatocellular injury from viruses or drugs is commonly associated with jaundice, but the transaminases would be elevated. In order for bilirubin to be excreted in the urine it must be conjugated, and therefore bilirubin is absent in the urine of patients with unconjugated hyperbilirubinemia.

252 to 254. **The answers are 252-b, 253-f, 254-d.** Pancreatitis typically causes severe abdominal pain that radiates into the back. It is almost always associated with nausea and vomiting. The most common etiology is heavy alcohol use. Other etiologies include gallstones, hyperlipidemia, certain medications (such as azathioprine and hydrochlorothiazide), trauma, and after endoscopic retrograde cholangiopancreatography (ERCP). Serum amylase and lipase are typically elevated. This patient is likely to have pancreatitis related to hypertriglyceridemia. Mild elevation of the amylase can also occur in renal failure, appendicitis, and mumps.

Intermittent mesenteric ischemia occurs from atherosclerotic obstruction of visceral arteries. Patients typically present with postprandial abdominal pain and weight loss ("intestinal angina"). Men are more commonly affected than women and usually have atherosclerotic disease elsewhere. Cigarette smoking is a risk factor. Diagnosis is usually made by Doppler ultrasound of the mesenteric vessels and confirmed by CT angiography. Treatment is usually interventional.

Acute intestinal obstruction is most often associated with adhesive bands from previous surgery. Hysterectomy and appendectomy are the most common preceding surgeries, although any operation associated with entry into the peritoneum can cause adhesions. The patient usually has the classic colicky pain associated with several pain-free minutes before the pain again builds up to maximum intensity. This kind of pain is much more commonly associated with intestinal obstruction than biliary or renal disease (so-called biliary and renal colic are often constant pains).

The pain of acute diverticulitis is usually steady and localized to the left lower quadrant. Acute cholecystitis begins with the severe but ill-localized upper abdominal pain of biliary colic; after the gallbladder wall becomes inflamed, the pain moves to the right upper quadrant and becomes more constant. Pain is the most characteristic symptom of irritable bowel syndrome; it is often cramping and ill-localized. Defecation often relieves the pain of IBS.

255 and 256. **The answers are 255-b, 256-e.** Cirrhosis is most commonly due to chronic alcohol ingestion or chronic hepatitis C infection (an RNA virus). An uncommon cause of cirrhosis is Wilson disease. In this condition a defect in the *ATP7B* gene results in defective excretion of copper. Copper accumulation in the liver can result in cirrhosis, and accumulation in the brain can result in tremor and psychiatric symptoms. Another uncommon cause of cirrhosis is hemochromatosis which is due to a defect in the *HFE* gene, a protein that regulates iron absorption. Patients with hemochromatosis have excessive iron stores and elevated levels of plasma iron, transferrin, and ferritin. These patients typically have arthralgias due to iron depositions in the synovium. Chronic iron deposition in the liver leads to cirrhosis, and iron deposition in the pancreas and gonads can result in diabetes and hypogonadism. Primary biliary cirrhosis is caused by immune-mediated destruction of interlobular bile ducts, and is most frequently seen in middle-age women with other rheumatologic conditions such as Sjögren syndrome, scleroderma, or the CREST syndrome. Patients typically present with fatigue and pruritus. Diagnosis is established by a positive antimitochondrial antibody. Cirrhosis can result from untreated infection with hepatitis B (a DNA virus) but not from hepatitis A (an RNA virus).

257 to 259. **The answers are 257-a, 258-e, 259-c.** The young African-American male patient with mild jaundice has unconjugated hyperbilirubinemia and anemia. Unconjugated bilirubin is bound to albumin in the circulation and is not excreted in the urine; hence the urine bilirubin level is negative. His jaundice may be secondary to G6PD deficiency with hemolysis precipitated by an offending antibiotic (sulfonamide or trimethoprim-sulfamethoxazole). These patients are unable to maintain an adequate level of reduced glutathione in their red blood cells when an antibiotic or other toxin causes oxidative stress to the red cells. The 55-year-old Hispanic man has nonalcoholic fatty liver disease (NAFLD). NAFLD is very common and is estimated to affect up to 20% of the U.S. population. The condition is more common in men than women and more common in whites than blacks. The condition is characterized by triglyceride accumulation in the hepatocytes (steatosis). The underlying pathophysiology is closely linked to insulin resistance and hence to obesity, diabetes, hyperlipidemia, and the metabolic syndrome. Most cases are discovered incidentally because of elevated transaminases. Patients may have nonspecific right upper quadrant discomfort and hepatomegaly. Abdominal ultrasound shows hyperechogenicity consistent with fatty infiltration. CT scan is also sensitive in diagnosing the condition (90%). Patients with NAFLD are at risk for progression to nonalcoholic steatohepatitis (NASH), which can lead to fibrosis and cirrhosis. The mainstay of treatment for NAFLD is lifestyle modification with increased exercise (hence increased insulin sensitivity) and weight loss. The young woman's case is most consistent with acute hepatitis—strikingly elevated hepatocellular enzymes and conjugated hyperbilirubinemia. Tenderness of the liver on palpation is common in acute hepatitis.

Pancreatic carcinoma causes painless obstructive jaundice with elevated alkaline phosphatase and normal transaminases. Crigler-Najjar and Gilbert syndromes are both caused by abnormalities in glucuronidation of bilirubin. They cause indirect hyperbilirubinemia without evidence of hemolysis or abnormalities of the other liver enzymes.

260 to 262.   The answers are 260-c, 261-b, 262-d. All of these patients have acute upper gastrointestinal bleeding, which is often characterized by emesis that looks like red blood or coffee grounds. Nonsteroidal anti-inflammatory drugs (NSAIDs), even over-the-counter brands, are common causes of GI bleeding. Preceding symptoms may be mild before the bleeding occurs. Cotreatment with misoprostol decreases GI bleeding but is expensive. Selective COX-2 inhibitors decrease the incidence of GI bleeding, but have been shown to increase cardiovascular events and to carry the same risk of renal dysfunction, edema, and blood pressure elevation as nonselective NSAIDs.

Erosion of the proximal end of a woven aortic graft into the distal duodenum or proximal jejunum can occur many years after surgery for abdominal aortic aneurysm. Often, the patient will have a smaller herald bleed, which is then followed by catastrophic bleeding. A high index of suspicion is necessary, as timely surgery can be lifesaving.

Mallory-Weiss tear occurs when there is a tear in the mucosa in the lower portion of the esophagus following retching.

Esophageal varices due to portal hypertension usually bleed without warning or preceding pain. Patients frequently have stigmata of cirrhosis (jaundice and spider angiomata) and portal hypertension (ascites and edema). Blood loss in both Mallory-Weiss tears and esophageal varices can be massive. Hereditary hemorrhagic telangiectasia or Osler-Weber-Rendu syndrome is a cause of nosebleeds, mild GI bleeding, and cutaneous or mucosal telangiectasias. Associated arteriovenous malformations can appear in the brain, lungs, liver, and intestine.

Dieulafoy lesion is a tortuous arteriole in the stomach that can erode and bleed; it can be difficult to find on endoscopy.

263 to 265. The answers are 263-b, 264-a, 265-c. Crohn disease can affect the entire GI tract from mouth to anus. Right lower quadrant pain, tenderness, and an inflammatory mass would suggest involvement of the terminal ileum. As opposed to ulcerative colitis (a pure mucosal disease), Crohn disease, with full-thickness involvement of the gut wall, can lead to fistula and deep abscess formation. Skip lesions (ie, segmental involvement) also suggest Crohn disease; granuloma formation on biopsies would also support the diagnosis of Crohn disease.

Although thought of a disease of young adults, ulcerative colitis has a second peak of incidence in the 60- to 80-year age group and should be considered in the differential diagnosis of diarrhea at any age. Colonic involvement starts in the rectum and proceeds toward the cecum in a continuous fashion (ie, no skip lesions). Inflammation is limited to the mucosa; so fistulas, deep abscesses, and granulomas are not seen.

Ischemic colitis usually occurs in the older age group. The ischemia is usually confined to the mucosa, so perforation is unusual. Pain is a prominent complaint and may mimic acute diverticulitis. The finding of segmental inflammation in watershed areas in the vascular distribution of the colon is characteristic. Most patients improve without surgical intervention.

Although acute diverticulitis is associated with lower abdominal pain and fever, diverticulosis is usually asymptomatic unless profuse rectal bleeding should occur. Amebic colitis is seen in emigrants from endemic areas and presents with bloody diarrhea. Tuberculomas are rare now that gastrointestinal disease from *Mycobacterium bovis* has been eradicated from domestic cattle in the United States. Tuberculomas are associated with fever, right lower quadrant pain, and hematochezia.

266 to 268. The answers are 266-e, 267-a, 268-d. Infection with *Salmonella* usually occurs by ingesting contaminated poultry or eggs, but has also been associated with handling turtles, lizards, and other reptiles. *Salmonella* gastroenteritis is often associated with fever and bloody diarrhea. Unless the patient is severely ill, antibiotic therapy is withheld because it can be associated with prolonged excretion of the organism in the stool.

Food-borne illness (food poisoning) is a very common cause of acute GI symptoms. This patient's short incubation period (indicating preformed toxin rather than bacterial proliferation in the gastrointestinal tract) as well as the prominent upper GI symptoms is characteristic of staphylococcal food poisoning.

Infection with certain *E coli* strains (generally associated with the production of Shiga toxin) can cause bloody diarrhea and fever. A particular strain (O157H7) commonly causes the hemolytic uremic syndrome; this pathogen can be transmitted by undercooked ground beef or by raw vegetables (eg, spinach) exposed to cow manure. Hemorrhagic diarrhea occurs more commonly in patients who have been treated with antibiotics. Although *C difficile* causes most cases of antibiotic-associated diarrhea, it would not account for the hemolytic anemia and acute kidney injury seen in this case.

Shigella dysenteriae causes acute bloody diarrhea, often with severe leukocytosis and clinical toxicity; person-to-person transmission is common. Amebiasis is an important cause of dysentery in developing nations. *Giardia* species cause chronic diarrhea, sometimes associated with foreign travel; since this organism is noninvasive, it does not cause bloody stools.

Suggested Readings

1. Kasper DL, Fauci AS, Hauser SL, Longo DL, Jameson LJ, Loscalzo J. *Harrison's Principles of Internal Medicine*. 19th ed. New York: McGraw-Hill; 2015. Chapters 53, 55, 57, 58, 59, 347, 348, 351, 352, 353, 358, 360, 362, 363, 365, 369.
2. American Gastroenterological Society Clinical Guidelines, available at: http://www.gastro.org/practice/medical-position-statements
3. American Association for the Study of Liver Diseases Practice Guidelines, available at: http://www.aasld.org/publications/practice-guidelines-0
4. Udell JA, Wang CS, Tinmouth J, et al. Does this patient with liver disease have cirrhosis? *JAMA*. 2012;307:832-842. doi: 10.1001/jama.2012.186.

Nephrology

Questions

269. A 76-year-old man presents to the emergency room. He had influenza and now complains of diffuse muscle pain and weakness. His medical history is remarkable for osteoarthritis for which he takes ibuprofen, and hypercholesterolemia for which he takes lovastatin. Physical examination reveals blood pressure of 130/90 with no orthostatic change. The only other finding is diffuse muscle tenderness. Laboratory data include

BUN: 30 mg/dL
Creatinine: 6 mg/dL
K: 6.0 mEq/L
Uric acid: 18 mg/dL
Ca: 6.5 mg/dL
PO_4: 7.5 mg/dL
UA: large blood, 2+ protein. Microscopic study shows muddy brown casts and 0 to 2 RBC/hpf (red blood cells/high power field).

Which of the following is the most likely diagnosis?

a. Nonsteroidal anti-inflammatory drug-induced acute kidney injury (AKI)
b. Volume depletion
c. Rhabdomyolysis-induced acute kidney injury
d. Urinary tract obstruction
e. Hypertensive nephrosclerosis

270. A 20-year-old man presents with obtundation. His medical history is unobtainable. Blood pressure is 120/70 without orthostatic change, and he is well perfused peripherally. The neurological examination is nonfocal. His laboratory values are as follows:

Na: 138 mEq/L
K: 4.2 mEq/L
HCO_3: 5 mEq/L
Cl: 104 mEq/L
Creatinine: 1.0 mg/dL
BUN: 14 mg/dL
Ca: 10 mg/dL
Arterial blood gas on room air: Po_2 96, Pco_2 15, pH 7.02
Blood glucose: 90 mg/dL
Urinalysis: Normal, without blood, protein, or crystals

Which of the following is the most likely acid-base disorder?

a. Pure normal anion-gap metabolic acidosis
b. Respiratory acidosis
c. Pure high anion-gap metabolic acidosis
d. Combined high anion-gap metabolic acidosis and respiratory alkalosis
e. Combined high anion-gap metabolic acidosis and respiratory acidosis

271. A 23-year-old woman with no other medical history was diagnosed with hypertension 6 months ago. She was initially treated with hydrochlorothiazide, followed by the addition of lisinopril, followed by a calcium channel blocker, but her blood pressure has not been well controlled. She assures the provider that she is taking all of her medicines. On examination her blood pressure is 165/105 in each arm, and 168/105 when checked by large cuff in the lower extremities. Her pulse is 60. Cardiac examination reveals an S_4 gallop but no murmurs. She has a soft mid-abdominal bruit. Distal pulses are intact and equal. She does not have hyperpigmentation, hirsutism, genital abnormalities, or unusual distribution of fat. Her sodium is 140, potassium 4.0, HCO_3 22, BUN 15, and creatinine 1.5. Which of the following is the most likely cause of her difficult-to-control hypertension?

a. Primary hyperaldosteronism (Conn syndrome)
b. Cushing syndrome
c. Congenital adrenal hyperplasia
d. Renal artery fibromuscular dysplasia
e. Coarctation of the aorta

272. A 67-year-old man with a history of gout presents with intense pain in his right great toe. He has a complex medical history, including hypertension, coronary artery disease, congestive heart failure, myelodysplasia, and chronic kidney disease with a baseline creatinine of 3.2 mg/dL and a uric acid level of 10 mg/dL. His medications include aspirin, simvastatin, clopidogrel, furosemide, amlodipine, and metoprolol. What is the best therapy in this situation?

a. Colchicine 1.2 mg po initially, followed by 0.6 mg 1 hour later
b. Allopurinol 100 mg po daily, titrated to uric acid less than 6 mg/dL
c. Prednisone 40 mg po daily
d. Naproxen 750 mg po once followed by 250 mg po tid
e. Probenecid 250 mg po bid

273. The doctor caring for the patient in the previous question forgot to test for uric acid, but the patient responded promptly to treatment ordered. The laboratory had saved serum from the time of admission; so the team ordered the uric acid level test after the fact and it returned with a value of 5 mg/dL (upper limit of normal is 6 mg/dL). In terms of pathophysiology, what is the most likely explanation?

a. The patient did not have gout initially.
b. Myelodysplastic syndrome causes a proximal renal tubular acidosis (RTA), which leads to uric acid wasting and hence hypouricemia.
c. The normal level can be explained by the fact that the gout attack caused an intense inflammatory reaction, including the production of uricosuric cytokines, thus lowering the serum level of uric acid.
d The lack of proper storage and handling of the serum specimen caused the uric acid level to be falsely low.
e. The patient was probably taking high-dose allopurinol at the time of admission, and he forgot to tell the admitting team this fact.

274. A 60-year-old diabetic woman develops angina and will need a coronary angiogram for evaluation of coronary artery disease. She has a creatinine of 2.2. Which of the following is the most effective in reducing the risk of contrast-induced nephropathy?

a. Administer mannitol immediately after the contrast is given.
b. Perform prophylactic hemodialysis after the procedure.
c. Give IV hydration with normal saline or sodium bicarbonate prior to and following the procedure.
d. Indomethacin 25 mg the morning of the procedure.
e. Dopamine infusion before and after the procedure.

275. A 47-year-old HIV-positive man is brought to the emergency room because of weakness. The patient has HIV nephropathy and adrenal insufficiency. He takes trimethoprim-sulfamethoxazole for PCP prophylaxis and is on triple-agent antiretroviral treatment. He was recently started on spironolactone for ascites due to alcoholic liver disease. Physical examination reveals normal vital signs, but his muscles are diffusely weak. Frequent extrasystoles are noted. He has mild ascites and 1+ peripheral edema. Laboratory studies show a serum creatinine of 2.5 with a potassium value of 7.3 mEq/L. ECG shows peaking of the T-waves and QRS widening to 0.14. What is the most important immediate treatment?

a. Sodium polystyrene sulfonate (Kayexalate)
b. Acute hemodialysis
c. IV normal saline
d. IV calcium gluconate
e. IV furosemide 80 mg stat

276. Once the above patient is stabilized and the T-waves have normalized, it is important to review the potential causes of his hyperkalemia and to take steps to prevent this from happening again. As you consider the pathophysiology of each confounding factor, which of the following statements is true?

a. Trimethoprim-sulfamethoxazole, which this patient was taking to prevent *Pneumocystis* infection, causes hypokalemia and therefore deterred this patient from presenting sooner.
b. Spironolactone, a commonly used diuretic for treating ascites in the setting of cirrhosis, acts as a competitive aldosterone inhibitor at the level of the collecting duct of the nephron, resulting in decreased potassium excretion and hyperkalemia.
c. This patient most likely had pseudohyperkalemia due to the use of a very small needle as well as rough handling of the specimen as it was transported to the laboratory, both of which caused hemolysis and release of potassium into the serum.
d. Once this patient is hospitalized he will likely receive heparin for the prevention of deep venous thrombosis. Heparin should help ameliorate the hyperkalemia in the ensuing days in the hospital.
e. The patient's reported adrenal insufficiency most likely did not affect aldosterone synthesis and hence potassium level by that mechanism.

277. An 85-year-old man who resides in a nursing home presents with a 3-day history of lower abdominal pain and increasing fatigue and lethargy. He is afebrile; his BP is 160/92, and RR 16. His lungs are clear and his heart examination normal. There is diffuse abdominal tenderness on palpation and a large area of fullness and dullness to percussion starting just below the umbilicus and extending to the suprapubic area. His serum sodium is 130 mEq/L, potassium 4.9 mEq/L, BUN 75 mg/dL, and creatinine is 3.5 mg/dL. His baseline BUN and creatinine were 25 and 1.3, respectively, as recently as 2 weeks ago. A Foley catheter is placed and 1200 cc of urine is obtained. What will be the likely clinical course for this patient with regard to his renal function?

a. His creatinine will continue to rise slowly for 2 to 3 more days.
b. His creatinine will return to 1.3 over the next week.
c. He will require dialysis within 24 hours.
d. He will produce minimal urinary output for at least 3 days.
e. His renal function is unlikely to show any improvement in the future and 3.5 will be his new baseline.

278. A 73-year-old man undergoes abdominal aortic aneurysm repair. According to the anesthesia record, he develops hypotension to 80/50 during the procedure; his blood pressure returns to normal with transfusion of four units of packed red blood cells. Postoperatively, his blood pressure is 110/70, heart rate is 110, surgical wound is clean, and a Foley catheter is in place. Over the next 2 days his urine output slowly decreases. His creatinine on postop day 3 is 3.5 mg/dL (baseline 1.2). His sodium is 140 mEq/L, K 4.6 mEq/L, and BUN 50 mg/dL. Hemoglobin and hematocrit are stable. Urinalysis shows occasional granular casts but otherwise is normal. Urine sodium is 50 mEq/L, urine osmolality is 290 mOsmol/L, and urine creatinine is 35 mg/dL. The fractional excretion of sodium (FeNa) based on these data is 3.5. What is the most likely cause of this patient's acute kidney injury?

a. Acute interstitial nephritis
b. Acute glomerulonephritis (GN)
c. Acute tubular necrosis
d. Prerenal azotemia
e. Contrast-induced nephropathy

279. A 25-year-old man is referred to you because of hematuria. He noticed brief reddening of the urine at the time of a recent respiratory infection. The gross hematuria resolved, but his physician found microscopic hematuria on two subsequent first-voided morning urine specimens. The patient is otherwise healthy; he does not smoke. His blood pressure is 114/72 and the physical examination is normal. The urinalysis shows 2+ protein and 10 to 15 RBC/hpf, with some dysmorphic erythrocytes. No WBC or casts are seen. What is the most likely cause of his hematuria?

a. Kidney stone
b. Renal cell carcinoma
c. Acute poststreptococcal glomerulonephritis
d. Chronic prostatitis
e. IgA nephropathy (Berger disease)

280. A 63-year-old woman with long-standing type 2 diabetes, hypertension, osteoarthritis, and controlled systolic congestive heart failure following a previous anterior myocardial infarction presents for a routine office visit. She denies any significant complaints. The patient faithfully takes her glargine insulin, lisinopril, carvedilol, furosemide, and aspirin. On examination her blood pressure is 122/82, pulse 85, RR 14, with clear lungs, regular heart beat, and 1+ bilateral pedal edema. You review the chart and find that her baseline creatinine is 1.5 mg/dL with an estimated glomerular filtration (GFR) rate of 42 mL/min. Her laboratory studies drawn early the morning of the visit returns as follows:

Na: 138 mEq/L
K: 6.0 mEq/L
HCO_3: 15 mEq/L
Cl: 120 mEq/L
BUN: 20 mg/dL
Creatinine: 1.8 mg/dL
Glucose: 183 mg/dL

You suspect she has a Type 4 renal tubular acidosis. What is the most common pathophysiologic scenario leading to this acid-base disturbance?

a. The combination of long-standing diabetes and hypertension has led to distal nephron dysfunction inhibiting both acid and potassium secretion.
b. The patient's heart failure has caused decreased renal perfusion resulting in the metabolic abnormalities.
c. The patient has been overtreated with diuretics leading to intravascular volume depletion and acidosis.
d. The patient's aspirin use has led to toxicity in the setting of acute kidney injury and hence the metabolic acidosis.
e. The patient's blood pressure has been overtreated with the combination of an ACE inhibitor and a beta-blocker, causing renal hypoperfusion and the noted metabolic derangements.

281. A 56-year-old man presents with hypertension and peripheral edema. He is otherwise healthy and takes no medications. Family history reveals that his father and a brother have kidney disease. His father was on hemodialysis before his death at age 68 of a stroke. Physical examination reveals BP 174/96 and AV nicking on funduscopic examination. He has a soft S_4 gallop. Bilateral flank masses measuring 16 cm in length are palpable. Urinalysis shows 15 to 20 RBC/hpf and trace protein but is otherwise normal; his serum creatinine is 2.4 mg/dL.

Which is the most likely long-term complication of his condition?

a. End-stage renal disease (ESRD) requiring dialysis or transplantation
b. Malignancy
c. Ruptured cerebral aneurysm
d. Biliary obstruction owing to cystic disease of the pancreas
e. Dementia

282. A 58-year-old female smoker with end-stage chronic obstructive pulmonary disease and osteoarthritis is on ipratropium bromide and albuterol inhalers, and hydrocodone-acetaminophen. She presents with respiratory distress for 2 days accompanied by increased thick, yellow sputum production, low grade fever, and increasing confusion. On examination she is mildly obtunded but arousable, BP 160/100, pulse 115/min, RR 30/min, O_2 saturation 84% on her usual 3 L/min nasal cannula oxygen. She is using accessory muscles to breath, has diffuse wheezing and rhonchi bilaterally, a prolonged expiratory phase, distant but regular heart sounds, and no peripheral edema.

Arterial blood gases (ABGs) on arrival are as follows: pH 7.20, Po_2 70 mm Hg, Pco_2 65 mm Hg, calculated HCO_3 29 mEq/L.

Electrolytes return shortly thereafter as follows: Na 140 mEq/L, K 5.1 mEq/L, HCO_3 29 mEq/L, Cl 100 mEq/L, BUN 20 mg/dL, creatinine 1.5 mg/dL, glucose 89 mg/dL.

After prompt initiation of noninvasive positive pressure ventilation (Bi-pap), blood cultures, toxicology screen, intravenous fluids, and IV antibiotics, you have time to consider the patient's metabolic situation. Choose the answer which best describes the acid-base condition and its etiology.

a. The patient has acute, severe respiratory acidosis caused by the sudden deterioration in her respiratory status.

b. The patient has an underlying metabolic acidosis caused by her renal insufficiency now compounded by a respiratory alkalosis.

c. The patient ingested abundant amounts of aspirin which caused a severe metabolic acidosis and respiratory failure.

d. The patient has a baseline chronic respiratory acidosis with metabolic compensation, now with a superimposed further respiratory acidosis caused by decreased ventilation.

e. The patient has become obtunded and her oral intake has decreased. Her elevated BUN and creatinine indicate she is volume-depleted, which explains her elevated serum bicarbonate level.

283. A 63-year-old man alcoholic with a 50-pack-year history of smoking presents to the emergency room with fatigue and confusion. Physical examination reveals a blood pressure of 110/70 with no orthostatic change. Heart, lung, and abdominal examinations are normal and there is no pedal edema. Laboratory data are as follows:

Na: 110 mEq/L
K: 3.7 mEq/L
Cl: 82 mEq/L
HCO_3: 20 mEq/L
Glucose: 100 mg/dL
BUN: 5 mg/dL
Creatinine: 0.7 mg/dL
Urinalysis: normal
Urine specific gravity: 1.016

Which of the following is the most likely diagnosis?

a. Volume depletion
b. Inappropriate secretion of antidiuretic hormone
c. Psychogenic polydipsia
d. Cirrhosis
e. Congestive heart failure

284. A 27-year-old alcoholic man presents with decreased appetite, mild generalized weakness, intermittent mild abdominal pain, perioral numbness, and some cramping of his hands and feet. His physical examination is initially normal. His laboratory returns with a sodium level of 140 mEq/L, potassium 4.0 mEq/L, calcium 6.9 mg/dL, albumin 3.5 g/dL, magnesium 0.7 mg/dL, and phosphorus 2.0 mg/dL. You go back to the patient and find that he has both a positive Trousseau and a positive Chvostek sign. Which of the following is the most likely cause of the hypocalcemia?

a. Poor dietary intake
b. Hypoalbuminemia
c. Pancreatitis
d. Decreased end-organ response to parathyroid hormone because of hypomagnesemia
e. Osteoporosis caused by hypogonadism

285. A 27-year-old woman presents to the emergency room with a panic attack. She appears healthy except for tachycardia and a respiratory rate of 30. Electrolytes include calcium 10.0 mg/dL, albumin 4.0 g/dL, phosphorus 0.8 mg/dL, and magnesium 1.5 mEq/L. Arterial blood gases include pH of 7.56, P_{CO_2} 21 mm Hg, and P_{O_2} 99 mm Hg. Which of the following is the most likely cause of the hypophosphatemia?

a. Hypomagnesemia
b. Hyperparathyroidism
c. Respiratory alkalosis with intracellular shift
d. Poor dietary intake
e. Vitamin D deficiency

286. A 50-year-old diabetic woman presents for follow-up of her hypertension. Her blood pressure is 152/96 in the office today and she brings in readings from home that are consistently in the same range over the past month. Her current medications are amlodipine 5 mg daily and hydrochlorothiazide 25 mg daily. The diuretic was added when she developed peripheral edema on the amlodipine; now she has only trace peripheral edema. A spot urine specimen shows 280 µg of albumin per mg creatinine (microalbuminuria is present if this value is between 30 and 300 µg/mg). What would be the best next therapeutic step in this patient?

a. Add clonidine.
b. Add a beta-blocker.
c. Increase the thiazide diuretic dose.
d. Add an alpha-blocker.
e. Add angiotensin-converting enzyme inhibitor or angiotensin receptor blocker.

287. A 29-year-old man with HIV, on a highly active antiretroviral therapy (HAART) regimen including the protease inhibitor indinavir, presents with severe edema and a serum creatinine of 2.0 mg/dL. He has had bone pain for 5 years and takes large amounts of acetaminophen with codeine, aspirin, and ibuprofen. He is on prophylactic trimethoprim-sulfamethoxazole. Blood pressure is 170/110; urinalysis shows 4+ protein, 5 to 10 RBC, 0 WBC; 24-hour urine protein is 6.2 g. The serum albumin is 1.9 g/dL (normal above 3.7). Which of the following is the most likely cause of his renal disease?

a. Indinavir toxicity
b. Analgesic nephropathy
c. Trimethoprim-sulfamethoxazole–induced interstitial nephritis
d. Focal segmental glomerulosclerosis
e. Renal artery stenosis

288. A 50-year-old diabetic, alcoholic man is brought to the emergency department by the police after they found him lying in a pool of his own urine on the side of the road downtown, not far from a bar. On examination he is obtunded, BP 110/70, pulse 120, respiratory rate 20, O_2 saturation 95% on room air, mouth is dry, lungs have crackles in the right axilla and right upper chest, heart is regular, abdomen somewhat tense but bowel sounds present, extremities without edema, and neurological examination nonfocal. Laboratory show:

Na: 122 mEq/L
K: 3.5 mEq/L
Cl: 100 mEq/L
HCO_3: 5 mEq/L
BUN: 40 m/dL
Cr: 1.8 mg/dL
Glucose: 800 mg/dL
Serum osmolality: Elevated
Serum ketones: Negative

What is the most likely cause of this patient's hyponatremia?

a. SIADH caused by the patient's delirium tremens
b. Primary polydipsia
c. Adrenal crisis in the setting of sepsis
d. Hyperglycemia-related hyponatremia
e. Pseudohyponatremia

289. A 39-year-old woman is admitted to the gynecology service for hysterectomy for symptomatic uterine fibroids. Postoperatively the patient develops an ileus accompanied by severe nausea and vomiting; ondansetron is piggybacked into an IV of D5½ normal saline running at 125 cc/h. On the second postoperative day the patient becomes drowsy and displays a few myoclonic jerks. Stat labs reveal Na 118, K 3.2, Cl 88 HCO_3 22, BUN 3, and creatinine 0.9. Urine studies for Na and osmolality are sent to the laboratory. What is the most appropriate next step?

a. Change the IV fluid to 0.9% (normal) saline and restrict free-water intake to 600 cc/d.
b. Change the ondansetron to promethazine, change the IV fluid to lactated Ringer solution, and recheck the Na in 4 hours.
c. Start 3% (hypertonic) saline, make the patient NPO, and transfer to the ICU.
d. Change the IV fluid to normal saline and give furosemide 40 mg IV stat.
e. Make the patient NPO and send for stat CT scan of the head to look for cerebral edema.

290. You evaluate a 48-year-old man for chronic renal insufficiency. He has a history of hypertension, osteoarthritis, and gout. He currently has no complaints. His medical regimen includes lisinopril 40 mg daily, hydrochlorothiazide 25 mg daily, allopurinol 300 mg daily, and acetaminophen for his joint pains. He does not smoke but drinks 8 oz of wine on a daily basis. Examination shows BP 146/86, pulse 76, a soft S_4 gallop, and mild peripheral edema. There is no abdominal bruit. His urinalysis (UA) reveals 1+ proteinuria and no cellular elements. Serum creatinine is 2.2 mg/dL and his estimated GFR from the MDRD formula is 42 mL/min. What is the most important element in preventing progression of his renal disease?

a. Discontinuing all alcohol consumption.
b. Discontinuing acetaminophen.
c. Adding a calcium channel blocker to improve blood pressure control.
d. Obtaining a CT renal arteriogram to exclude renal artery stenosis.
e. Changing the lisinopril to losartan.

Questions 291 to 293

Match the clinical presentation with the likely cause of the patient's acute kidney injury. Each lettered option may be used once, more than once, or not at all.

a. Prerenal azotemia because of intravascular volume depletion
b. Ischemia-induced acute tubular necrosis
c. Nephrotoxin-induced acute tubular necrosis
d. Acute interstitial nephritis
e. Postrenal azotemia because of obstructive uropathy
f. Postinfectious glomerulonephritis

291. A patient is admitted to the hospital with a nursing-home–acquired pneumonia. His blood pressure is normal and the extremities well-perfused. Admission creatinine is 1.2 mg/dL. UA is clear. The patient is treated on the floor with piperacillin/tazobactam and improves clinically. On the fourth hospital day, the patient notes a nonpruritic rash over the abdomen. The creatinine has risen to 2.2 mg/dL. The urinalysis shows 2+ protein, 10 to 15 WBC/hpf, and no casts or RBCs.

292. A 62-year-old man is admitted with pneumonia and severe sepsis. Vasopressors are required to maintain peripheral perfusion, and mechanical ventilation is needed because of acute respiratory distress syndrome (ARDS). Admission creatinine is 1.0 mg/dL but rises by the second hospital day to 2.2 mg/dL. Urine output is 300 cc/24 h. UA shows renal tubular epithelial cells and some muddy brown casts. The fractional excretion of sodium is 3.45.

293. An 87-year-old woman is admitted with acute delirium, nausea, and vomiting for 1 day from a local nursing home. She has a history of early stage Alzheimer's dementia, hypertension, osteoarthritis, and hypothyroidism. Admission creatinine is 3.8 mg/dL. She is found to be clinically dehydrated and to have >100 WBC in her urine along with nitrite positive and 3+ bacteria on her urinalysis. She responds to ceftriaxone and intravenous hydration; by the next day she is producing adequate quantities of urine, her mentation has improved some, and her creatinine is 2.0 mg/dL.

Questions 294 to 296

Match the clinical and microscopic presentation with the correct primary glomerular disease. Each lettered option may be used once, more than once, or not at all.

a. Minimal change disease
b. IgA nephropathy
c. Focal and segmental glomerulosclerosis
d. Anti-glomerular basement membrane disease
e. Membranous nephropathy
f. Membranoproliferative glomerulonephritis

294. A 50-year-old white man presents with mild hypertension, nephrotic syndrome, microscopic hematuria, and venous thromboses (including renal vein thrombosis). Renal biopsy reveals a thickened glomerular basement membrane with subepithelial immunoglobulin deposition.

295. A 19-year-old white man presents with hypertension, nephrotic syndrome, mild renal insufficiency, RBC casts in urine, and depressed third component of complement (C3). Renal biopsy shows thickened basement membranes and increased cellular elements. Electron microscopy shows dense deposits within the basement membrane.

296. A 43-year-old woman complains of fatigue and swelling of her legs. She has no history of lymphadenopathy, night sweats, or weight loss. On examination she has a slightly puffy face and her blood pressure is 150/95. She has no adenopathy, her lungs are clear, her heart is normal, and she has 2+ pitting edema to the mid-calf bilaterally. Her creatinine is 0.8 and her urinalysis shows 3+ protein. Her 24-hour urine protein is 3.9 g. Renal biopsy results show normal light microscopy and no deposits by immuno-fluorescent microscopy. Electron microscopy shows effacement of the foot processes.

Questions 297 to 299

Match the presentation with the most likely systemic disease. Each lettered option may be used once, more than once, or not at all.

a. Macroscopic (classic) polyarteritis nodosa
b. Microscopic polyangiitis
c. Granulomatosis with polyangiitis (Wegener granulomatosis)
d. Churg-Strauss syndrome
e. Cryoglobulinemic vasculitis
f. Lupus nephritis

297. A 66-year-old man presents with severe hypertension and abdominal pain. He has low-grade fever and livedo reticularis over the lower extremities. Neurological examination shows a right peroneal neuropathy and sensory loss in the left radial nerve distribution, consistent with mononeuritis multiplex. UA reveals 1+ proteinuria and 15 to 20 RBC/hpf.

298. A 75-year-old man presents with a 6-month history of nasal congestion, mild epistaxis, and sinus tenderness. He develops a cough and peripheral edema. CT scan of the sinuses shows evidence of chronic sinusitis, and the chest x-ray reveals several nodular densities, one with early cavitation. His serum creatinine has risen from 1.1 to 2.7 mg/dL over the past 3 weeks. The UA shows 2+ protein and moderate hematuria.

299. A 30-year-old African-American woman presents with fatigue, hypertension, symmetric arthritis, a mildly elevated creatinine, nephrotic range proteinuria, and red cell casts in her urinalysis. Both C3 and C4 complement levels are low.

Nephrology

Answers

269. The answer is c. Rhabdomyolysis-induced AKI is characterized by hyperkalemia, hyperphosphatemia, and hyperuricemia, all caused by release of intracellular muscle products. The high phosphorus level causes hypocalcemia. The BUN/creatinine ratio, normally 10/1, is reduced because of release of muscle creatine, which is converted to creatinine. The load of creatinine to be excreted by the failing kidney therefore exceeds the urea load, which is little changed. The presence of "blood" on the dipstick determination is caused by myoglobinuria. The dipstick registers red blood cells, hemoglobin (eg, from intravascular hemolysis), and myoglobin as "blood." Trauma, medications (especially statins), infectious processes (influenza, sepsis), and extreme muscular exertion (seizures, exertional heat stroke) are common causes.

All nonsteroidal agents may cause decreased renal function. Usually this is attributed to decreased blood flow—less commonly, to drug-induced interstitial nephritis. The laboratory abnormalities in this case do not suggest decreased blood flow or interstitial nephritis. However, stopping the ibuprofen would be prudent. The absence of orthostatic hypotension makes the diagnosis of volume depletion very unlikely, and the BUN/creatinine ratio is often elevated in prerenal azotemia. Nothing on history, physical examination, or electrolyte abnormalities suggests obstruction. However, in a 76-year-old man, a renal sonogram to rule out occult obstruction would be reasonable. Hypertensive nephrosclerosis causes chronic rather than acute renal insufficiency and would not account for the electrolyte abnormalities.

270. The answer is c. The first step in analyzing an acid-base disturbance is simply to look at the pH. This patient has an acidosis. Then look at the HCO_3 and the Pco_2 to determine the primary disturbance; that is, is it a metabolic acidosis or a respiratory acidosis? The serum HCO_3 has decreased from 24 to 5 mEq/L, so this must be a metabolic acidosis. The Pco_2 is below the normal value of 40 mm, so this *cannot* be a respiratory acidosis (the Pco_2 would be above 40 in a respiratory acidosis). The first two steps are straightforward and unambiguous.

The third (and most difficult) step is to assess the compensatory response. This patient has a metabolic acidosis, so you need to assess the respiratory compensation. That is to say, has the Pco_2 decreased appropriately to compensate for the metabolic acidosis? The normal compensatory response in metabolic acidosis is for the Pco_2 to decrease by 1 to 1.5 mm Hg for each 1-mEq decrease in HCO_3. This patient's 19 mEq/L drop in bicarbonate is matched by a 25-mm drop in the Pco_2. Hence, this is a compensated metabolic acidosis. Another method of assessing compensation in a metabolic acidosis is to use the Winters formula, which says that the appropriate Pco_2 equals 1.5 (HCO_3) + 8. This would give an appropriate Pco_2 of 15.5, very close to the measured Pco_2. Again, the compensatory response is appropriate for the degree of acidosis; the patient does not have a respiratory acid-base disorder.

The fourth step is to calculate the anion gap. The normal anion gap (Na− [Cl + HCO_3]) is 8 to 10 mEq/L; in this case the value is 29 mEq/L. Therefore, this is a wide anion-gap metabolic acidosis with appropriate respiratory compensation. A brief differential of anion-gap metabolic acidosis is as follows:

Diabetic ketoacidosis
Lactic acidosis
Alcoholic ketoacidosis
Toxic alcohol (methanol, ethylene glycol) ingestion
Salicylate intoxication
Renal failure

271. The answer is d. This patient is abnormally young to have essential hypertension, and the renal bruit is highly suggestive of a secondary cause of the condition: renal artery stenosis caused by fibromuscular dysplasia (FMD). FMD is more common in young females (85%–90% of patients are women). The exact etiology of the condition is unknown, but renal artery stenosis causing hypertension is a common presentation. Renal angiography is the diagnostic modality of choice, although duplex ultrasonography, CT angiography, and MR angiography can also be utilized. Etiologies that can mimic fibromuscular dysplasia include atherosclerosis and vasculitis. The patient has no physical findings to make one suspect Cushing syndrome (abnormal fat distribution, ecchymoses, hirsutism, etc), congenital adrenal hyperplasia (virilization), or coarctation of the aorta (BP lower in legs than in arm). She does not have the metabolic alkalosis and hypokalemia of primary hyperaldosteronism.

272. The answer is c. The first priority in treating acute gout is to control the inflammation. Nonsteroidal anti-inflammatory agents or colchicine are usually used first line for acute gout; however, this patient has several contraindications (chronic kidney disease and myelodysplasia, respectively) to their use. Prednisone is very effective at treating acute gout in this situation and is the best choice given this patient's comorbidities. Intra-articular injection of the affected joint with steroids is also effective but requires special expertise to perform the procedure. Colchicine is less well tolerated in the elderly and is contraindicated in patients with myelodysplasia. Allopurinol, febuxostat, and probenecid are avoided in acute gout. Paradoxically, these agents, which lower serum uric acid levels in the long term, can cause worsening of acute gout. If the patient goes on to have numerous symptomatic episodes of gout or if tophaceous disease should develop, allopurinol, or febuxostat can be started. Probenecid, a uricosuric agent, is ineffective in the setting of chronic kidney disease.

NSAIDs are contraindicated in this case due to the patient's poor renal function as indicated by his creatinine of 3.2.

273. The answer is c. Cytokines produced during an acute gout attack are uricosuric and can cause a reduction in serum uric acid levels, sometimes into the normal range. This should not deter one from making the diagnosis of acute gout. Measuring the uric acid level several weeks after the acute attack will give a more accurate sense of the true uric acid level and can help guide further treatment. Myelodysplastic syndrome (MDS) is not associated with hypouricemia; some diseases such as multiple myeloma and cadmium poisoning can cause proximal tubule dysfunction (Fanconi syndrome) and uric acid wasting by the kidney, but MDS is not one of them. Uric acid is stable and can be measured accurately in the serum even after storage. Allopurinol is certainly effective and lowering the uric acid level of a patient but must be used very cautiously in the setting of chronic kidney disease due to potential toxicity; hence it is unlikely the patient was taking "high doses" as mentioned in answer e.

274. The answer is c. Contrast agents harm the kidney by causing the production of oxygen radicals and by causing vasoconstriction, both of which can lead to acute kidney injury. Patients with underlying kidney disease at baseline, those with diabetes, congestive heart failure, multiple myeloma, and dehydration are at greatest risk of this complication. Prehydration with IV normal saline or bicarbonate has been proven to decrease the risk of contrast nephropathy. *N*-acetylcysteine is also used by some clinicians for prevention, though studies have not been as convincing as those using saline or bicarbonate. Mannitol, dopamine, and prophylactic hemodialysis have been studied and found ineffective in preventing contrast nephropathy. Indomethacin would cause further vasoconstriction and is contraindicated in patients with renal insufficiency.

275. The answer is d. This patient has life-threatening hyperkalemia as suggested by the ECG changes in association with documented hyperkalemia. Death can occur within minutes as a result of ventricular fibrillation, and immediate treatment is mandatory. Intravenous calcium is given to combat the membrane effects of the hyperkalemia, and measures to shift potassium acutely into the cells must be instituted as well. IV regular insulin 10 units and (unless the patient is already hyperglycemic) IV glucose (usually 25 g) can lower the serum potassium level by 0.5 to 1.0 mEq/L. Nebulized albuterol is often used and is probably more effective than IV sodium bicarbonate. It is crucial to remember that measures to promote potassium loss from the body (Kayexalate, furosemide, or dialysis), although important in the long run, take hours to work. These measures will not promptly counteract the membrane irritability of hyperkalemia. IV normal saline will not lower the serum potassium level.

276. The answer is b. Spironolactone, a potassium sparing diuretic by way of competitive inhibition of aldosterone at the collecting duct of the nephron, can lead to significant hyperkalemia in the setting of chronic kidney disease. Trimethoprim-sulfamethoxazole can also cause hyperkalemia by interfering with potassium exchange in the distal nephron. Heparin, including low-molecular-weight types, directly affects the zona glomerulosa of the kidney, reducing aldosterone production; it can lead to severe hyperkalemia in patients with already damaged kidneys. Adrenal insufficiency also leads to decreased aldosterone synthesis and hyperkalemia. Pseudohyperkalemia occurs precisely as described in answer c, however, this patient had clinical signs and ECG changes consistent with true hyperkalemia.

277. The answer is b. This patient has obstructive uropathy. With relief of the obstruction due to an enlarged prostate, the likely cause of his bilateral obstruction, renal function will return to baseline over the ensuing week. If the obstruction had been present for more than 1 to 2 weeks, recovery may be only partial. Obstruction that has lasted several weeks often causes irreversible damage. A nuclear medicine renal scan performed following relief of the obstruction may give an indication of the prognosis. Relief of bilateral obstruction is associated with a post obstructive diuresis. Urine output in this situation can be brisk and may require careful attention to volume status of the patient. In most patients, however, this is associated with appropriate excretion of retained salt and water.

278. The answer is c. This patient with known atherosclerotic disease and a minimally elevated baseline creatinine has suffered a period of hypotension and hence renal hypoperfusion. By calculating the fractional excretion of sodium (FeNa) using the data that have been provided (FeNa = Urine sodium • plasma creatinine • 100/plasma sodium • urine creatinine), as shown in the equation below:

$$FeNa = \frac{U_{Na} \times P_{Cr} \times 100}{P_{Na} \times U_{Cr}}$$

One can feel more comfortable distinguishing between prerenal azotemia and acute tubular necrosis. If the FeNa is less than 1, the patient likely has prerenal azotemia. If it is over 2, it is more likely that the patient has acute tubular necrosis or some other intrinsic renal disease. The clinical scenario of this patient, along with the high FeNa and the granular (sometimes called "muddy brown") casts in the urine, all point toward acute tubular necrosis (ATN). Interstitial nephritis more commonly occurs in patients following exposure to certain medications and typically is associated with white blood cells (especially eosinophils) in the urine. Glomerulonephritis is unlikely due to the hypotension and the lack of red cell casts on the urinalysis. This patient may have had recent exposure to a contrast agent, but that has not been mentioned.

279. The answer is e. Dysmorphic erythrocytes and proteinuria suggest a glomerular source of hematuria. The commonest causes of glomerular hematuria in this population are IgA nephropathy (Berger disease) and thin basement membrane disease. Berger disease can cause hypertension or even renal insufficiency; thin basement membrane disease is a benign condition. Berger disease is associated with IgA deposits in the mesangium. Patients with IgA nephropathy often have an exacerbation of their hematuria at the time of upper respiratory illnesses.

Although urological cancers, kidney stones, and prostatitis are important causes of hematuria (especially in an older or symptomatic patient), they would not cause dysmorphic erythrocytes or protein in the urine. Acute glomerulonephritis usually occurs a week or two *after* the sore throat (ie, to give enough time for vigorous antibody production against the streptococcal antigens). The condition is usually symptomatic (hypertension, periorbital edema) and is associated with red blood cell casts and an active urinary sediment. Poststreptococcal GN is now a rare condition in the adult population of developed nations.

280. The answer is a. Type 4 renal tubular acidosis occurs when there is distal nephron dysfunction leading to disproportionate levels of hyperkalemia and acidosis compared to the degree of kidney disease encountered. This is most commonly seen in patients with long-standing diabetes and can be exacerbated by the use of nonsteroidals, trimethoprim-sulfamethoxazole and angiotensin-converting enzyme inhibitors. A patient with congestive heart failure and renal hypoperfusion can develop prerenal azotemia, but you would expect clinical evidence of decompensated heart failure and an elevated BUN to creatinine ratio (well above 10/1). A patient who has been overdiuresed will tend to have hypokalemia, a higher BUN/Cr ratio and a contraction alkalosis. Salicylate poisoning typically requires a significant ingestion (not mentioned in this question) and causes a wide-anion gap metabolic acidosis. Use of ACE inhibitors can lead to hyperkalemia but neither ACE inhibitors nor beta-blockers typically lead to a Type 4 RTA.

281. The answer is a. This patient has adult polycystic kidney disease (APCKD), an autosomal dominant condition. It is the commonest genetic renal disease causing ESRD and often presents with hypertension, hematuria, and large palpable kidneys. Imaging studies would confirm the diagnosis by showing numerous bilateral renal cortical cysts. Cysts are often seen in the liver and pancreas but rarely cause symptoms. Most patients progress to end-stage renal disease despite meticulous blood pressure control with ACE inhibitors or angiotensin receptor blockers.

Malignancy and dementia are not seen with increased incidence in APCKD patients. About 10% of patients with APCKD harbor berry aneurysms in the circle of Willis; a ruptured berry aneurysm may have accounted for his father's stroke. APCKD patients also have an increased incidence of abdominal and thoracic aneurysms as well as diverticulosis. The abnormal gene, on chromosome 16 in 85% of patients, appears to encode a structural protein that helps keep the renal tubules open and unobstructed. This same protein provides strength to the walls of arteries and other epithelial structures (pancreatic ductules, bile ductules, and colon).

282. The answer is d. Patients with severe COPD often have a baseline chronic respiratory acidosis with a P_{CO_2} in the 50 to 60 mm Hg range.

They are unable to ventilate sufficiently to correct the acidotic situation this creates. The kidney then compensates by retaining HCO_3. This results in a new steady state in which the patient has a near-normal pH on their blood gas despite the chronically elevated CO_2. In this question the further deterioration in the patient's respiratory status due to COPD exacerbation has caused further CO_2 retention and a superimposed acute respiratory acidosis on top of the chronic respiratory acidosis. Salicylate overdose normally causes an anion gap acidosis and the AG is normal here. Volume depletion, especially due to recurrent vomiting, can lead to a contraction alkalosis, but this patient's acidosis indicates that the elevated bicarbonate level is caused by renal compensation for her chronic CO_2 retention.

283. The answer is b. Inappropriate secretion of antidiuretic hormone is suggested in a patient without clinical evidence of volume depletion or an edematous (ie, salt-retaining) condition. This syndrome may be idiopathic, associated with certain pulmonary and intracranial pathologies, resulting from endocrine disorders (eg, hypothyroidism), or drug-induced (eg, many psychotropic agents). Volume depletion is unlikely in the absence of orthostatic hypotension. Psychogenic polydipsia requires the ingestion of huge quantities of water to overcome the kidneys' ability to excrete a free-water load and would be associated with a very dilute urine (ie, urine specific gravity of 1.001 or 1.002). Cirrhosis is unlikely in the absence of ascites and edema. Congestive heart failure can cause hyponatremia but would be associated with edema and evidence of venous congestion.

284. The answer is d. One of the commonest causes of hypocalcemia is impaired parathormone (PTH) production. Hypomagnesemia causes decreased production of PTH as well as decreased end-organ response to the hormone. Alcohol causes increased urinary losses of magnesium which then leads to the mentioned effects on PTH and ultimately to hypocalcemia. Poor dietary intake and osteoporosis do not lead to hypocalcemia unless the patient has vitamin D deficiency. Routine calcium levels are not accurate in the setting of a low albumin. To estimate the true calcium level, one may add 0.8 mg/dL to the observed calcium level for every 1 g/dL reduction in the albumin level (from 4 used as normal). In this case, the albumin is not far from 4 and hence the calculation would change the low calcium level very little. An ionized calcium level is consistent and accurate regardless of the albumin level.

While pancreatitis can cause hypocalcemia, this patient's presentation does not suggest the condition.

285. The answer is c. Respiratory alkalosis is one of the commonest causes of hypophosphatemia; it results from shift of phosphate from the extracellular to the intracellular space. Hypomagnesemia alone would increase phosphorus by decreasing parathormone effect. Hyperparathyroidism can decrease phosphorus but would cause hypercalcemia. Severe hypophosphatemia is seen with malnutrition, especially during the refeeding stage when carbohydrate intake causes phosphate to shift into the intracellular space. Such patients have clear clinical evidence of malnutrition. In addition, malnutrition almost always causes hypoalbuminemia. Vitamin D deficiency is uncommon in this age group and would be associated with hypocalcemia.

286. The answer is e. By a variety of mechanisms, angiotensin-converting enzyme inhibitors and angiotensin receptor blockers help preserve renal function in diabetes. Both classes of medication can cause hyperkalemia, so it is important to monitor serum potassium after initiation. A significant increase in serum creatinine may suggest the presence of renovascular hypertension. A common side effect of ACE inhibitors is a dry cough. A less frequent side effect would be angioedema. Clonidine has not been shown to slow the progression of diabetic renal disease, and often causes orthostatic hypotension, constipation, and erectile dysfunction. Although many diabetic patients receive beta-blockers because of coronary disease, these are not first-line drugs for preventing progression of renal failure. Because of low cost and proven efficacy, thiazide diuretics remain a good choice for the general population, but do not have a specific effect on the progression of renal disease. Alpha-blockers are fourth-line agents for the treatment of hypertension and do not have renal-preserving effect in diabetes.

287. The answer is d. Although many glomerular lesions occur in association with HIV, focal segmental glomerulosclerosis (FSGS) is by far the commonest etiology of this patient's nephrotic syndrome. While FSGS is more common in intravenous drug users with HIV, the lesion is different from so-called heroin nephropathy. Indinavir toxicity may cause tubular obstruction by crystals and is a cause of renal stones, but does not cause nephrotic syndrome. Analgesic nephropathy is a frequently unrecognized cause of occult renal failure. This entity requires at least 10 years of high-level analgesic use and may cause renal colic owing to papillary necrosis.

Analgesic abuse nephropathy, however, is an interstitial disease and does not cause nephrotic range proteinuria. Trimethoprim-sulfamethoxazole may cause acute interstitial nephritis, but the patient does not have fever, rash, WBC casts, or eosinophils in the urinalysis. Again, interstitial diseases do not cause high-level proteinuria. Bilateral renal artery stenosis would be rare at this age and is associated with a normal urinalysis.

288. The answer is d. This patient is in a hyperosmolar state due to his uncontrolled type II diabetes and recent alcohol ingestion. Severe hyperglycemia pulls free water from the cell, leaving the plasma hyponatremic. Free water will return to the intracellular space as the hyperglycemia is reversed with appropriate therapy. The rough calculation to predict what the sodium will be once the hyperglycemia is corrected is to subtract 2 mEq/L from a "normal" sodium of 140 for every 100 mg/dL elevation of glucose over 100 observed in the patient's laboratories. In this case the patient's glucose is 700 over 100 therefore 7 times 2 (mEq for every 100) = 14 or a predicted sodium of 136 mEq/L (normal). SIADH, psychogenic polydipsia, and adrenal insufficiency can cause hyponatremia but would be associated with low serum osmolality. Pseudohyponatremia would be associated with normal osmolality.

289. The answer is c. The patient has acute symptomatic hyponatremia, a life-threatening condition. Symptomatic hyponatremia should be treated with hypertonic saline. This patient is at high risk of seizure and respiratory arrest, the main cause of permanent CNS damage in hyponatremia. ICU care, with frequent monitoring of the serum sodium level and CNS status, is critical. Once the Na has risen 4 to 6 mEq/L and the symptoms have improved, hypertonic saline can be discontinued; the rate of correction should not exceed 10 mEq/L in the first 24 hours. Less aggressive methods of treating her free-water overload, such as fluid restriction alone or in combination with furosemide are not appropriate for this acute emergency. Isotonic fluids such as normal saline and lactated Ringer solution are useful in volume depletion but will *not* treat this patient's free-water excess. Postoperative hyponatremia is particularly common in premenopausal women. The nausea and pain sometimes associated with surgery are very potent stimulators of vasopressin (ADH) release by the neurohypophysis. If hypotonic fluids are used at all in this setting, the serum sodium level should be closely monitored, and isotonic fluids used if there is any trend toward free-water retention (ie, hyponatremia).

290. The answer is c. This patient has stage III chronic kidney disease (estimated GFR 30–60 mL/min/M2). At this stage it is crucial for the internist to prevent progression to end-stage renal disease. In 2014, the long awaited 8th Joint National Committee (JNC 8) recommended blood pressure targets for all patients (less than 65 years of age) to be less than 140 systolic and less than 90 diastolic. Some nephrology groups recommend a goal of less than 130/80 for patients with proteinuria or microalbuminuria in an effort to reduce progression. The patient is on maximal doses of thiazide and angiotensin-converting inhibitor (ACEI), so the addition of a calcium channel blocker is appropriate. Other important management issues include avoiding nephrotoxins (such as NSAIDs and IV contrast agents), if possible, modest dietary protein restriction, and atherosclerotic risk factor management. If the patient progresses to stage IV CKD (estimated GFR 15-30 mL/min), he should be referred to a nephrologist.

Modest ethanol consumption is not a renal or cardiovascular risk factor and need not be modified unless you believe the patient is consuming much more alcohol than he admits. Acetaminophen in usual therapeutic doses is the safest agent to control DJD pain and certainly is preferable to nonsteroidals. The absence of an abdominal bruit and the fact that he has not had rapid worsening of renal function despite treatment with an ACEI makes renal artery stenosis unlikely. In addition, randomized trials have shown that medical management is not inferior to stenting of renal artery stenosis lesions. Angiotensin receptor blockers (such as losartan) can be substituted for ACEIs if side effects such as cough occur, but ARBs have no advantage over ACEIs in preventing progression of CKD. The critical element is tighter blood pressure control.

291 to 293. The answers are 291-d, 292-b, 293-a. Acute kidney injury in adults usually occurs during hospitalization for other illness. The history (in particular, exposure to nephrotoxins including intravenous contrast agents), physical examination (in particular, assessment of volume status and search for allergic manifestations such as skin rash), and urine studies will usually establish the diagnosis. The fractional excretion of sodium may demonstrate renal underperfusion if this is not clear from the clinical setting. If the kidneys are underperfused from volume depletion, third space losses, or poor cardiac output, the kidneys will retain salt and water, and the fractional excretion of sodium (FENa) will be low. In the cases presented here, the clinical setting suggests the diagnosis.

Interstitial nephritis typically occurs as an allergic reaction to antibiotics, particularly beta-lactams and sulfa derivatives. So-called tubular proteinuria is modest (<1 g/24 h), albuminuria is minimal, and the nephrotic syndrome does not occur. Pyuria is usually present. The commonest cause of acute renal failure is acute tubular necrosis. The FENa is usually above two and muddy brown cases may be present on the urinalysis. Ischemia (often owing to sepsis) and nephrotoxins are the usual causes.

The patient with delirium and dehydration showed marked elevation in creatinine that improved remarkably within 24 hours of adequate volume repletion. This is typical of prerenal azotemia secondary to intravascular volume depletion.

Obstructive uropathy can occur acutely, particularly in the setting of bladder outlet obstruction (BPH) or neurogenic bladder (as can occur in diabetes). The patient will often have difficulty voiding and the urinalysis will be unremarkable. Complete anuria or fluctuations from oliguria to polyuria also suggest the diagnosis. Bladder catheterization or renal sonography is diagnostic. Glomerulonephritis rarely occurs during hospitalization for unrelated acute illness.

294 to 296. The answers are 294-e, 295-f, 296-a. Glomerular diseases present with proteinuria and sometimes with an active urinary sediment (dysmorphic red cells, white blood cells, and red cell casts). Many patients have the nephrotic syndrome. Patients who present with an active sediment, hypertension, and worsening renal function without nephrotic-range proteinuria and hypoalbuminemia are said to have the nephritic syndrome. Finally, some patients (eg, the usual patient with IgA nephropathy) will have asymptomatic proteinuria or hematuria. Serological studies, complement levels, and, often, renal biopsy will be necessary to establish a definite diagnosis and to adequately plan treatment.

Membranous nephropathy is the commonest cause of idiopathic nephrotic syndrome in adults. One-third of cases improve spontaneously, one-third remains stable, and one-third progress to end-stage renal disease if untreated. The condition is fairly responsive to corticosteroid and cytotoxic therapy. Membranoproliferative glomerulonephritis is an uncommon cause of idiopathic nephrotic syndrome in adults. Depressed C3 is caused by an autoantibody that directly activates the third component of complement. A progressive clinical course and erratic response to therapy are typical.

Minimal change disease is the cause of nephrotic syndrome in about 15% of adults and 70% to 90% of children. While it often presents as primary renal disease, it is also seen in association with other conditions such as NSAID use with concomitant interstitial nephritis and Hodgkin disease. Clinically, patients present as described with sudden onset of edema, nephrotic syndrome, and amorphous urinary sediment on the urinalysis. Most (70%) adults achieve remission of the disease with the use of prednisone; cyclophosphamide, chlorambucil, or mycophenolate mofetil may be required in refractory cases. Relapses can occur but are less common in adults than in children. While children often do not require a biopsy if they respond to high-dose steroids, most adults do undergo biopsy to confirm the etiology. Renal biopsy and electron microscopy are exactly as described in the question.

IgA nephropathy is the commonest glomerular disease in adults but rarely causes nephrotic syndrome. Focal segmental glomerulosclerosis is often associated with drug use or AIDS. Anti-glomerular basement membrane (anti-GBM) disease causes a nephritic picture with hematuria and rapidly progressive renal insufficiency. Light microscopy often reveals crescent formation, and immunofluorescence shows linear IgG staining of the GBM.

297 to 299. The answers are 297-a, 298-c, 299-f. Renal involvement in systemic vasculitis is common and can lead to serious morbidity, including end-stage renal disease. The pattern of renal disease can be diagnostically useful. Macroscopic polyarteritis nodosa is a vasculitis of medium-sized blood vessels that causes renal artery aneurysms (severe hypertension), abdominal aneurysms (abdominal pain), and ischemic damage to skin and peripheral nerves. Patients are most commonly older males and anyone who is hepatitis B-surface-antigen-positive. Microscopic polyangiitis is a different disease entirely. It is often associated with lung involvement and alveolar hemorrhage (pulmonary involvement is rare in classic PAN) and small-vessel (ie, glomerular) renal involvement rather than the arcuate artery aneurysms that are seen on angiography in classic PAN. Granulomatosis with polyangiitis (Wegener granulomatosis) is one of the most common of the vasculitides. It usually occurs in older males and typically starts with chronic sinusitis. Pulmonary and renal involvements then develop. A positive c-cytoplasmic antineutrophil cytoplasmic antibody (ANCA) test, associated with antibodies against proteinase 3, is an important diagnostic clue. Perinuclear or p-ANCA positivity is caused by antibodies to myeloperoxidase and can be seen in other vasculitic syndromes.

Lupus nephritis is a common and serious complication of systemic lupus erythematosus. Up to 50% of patients have evidence of renal disease at the time of diagnosis. Renal damage is a result of circulating immune complex deposition which leads to activation of the complement cascade, leukocyte infiltration, and release of cytokines. The clinical signs are as described with nephrotic range proteinuria, hematuria, hypertension, and some degree of renal insufficiency. Red cell casts on the urinalysis are common. Hypocomplementemia is common in acute disease. Renal biopsy is the most reliable way of identifying the condition and the severity is classified from class I (minimal mesangial) to class VI (sclerotic nephritis). Other kidney diseases with low complement levels include post-infectious glomerulonephritis, membranoproliferative glomerulonephritis, mixed cryoglobulinemia, serum sickness, atheroembolic renal disease, hemolytic uremic syndrome, and thrombotic thrombocytopenic purpura.

Microscopic polyangiitis causes renal and pulmonary inflammation. It should be distinguished from polyarteritis nodosa, which rarely affects the lungs. Churg-Strauss syndrome is a vasculitic illness that usually occurs in patients with poorly controlled asthma; eosinophilia and pulmonary involvement are prominent. Cryoglobulinemia causes renal disease and a small vessel cutaneous vasculitis. Seventy percent of cases occur in the setting of active hepatitis C.

Suggested Readings

1. Kasper DL, Fauci AS, Hauser SL, Longo DL, Jameson LJ, Loscalzo J. *Harrison's Principles of Internal Medicine*. 19th ed. New York: McGraw-Hill; 2015. Chapters 61, 63, 66, 334, 335, 338.

2. McKean SC, Ross JJ, Dressler DD, Brotman DJ, Ginsberg JS. *Principles and Practice of Hospital Medicine*. New York: McGraw-Hill; 2012. Section 17: Renal (Chapters 245-253).

3. Stern S, Cifu AS, Altkorn D. *Symptom to Diagnosis: An Evidence-Based Guide*. 2nd ed. New York: McGraw-Hill; 2010. Chapters 4, 21, 28.

4. Lerma EV, Berns JS, Nissenson AR. *Current Diagnosis & Treatment: Nephrology & Hypertension*. New York: McGraw-Hill; 2009.

5. Clinical Practice Guidelines in Nephrology, available at: http://www.kdigo.org/clinical_practice_guidelines/pdf/KDIGO%20AKI%20Guideline.pdf

6. Chawla LS, Eggers PW, Star RA, Kimmel PL. Acute kidney injury and chronic kidney disease as interconnected syndromes (review). *N Engl J Med*. 2014;371:58-66.

7. Roumelioti ME, Unruh M. Update in nephrology. *Ann Intern Med*. 2014;161:54-57.

Hematology and Oncology

Questions

300. A 55-year-old man is being evaluated for constipation. There is no history of prior gastrectomy or of upper GI symptoms. Hemoglobin is 10 g/dL, mean corpuscular volume (MCV) is 72 fL, serum iron is 4 µg/dL (normal 50-150 µg/dL), iron-binding capacity is 450 µg/dL (normal 250-370 µg/dL), saturation is 1% (normal 20%-45%), and ferritin is 10 µg/L (normal 15-400 µg/L). Which of the following is the best next step in the evaluation of this patient's anemia?

a. Red blood cell folate
b. Serum lead level
c. Colonoscopy
d. Bone marrow examination
e. Hemoglobin electrophoresis with A2 and F levels

301. A 50-year-old woman complains of pain and swelling in her proximal interphalangeal joints, both wrists, and both knees. She complains of morning stiffness. She had a hysterectomy 10 years ago. Physical examination shows swelling and synovial thickening of the proximal interphalangeal (PIP) joints. Hemoglobin is 10.3 g/dL, MCV is 80 fL, serum iron is 28 µg/dL, iron-binding capacity is 200 µg/dL (normal 250-370 µg/dL), and saturation is 14%. Which of the following is the most likely explanation for this woman's anemia?

a. Occult blood loss
b. Vitamin deficiency
c. Anemia of chronic disease
d. Sideroblastic anemia
e. Occult renal disease

302. A 35-year-old woman presents with several days of increasing fatigue and shortness of breath on exertion. She was recently diagnosed with *Mycoplasma pneumoniae*. Physical examination reveals BP 113/67, HR 114 beats/min, and respiratory rate 20 breaths/min. She appears icteric and in mild respiratory distress. Her hemoglobin is 9.0 g/dL and MCV is 110. Which of the following is the best next diagnostic test?

a. Serum protein electrophoresis
b. Flow cytometry
c. Peripheral blood smear
d. Glucose-6-PD level
e. Bone marrow biopsy

303. A 26-year-old woman is evaluated in the ER for diffuse abdominal pain and nausea. The pain started 1 day ago and is currently at its maximum intensity. She denies fever but has noticed constipation and dark urine. She had similar episodes in the past and underwent appendectomy and cho-lecystectomy on two different occasions. On physical examination, she is tachycardic with diffuse abdominal tenderness but no rebound tenderness. Her bowel sounds are slightly sluggish. On neurological examination, she has decreased sensation to fine and crude touch in both lower extremities up to her knees. Her hemoglobin, WBC, and platelet count are normal. She has mild transaminitis with alanine transaminase (ALT) 123 IU/L, aspartate transaminase (AST) 160 IU/L, and alkaline phosphatase (ALP) 122 IU/L. Urine is red but urine dipstick is negative for blood, leukocyte esterase, nitrite, glucose, or protein. Urine porphobilinogen and total porphyrin level are elevated, plasma porphyrin level is normal. What is the most likely explanation of her recurrent symptoms?

a. Variegate porphyria
b. Thalassemia
c. Acute intermittent porphyria
d. Porphyria cutanea tarda
e. Autoimmune hepatitis

304. A 64-year-old man complains of cough, increasing shortness of breath, and headache for the past 3 weeks. He has mild hypertension for which he takes hydrochlorothiazide; he has smoked 1 pack of cigarettes a day for 40 years. On examination you notice facial plethora and jugular venous distension to the angle of the jaw. He has prominent veins over the anterior chest and a firm to hard right supraclavicular lymph node. Cardiac examination is normal and lungs are without rales. Peripheral edema is absent. What is the most likely cause of his condition?

a. Long-standing hypertension
b. Gastric carcinoma
c. Emphysema
d. Lung cancer
e. Nephrotic syndrome

305. A 38-year-old woman presents with a 3-day history of fever and confusion. She was previously healthy and is taking no medications. She has not had diarrhea or rectal bleeding. She has a temperature of 38°C (100.4°F) and a blood pressure of 145/85. Splenomegaly is absent. She has no petechiae but does have evidence of early digital gangrene of the right second finger. Except for confusion the neurological examination is normal. Her laboratory studies reveal the following:

Hemoglobin: 8.7 g/dL
Platelet count: 25,000/µL
Peripheral smear: numerous fragmented RBCs, few platelets
LDH: 562 IU/L (normal <180)
Creatinine: 2.7 mg/dL
Liver enzymes: normal
Prothrombin time/PTT/fibrinogen levels: normal

What is the most likely pathogenesis of her condition?

a. Disseminated intravascular coagulation
b. Antiplatelet antibodies
c. Failure to cleave von Willebrand factor multimers
d. Shiga toxin-induced endothelial damage
e. Cirrhosis with sequestration of erythrocytes and platelets in the spleen

306. A 60-year-old man develops numbness of the feet. On physical examination he has lost proprioception in the lower extremities and is noticed to have a wide based gait with a positive Romberg sign. His medical history includes hypertension, hypothyroidism, and previous gastrectomy for gastric cancer. The peripheral blood smear is shown in the following figure. What is the most likely cause of his symptoms?

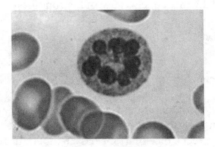

Reproduced, with permission, from Lichtman MA, Shafer JA, Felgar RE, et al. *Lichtman's Atlas of Hematology*. New York, NY: McGraw-Hill Education, 2007. www.accessmedicine. com. Figure II.C.23.

a. Folic acid deficiency
b. Vitamin B_{12} deficiency
c. Vitamin K deficiency
d. Iron deficiency
e. Thiamine deficiency

307. A 60-year-old man presents with vague left upper quadrant abdominal fullness. He also has fatigue, malaise, and weight loss. Physical examination reveals splenomegaly but no peripheral lymphadenopathy. CBC shows

Hb: 12 g/dL (normal 14-18)
Leukocytes: 40,000/µL (normal 4300-10,800) with increased basophils and myelocytes but no blast forms
Platelet count: 500,000/µL (normal 150,000-400,000)
Bone marrow biopsy shows hypercellular marrow. Chromosomal study is shown in the figure below.

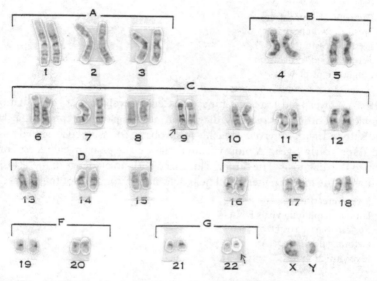

Reproduced, with permission, from Kantarjian HM, Wolff RA, Koller CA. *MD Anderson Manual of Medical Oncology.* New York, NY: McGraw-Hill Education, 2006. Figure 4-1.

Which of the following is the most likely diagnosis?

a. Acute myeloid leukemia
b. Chronic myeloid leukemia
c. Chronic lymphocytic leukemia
d. Acute lymphocytic leukemia
e. Myelodysplastic syndrome

308. A 25-year-old woman complains of persistent bleeding for 5 days after a dental extraction. She has noticed easy bruisability since childhood, and was given a blood transfusion at age 17 because of prolonged bleeding after an apparently minor cut. She denies ecchymoses or bleeding into joints. Her father has noticed similar symptoms but has not sought medical care. Physical examination is normal except for mild oozing from the dental site. She does not have splenomegaly or enlarged lymph nodes. Her CBC is normal, with a platelet count of 230,000. Her prothrombin time is normal, but the partial thromboplastin time is mildly prolonged. The bleeding time is 12 minutes (normal 3-9 minutes). What is most appropriate way to control her bleeding?

a. Factor VIII concentrate
b. Fresh frozen plasma
c. Desmopressin (DDAVP)
d. Whole blood transfusion
e. Single donor platelets

309. A 42-year-old man of Chinese descent is evaluated at the radiation oncologist's office for recently diagnosed nasopharyngeal carcinoma. He had suffered symptoms of headache, nasal obstruction, and occasional nose bleed for nearly 1 year. A biopsy from a mass at the pharyngeal recess confirmed the diagnosis. The tumor is localized with no evidence of metastasis. Which of the following tests will help determine prognosis of the disease?

a. Serum creatinine
b. Human papilloma virus DNA
c. Epstein-Barr virus DNA
d. Cytomegalovirus DNA
e. Liver function tests

310. A 38-year-old woman presents with repeated episodes of sore throat. She is on no medications, does not use ethanol, and has no history of renal disease. Physical examination is normal. Hb is 9.0 g/dL, MCV is 85 fL (normal), white blood cell count is 2000/μL, and platelet count is 30,000/μL. Which of the following is the best approach to diagnosis?

a. Erythropoietin level
b. Serum B_{12}
c. Bone marrow biopsy
d. Liver spleen scan
e. Therapeutic trial of corticosteroids

311. A 31-year-old woman is evaluated by her primary care physician for an annual health checkup. During her visit, she expresses concern regarding her risk of ovarian cancer, as one of her close friends was recently diagnosed with advanced ovarian cancer. She works as a software engineer in an IT firm, smokes 6 to 8 cigarettes per day, and has no family history of ovarian, breast, or colon cancer. She appears healthy, and her physical examination is unremarkable. What is the best screening option for the patient?

a. CA-125
b. Transvaginal pelvic ultrasonography
c. *BRCA-1* and *BRCA-2* mutation analysis
d. Pelvic CT scan
e. No screening is required

312. A 52-year-old man with cirrhosis resulting from chronic hepatitis C presents with increasing right upper quadrant pain, anorexia, and 15-lb weight loss. The patient is mildly icteric and has moderate ascites. A friction rub is heard over the liver. Abdominal paracentesis reveals blood-tinged fluid, and CT scan shows a 4-cm solid mass in the right lobe of the liver. Which of the following is the most important initial diagnostic study?

a. Serum α-fetoprotein level
b. Colonoscopy to search for a primary neoplasm
c. Measurement of hepatitis C viral RNA
d. Upper GI endoscopy
e. Positron emission tomography (PET) scan

313. A 60-year-old man presents with dull aching pain in the right flank. Physical examination reveals a firm mass that does not move with inspiration. Laboratory studies show normal BUN, creatinine, and electrolytes. Urinalysis (UA) shows hematuria. Hemoglobin is elevated at 18 g/dL and serum calcium is 11 mg/dL. What is the most likely diagnosis?

a. Polycystic kidney disease
b. Pheochromocytoma
c. Adrenal carcinoma
d. Renal adenomyolipoma
e. Renal cell carcinoma

314. A 64-year-old woman who is receiving chemotherapy for metastatic breast cancer has been treating midthoracic pain with acetaminophen. Over the past few days she has become weak and unsteady on her feet. On the day of admission she develops urinary incontinence. Physical examination reveals fist percussion tenderness over T8 and moderate symmetric muscle weakness in the legs. Anal sphincter tone is reduced. Which of the following diagnostic studies is most important to order?

a. Serum calcium
b. Bone scan
c. Plain radiographs of the thoracic spine
d. MRI scan of the spine
e. Electromyogram with nerve conduction studies

315. A 20-year-old man finds an asymptomatic mass in his scrotum. He denies fever, dysuria, or hematospermia. Which of the following is the most appropriate first step in evaluating this mass?

a. Palpation and transillumination
b. HCG and α-fetoprotein
c. Scrotal ultrasonography
d. Evaluation for inguinal adenopathy
e. Referral for inguinal orchiectomy

316. A 65-year-old man presents with painless hematuria. He has a 45-year history of tobacco use. He denies fever, chills, and dysuria. General physical examination is unremarkable. On rectal examination, the prostate is small, nonnodular, and nontender. A urinalysis shows 100 red blood cells per high-power field. No white cells or protein are present. Three months ago, the patient had an abdominal ultrasound for right upper quadrant pain; on review, both kidneys were normal. Which of the following is the most useful diagnostic test at this time?

a. Urine culture and sensitivity
b. Prostate-specific antigen (PSA)
c. Bladder scan
d. Cystoscopy and retrograde pyelography
e. CT scan of the kidneys

317. A 43-year-old woman complains of fatigue and night sweats associated with itching for 2 months. On physical examination, there is diffuse nontender lymphadenopathy, including small supraclavicular, epitrochlear, and scalene nodes. CBC and chemistry studies (including liver enzymes) are normal. Chest x-ray shows hilar lymphadenopathy. Which of the following is the best next step in evaluation?

a. Excisional lymph node biopsy
b. Monospot test
c. Toxoplasmosis IgG serology
d. Serum angiotensin-converting enzyme level
e. Percutaneous aspiration biopsy of the largest lymph node

318. A 19-year-old woman presents for evaluation of a nontender left axillary lymph node. She is asymptomatic and denies weight loss or night sweats. Examination reveals three rubbery firm nontender nodes in the axilla, the largest 3 cm in diameter. No other lymphadenopathy is noted; the spleen is not enlarged. Lymph node biopsy, however, reveals mixed-cellularity Hodgkin lymphoma. Liver function tests are normal. Which of the following is the best next step in evaluation?

a. Bone marrow biopsy
b. Liver biopsy
c. Staging laparotomy
d. Erythrocyte sedimentation rate (ESR)
e. CT scan of chest, abdomen, and pelvis

319. A 69-year-old African-American man presents with weight loss and back pain. Over the past 2 months he has developed hyperglycemia with a fasting glucose of 153 mg/dL. He does not have nocturia. His appetite is decreased, and he has noticed mild constipation. The back pain is constant and keeps him awake at night. On examination he appears cachectic and pale. He does not have scleral icterus. Laboratory studies reveal a mild normochromic anemia. Liver and kidney function studies are normal. What diagnostic study is most likely to reveal the cause of his symptoms?

a. CT scan of the abdomen with IV contrast
b. Glucose tolerance test
c. Colonoscopy
d. Stool studies for malabsorption
e. Whole body PET scan

320. A 75-year-old man with a history of adenocarcinoma of the prostate treated with radical prostatectomy presents with pain in the left hip. The pain awakens him at night and has become increasingly severe over the past 3 weeks. Plain radiographs show numerous bilateral osteoblastic lesions in the hip and sacrum, and the prostate-specific antigen level is 83 µg/mL (normal 0-4). Which of the following is the treatment of choice?

a. Observation
b. Radiation therapy
c. Estrogen therapy
d. Gonadotropin-releasing hormone (GnRH) analogue
e. Chemotherapy

321. A 73-year-old woman is admitted for deep venous thrombosis and concern for pulmonary embolism. She has a history of type 2 diabetes mellitus, hypertension, and coronary artery disease. She had been admitted for a three-vessel coronary artery bypass graft (CABG) 2 weeks prior to this admission. She did well and was dismissed 5 days after the procedure. Pain and swelling of the right leg began 2 days before the present admission; she has noticed mild dyspnea but no chest pain. The clinical suspicion of deep vein thrombosis (DVT) is confirmed by a venous Doppler, and the patient is started on unfractionated heparin. Her initial laboratory studies, including CBC, are normal.

The next day her pain has improved, and helical CT scan of the chest reveals no evidence of pulmonary embolism. She is instructed in the use of low-molecular-weight heparin (LMWH) and warfarin; she is eager to go home. Her serum creatinine is normal. Her predischarge CBC shows no anemia, but the platelet count has dropped to 74,000. An assay for antibodies to heparin-platelet factor 4 complexes is ordered. What is the best next step in her management?

a. Dismiss the patient on low-molecular heparin, warfarin, and close outpatient follow-up.
b. Obtain a liver-spleen scan to look for platelet sequestration.
c. Discontinue all forms of heparin, continue warfarin, and add aspirin 162 mg daily until INR becomes therapeutic.
d. Keep the patient in the hospital, discontinue unfractionated heparin, add low-molecular-weight heparin, and monitor the platelet count daily.
e. Keep the patient in the hospital, discontinue all forms of heparin, and start the patient on lepirudin by intravenous infusion.

322. A 26-year-old healthy man comes to your clinic for an annual wellness examination. He does not take any medications. He smokes half pack of cigarettes daily. He tells you that his father died of colon cancer at the age of 45. He also has a 25-year-old cousin who recently had colonoscopy for rectal bleeding was found to have multiple polyps and is scheduled for total colectomy. Your patient wants to know if he can inherit colon cancer and if there is a way to find out if he is at risk. You talk to him about how some cancers can be caused by genetic mutations. For what genetic mutation is this patient at highest risk?

a. *MEN1*
b. *RET*
c. *APC*
d. *MSH*
e. *BRCA*

323. A patient with bacterial endocarditis develops thrombophlebitis while hospitalized. His course in the hospital is uncomplicated. On discharge he is treated with penicillin, rifampin, and warfarin. Therapeutic prothrombin levels are obtained on 15 mg/d of warfarin. After 2 weeks, the penicillin and rifampin are discontinued. Which of the following is the best next step in management of this patient?

a. Cautiously increase warfarin dosage
b. Continue warfarin at 15 mg/d for about 6 months
c. Reduce warfarin dosage
d. Stop warfarin therapy
e. Restrict dietary vitamin K

324. A 65-year-old man with diabetes mellitus, bronzed skin, and cirrhosis of the liver is being treated for hemochromatosis previously confirmed by liver biopsy. The patient experiences increasing right upper quadrant pain, and his serum alkaline phosphatase is now elevated. There is a 15-lb weight loss. Which of the following is the best next step in management?

a. Increase frequency of phlebotomy for worsening hemochromatosis
b. Obtain α-fetoprotein level and CT scan to rule out hepatocellular carcinoma
c. Obtain hepatitis B serology
d. Obtain antimitochondrial antibody to rule out primary biliary cirrhosis
e. Check a serum ferritin level

325. A 66-year-old postmenopausal woman presents with a painless breast mass and is found to have a 3-cm infiltrating ductal breast cancer. Sentinel node sampling reveals metastatic cancer in the sentinel node; a formal axillary node dissection shows that 4 of 13 nodes are involved by the malignant process. Both estrogen and progesterone receptor are expressed in the tumor. There is no evidence of metastatic disease outside the axilla. In addition to lumpectomy and radiation therapy to the breast and axilla, what should her treatment include next?

a. No further treatment at this time
b. Radiation therapy to the internal mammary nodes
c. Platinum-based adjuvant chemotherapy
d. Bilateral oophorectomy
e. Adjuvant hormonal therapy (aromatase inhibitor or tamoxifen)

326. A 68-year-old man is evaluated in ER for generalized weakness. He also has shortness of breath and cough with productive sputum for 6 days. Two months ago, he had been treated with levofloxacin for community-acquired pneumonia. He works as a volunteer in a local church. He does not have a history of excessive alcohol consumption or recreational drug use. On physical examination, his blood pressure is 132/87 mm of Hg, pulse 107/min, temperature 38°C (100°F), and respiratory rate 22/min. He looks pale and has mild crackles in right base. No lymphadenopathy or hepatosplenomegaly is appreciated. Neurological examination is normal. Laboratory results reveal: hemoglobin 8.6 gm/dL, hematocrit 28, MCV 106 fL, leukocyte count 3600/μL, platelet count 71,000/μL, ferritin 68 ng/mL, iron 156 μg/dL, transferrin saturation 48%, aPTT 32s, INR 1.1, total protein 6.2 g/dL, albumin 3.8 g/dL, LDH 128 u/L (normal), and total bilirubin 1.5 mg/dL. Peripheral blood film examination reveals evidence of dysplasia in the red and white blood cell series. A chest x-ray reveals right basilar infiltrate; a CT scan of the abdomen is negative for any significant visceral abnormality. What is the next best step to diagnose the hematological abnormality?

a. Liver biopsy
b. Bone marrow biopsy
c. Hemoglobin electrophoresis
d. *JAK2* mutation analysis
e. Methylmalonic acid measurement

327. A 47-year-old woman complains of fatigue, weight loss, and itching after taking a hot shower. Physical examination shows plethoric facies and an enlarged spleen, which descends 6 cm below the left costal margin. Her white cell count is 17,000 with a normal differential, the platelet count is 560,000, and hemoglobin is 18.7. Liver enzymes and electrolytes are normal; the serum uric acid level is mildly elevated. What is the most likely underlying process?

a. Myelodysplastic syndrome
b. Myeloproliferative syndrome
c. Paraneoplastic syndrome
d. Cushing syndrome
e. Gaisböck syndrome

328. A 20-year-old black man presents to the emergency room complaining of diffuse bone pain and requesting narcotics for his sickle cell crisis. Which of the following physical examination features would suggest an alternative diagnosis to sickle cell anemia (hemoglobin SS)?

a. Scleral icterus
b. Systolic murmur
c. Splenomegaly
d. Ankle ulcers
e. Leukocytosis

329. A 30-year-old black man plans a trip to India and is advised to take prophylaxis for malaria. Three days after beginning treatment, he develops pallor, fatigue, and jaundice. Hematocrit is 30% (it had been 43%) and reticulocyte count is 7%. He stops taking the medication. The next step in treatment should consist of which of the following?

a. Splenectomy
b. Administration of methylene blue
c. Administration of vitamin E
d. Exchange transfusions
e. No additional treatment is required

330. A 26-year-old man complains of heaviness in the left testicle. There has been no recent trauma. Physical examination reveals a 3-cm painless firm mass that clearly arises from the testicle. The physical examination is otherwise unremarkable. Abdominal CT scan shows matted periaortic lymphadenopathy, with the largest node approximately 3.5 cm in size. CT of the chest shows no abnormalities. In addition to urological referral, what should be the next diagnostic study?

a. Needle aspiration biopsy of the retroperitoneal mass
b. Needle aspiration of the testicular mass
c. Measurement of α-fetoprotein, β-hCG, and lactate dehydrogenase (LDH)
d. Positron emission tomography (PET) scan
e. Measurement of carcinoembryonic antigen (CEA) and α-fetoprotein

331. A 50-year-old man presents with 3 days of fever, diffuse bone pain, and extreme weakness. He denies any sick contacts. On examination, there is conjunctival pallor, dried blood on the nasal mucosa, and petechiae on both lower extremities. There is no lymphadenopathy or hepatosplenomegaly. CBC shows hemoglobin 7.9 g/dL, leukocyte count 23,600, and platelet count 14,000. Urinalysis and chest x-ray are normal. The peripheral blood smear is shown in the following figure. What is the most likely diagnosis?

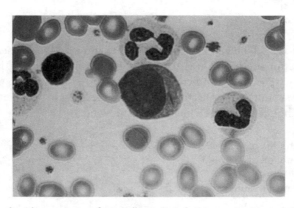

Reproduced, with permission, from Hillman R, Ault K, Leporrier M, et al. *Hematology in Clinical Practice.* 5th ed. New York, NY: McGraw-Hill Education, 2010. Figure 18-2B.

a. Multiple myeloma
b. Myelofibrosis
c. Acute myeloid leukemia (AML)
d. Chronic myeloid leukemia (CML)
e. Acute lymphocytic leukemia (ALL)

332. A 70-year-old intensive care unit patient complains of fever and shaking chills. The patient develops hypotension, and blood cultures are positive for gram-negative bacilli. The patient begins bleeding from venipuncture sites and around his Foley catheter. Laboratory studies are as follows:

Hct: 38%
WBC: 15,000/μL
Platelet count: 40,000/μL (normal 150,000-400,000)
Peripheral blood smear: fragmented RBCs
PT: elevated
PTT: elevated
Plasma fibrinogen: 70 mg/dL (normal 200-400)

Which of the following is the best course of therapy in this patient?

a. Begin heparin
b. Treat underlying disease
c. Begin plasmapheresis
d. Give vitamin K
e. Begin red blood cell transfusion

333. A 30-year-old woman with Graves disease has been started on pro-pylthiouracil. She complains of low-grade fever, chills, and sore throat. Which of the following is the most important initial step in evaluating this patient's fever?

a. Serum TSH
b. Serum T_3 by RIA
c. CBC with differential
d. Chest x-ray
e. Blood cultures

334. A 62-year-old woman has noted fever to 38.3°C (101°F) every evening for the past 3 weeks, associated with night sweats and a 15-lb weight loss. Physical examination reveals matted supraclavicular lymph nodes on the right; the largest node is 3.5 cm in diameter. She also has firm rubbery right axillary and bilateral inguinal nodes. Excisional biopsy of one of the nodes shows diffuse replacement of the nodal architecture with large neoplastic cells which stain positively for B-cell markers. No Reed-Sternberg cells are seen. Which statement most accurately reflects her prognosis?

a.   This is an indolent process which will respond to corticosteroids.
b.   This is an aggressive neoplasm which responds poorly to chemotherapy and will likely be fatal in 6 months or less.
c.   This is an aggressive neoplasm, but it may be cured with chemotherapy in up to 60% of the cases.
d.   The neoplasm often responds to chemotherapy but almost always relapses.
e.   Radiation therapy is curative.

335. A 37-year-old woman presents for evaluation of a self-discovered breast mass. There is no family history of breast cancer; she is otherwise healthy. Examination reveals a 1.5-cm area of firmness in the right upper outer quadrant. No skin changes or axillary lymphadenopathy are noted. Ultrasonography reveals a solid lesion; a mammogram is ordered and is normal. Which of the following is the most appropriate next step in management?

a.   Refer the patient for further evaluation to a surgeon or comprehensive breast radiologist.
b.   Reevaluate the patient in 6 months.
c.   Give oral contraceptives to decrease ovulation and help shrink the lesion.
d.   Recommend tamoxifen to decrease her chance of developing cancer.
e.   Reassure the patient.

336. A 60-year-old woman develops deep venous thrombosis after a 14-hour plane flight from New Zealand. The diagnosis is confirmed by a venous Doppler. There is no evidence of pulmonary embolism, and she is started on subcutaneous low-molecular-weight heparin. She has no family history of venous thrombosis, and she is on no medications that would increase her risk of clotting. In addition to routine monitoring of coagulation parameters and a CBC, what diagnostic tests should be ordered next?

a.   Functional test for factor V Leiden (activated protein C resistance)
b.   Protein C, protein S, and antithrombin III levels
c.   Antiphospholipid antibody test
d.   Genetic testing for prothrombin *G20210A* gene mutation
e.   No further testing

Questions 337 to 339

Match the most appropriate answer for each following question. Each lettered option may be used once, more than once, or not at all.

a. Rivaroxaban
b. Low-molecular-weight heparin
c. Warfarin
d. Low dose aspirin (81 mg/d)
e. Inferior vena cava filter placement
f. Antithrombin III level
g. Factor V Leiden gene mutation analysis

337. A 62-year-old man is evaluated in the ER for sudden onset of swelling of the right calf with pain for past 2 days. The patient noticed the swelling after he woke up from sleep and had pain while walking. He cannot recollect any history of trauma, denies any recent travel, and has never had a blood clot in the past His medical history is remarkable for hypertension, adequately controlled with lisinopril, and stage-III squamous cell carcinoma of the lung for which he recently completed six cycles of chemotherapy. On physical examination, there is tender swelling of the right calf without erythema. His D-dimer is 640 ng/mL. Venous Doppler of the right leg reveals occlusive thrombi in the deep veins. A plan is made to initiate anticoagulation and to extend the treatment for 6 months.

What will be the drug of choice for anticoagulation for this patient?

338. A 27-year-old woman is evaluated in the ER for sudden onset shortness of breath for 3 hours. The patient mentions that she was sleeping last night peacefully and woke up with breathing difficulty. She denies fever, chills, cough, nausea, vomiting, chest trauma, or any other unusual symptoms prior to the onset of her dyspnea. There is no history of recent travel or prolonged immobility. She does not smoke, drink alcohol, or use recreational drugs. She is not on oral contraceptive pills. She mentions, however, that 2 years ago she had an episode of deep vein thrombosis in her right leg for which she was on Coumadin (warfarin) for 3 months. Her mother was diagnosed with unprovoked DVT twice in her lifetime.

Her blood pressure is 142/88 mm Hg, pulse 112/min, temperature 36.6°C (98°F), respiratory rate 22/min, and oxygen saturation 91% on room air. Her lungs are clear, and the rest of the physical examination is normal. CT angiogram of the chest reveals right-sided pulmonary embolism. She is started on weight-based low-molecular-weight heparin therapy.

Which additional test(s) should be ordered to detect an underlying hypercoagulable disorder?

339. A 56-year-old man is evaluated for recent onset painful skin lesion which involves his abdominal wall. The lesion started 3 days ago as a small erythematous macule which has gradually increased in size to a large purpuric lesion with bulla formation. He is afebrile and does not recall any trauma. His medical history is significant for atrial fibrillation; he was recently switched from rivaroxaban to warfarin due to the high cost of rivaroxaban.

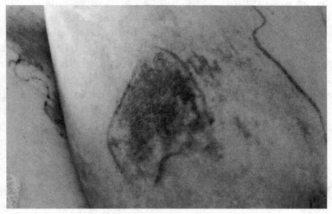

Reproduced, with permission, from Lichtman MA, Kipps TJ, Seligsohn U, et al. *Williams Hematology.* 8th ed. New York: McGraw-Hill Education, 2010. Figure 123-6.

What is the most probable cause of the condition?

Questions 340 to 342

Match the most appropriate answer for each following question. Each lettered option may be used once, more than once, or not at all.

a. Multiple myeloma
b. Smoldering multiple myeloma
c. Monoclonal gammopathy of undetermined significance
d. Waldenström macroglobulinemia
e. Nonsecretory myeloma

340. A 70-year-old man complains of 2 months of low back pain and fatigue. He has developed fever with purulent sputum production. On physical examination, he has pain over several vertebrae and rales at the left base. Laboratory results are as follows:

Hemoglobin: 7 g/dL
MCV: 89 fL (normal 86-98)
Leukocyte count: 12,000/mL
BUN: 44 mg/dL
Creatinine: 3.2 mg/dL
Ca: 11.5 mg/dL

Chest x-ray indicates left lower lobe infiltrate. A peripheral smear is shown in the following figure.

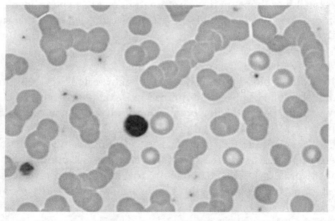

Reproduced, with permission, from Longo DL, Fauci AS, Kasper DL, et al. *Harrison's Principles of Internal Medicine*. 18th ed. New York: McGraw-Hill Education, 2012. Figure e17-9.

341. A 64-year-old man is evaluated in the ER for generalized fatigue, headache, and blurring of vision for 3 months. The patient mentions that he occasionally has vertigo and dizziness which are not associated with any change in posture. He has no history of vomiting or diarrhea. He recently has noticed occasional gum bleeding and dried blood in his nose. His medical history is only significant for asthma which is well controlled. On physical examination, cranial nerves are intact but there is decreased sensation to both fine and crude touch on both lower extremities extending up to his knees. Funduscopic examination shows dilated tortuous retinal veins with some hemorrhages. Liver and spleen are enlarged, and there is mild peripheral lymphadenopathy. The lab work up reveals hemoglobin 7.6 gm/dL, hematocrit 25, leukocyte count 4500/μL, and platelet 149,000/μL. Total protein 8.2 g/dL, albumin 3.4 g/dL, BUN 16 mg/dL, and creatinine 0.75 mg/dL. Serum protein electrophoresis reveals a sharp, narrow spike of monoclonal IgM; bone marrow examination reveals hypercellular marrow with more than 10% lymphoid and plasmacytoid cells. A skeletal survey is negative for lytic lesions.

342. A 71-year-old man is evaluated in the ER for a recent finding of high ESR in a routine blood test. He has history of hypertension, well controlled with metoprolol. His physical examination is completely normal. His laboratory workup reveals hemoglobin 12.6 gm/dL, leukocyte count 8500/μL, and platelet 265,000/μL. Total protein 6.2 g/dL, albumin 3.4 g/dL, BUN 16 mg/dL, creatinine 0.75 mg/dL, and calcium 9.2 mg/dL. Serum protein electrophoresis reveals a sharp, narrow spike, serum immunofixation reveals M-protein 1.2 gm/dL, bone marrow examination reveals less than 10% of monoclonal plasma cells. A skeletal survey is negative for any lytic lesions.

Questions 343 and 344

Match the most appropriate answer for each of the following question. Each lettered option may be used once, more than once, or not at all.

a. Trousseau syndrome
b. Sézary syndrome
c. Syndrome of inappropriate antidiuretic hormone
d. Tumor lysis syndrome
e. Lambert-Eaton myasthenic syndrome
f. Opsoclonus-myoclonus

343. A 62-year-old man is evaluated in the ER for drowsiness and generalized weakness for the past 4 weeks. He is brought to the hospital by EMS after he experienced a tonic clonic seizure in a local restaurant. His medical history is positive for HTN and gout, for which he takes metoprolol and allopurinol. He has smoked 1 pack per day for nearly 40 years, with no alcohol or recreational drug abuse. He noticed nearly 20 lb weight loss in past 2 months. Physical examination is normal. Laboratory tests reveal hemoglobin 10.2 gm/dL, leukocyte count 9500/μL, and platelet 171,000/μl. Serum sodium is 122 mEq/L, potassium 3.8 mEq/L, blood urea nitrogen (BUN) 26 mg/dL, and creatinine 0.9 mg/dL. Additional laboratory findings include serum osmolality 258 mOsm/kg, urine osmolality 300 mOsm/kg, and urine sodium 48 mmol/L. TSH and cortisol levels are normal.

344. A 66-year-old man is evaluated in the ER for nausea, vomiting, poor appetite, lethargy, and muscle cramps for past 2 days. He has vomited six times in past 2 days without any blood. He denies fever. His medical history is significant for non-Hodgkin lymphoma diagnosed 3 months ago; he recently completed the fourth cycle of chemotherapy. On physical examination, he appears quite ill and dehydrated. Laboratory studies reveal serum sodium 132 mEq/L, potassium 6.4 mEq/L, bicarbonate 17 mEq/L, uric acid 13.2 mg/dL, phosphorus 6.8 mg/dL, and calcium 6.8 mg/dL.

Questions 345 to 347

Match the most appropriate answer for each following question. Each lettered option may be used once, more than once, or not at all.

a. Acute lymphoblastic leukemia
b. Immune thrombocytopenic purpura
c. Leukemoid reaction
d. Chronic lymphocytic leukemia
e. Hemophilia
f. Thrombotic thrombocytopenic purpura

345. A 69-year-old man is evaluated in the ER for new appearance of a knot on the left side of his neck. The patient also mentions generalized weakness, malaise, and poor appetite for past six weeks. He is afebrile. Physical examination reveals nontender generalized lymphadenopathy with the largest node in the left cervical chain measuring 3.5 cm. There is mild hepatosplenomegaly. Initial laboratory data show hemoglobin 12.8 gm/dL, hematocrit 38, MCV 86 fL, leukocyte count 55,000/μL, and platelet 221,000/μL. A peripheral smear examination reveals small, mature appearing lymphocytes with a dense nucleus. Bone marrow examination reveals hypercellular marrow with monotonous infiltration of marrow with small rounded lymphocytes. What is the most probable diagnosis?

346. A 28-year-old man is evaluated in the primary care office for new onset rash on both legs for 1 week. He is a healthy person with no past medical illness, and is not taking any medications. There is no history of recent fever but he has noticed occasional gum bleeding and one episode of nose bleed 4 days ago. He does not smoke, drinks alcohol only socially, and does not use any recreational drug. On physical examination, he is a healthy appearing man with no lymphadenopathy or hepatosplenomegaly. Laboratory studies reveal hemoglobin 14.8 gm/dL, hematocrit 42, MCV 86 fL, leukocyte count 6,000/μL, and platelet 22,000/μL. Liver function and renal function studies are normal. Peripheral smear reveals decrease in platelet count and no red cell abnormalities. What is the most probable diagnosis?

347. A 21-year-old man is evaluated in a family physician's office for swelling of the left knee joint. He recently emigrated from Africa. His medical history is negative, and family history cannot be obtained since he was adopted in childhood. Upon questioning, he mentions that he occasionally has bruises after minor trauma and had a similar left knee swelling 2 years ago. Currently he does not have any fever. On examination, he is healthy looking man without any distress. The left knee is swollen, hot, and tender to palpation with restricted active and passive movements. Initial blood workup shows hemoglobin 12.8 gm/dL, leukocyte count 9000/μL, and platelet 322,000/μL; bleeding time (BT) is normal, prothrombin time (PT) is normal, but activated partial thromboplastic time (aPTT) is prolonged. What is the most probable diagnosis?

Hematology and Oncology

Answers

300. The answer is c. The patient has a microcytic anemia. A low serum iron, low ferritin, and high iron-binding capacity are diagnostic of iron-deficiency anemia. Most iron-deficiency anemia is explained by blood loss. The patient's symptoms of constipation point to blood loss from the lower GI tract. Colonoscopy would be the highest-yield procedure. Barium enema misses 50% of polyps and a significant minority of colon cancers. Even patients without GI symptoms who have no obvious explanation (such as menstrual blood loss or multiple prior pregnancies in women) for their iron deficiency should be worked up for GI blood loss. Folate deficiency presents as a megaloblastic anemia with macrocytosis (large, oval-shaped red cells) and hypersegmentation of the polymorphonuclear leukocytes. Lead poisoning can cause a microcytic hypochromic anemia, but this would not be associated with the abnormal iron studies and low ferritin seen in this patient. Basophilic stippling or target cells seen on the peripheral blood smear would be important clues to the presence of lead poisoning. Although a bone marrow examination will prove the diagnosis by the absence of stainable iron in the marrow, the diagnosis of iron deficiency is clear from the serum studies. Thalassemia (diagnosed by hemoglobin electrophoresis) is not associated with abnormal iron studies. The most important issue is now to find the source of the iron loss.

301. The answer is c. Patients with chronic inflammatory or neoplastic disease often develop anemia of chronic disease. Cytokines produced by inflammation cause a block in the normal recirculation of iron from reticuloendothelial cells (which pick up the iron from senescent red blood cells) to the red cell precursors (normoblasts). The peptide hepcidin is felt to be the main mediator of the effect. This defect in iron reutilization causes a drop in the serum iron concentration and a normocytic or mildly microcytic anemia. The inflammatory reaction, however, also decreases the iron-binding capacity (as opposed to iron-deficiency anemia, where the iron-binding capacity is elevated), so the saturation is usually between 10% and 20%. The anemia is rarely severe (Hgb rarely <8.5 g/dL). The hemoglobin and hematocrit will improve if the underlying process is treated. Diseases not associated with inflammation or neoplasia (ie, diabetes, hypertension, etc.) do not cause anemia of chronic disease. Blood loss causes a lower serum iron level, an elevated iron-binding capacity, and a lower iron saturation. The serum ferritin (low in iron deficiency, normal or high in anemia of chronic disease) will usually clarify this situation. Vitamin B_{12} and folate deficiencies are associated with macrocytic anemia. Sideroblastic anemia can be either microcytic or macrocytic (occasionally with a dimorphic population of cells, some small and some large), but is associated with an elevated iron level. In addition, this patient's history (which suggests an inflammatory polyarthritis) would not be consistent with sideroblastic anemia. The diagnosis of sideroblastic anemia is made by demonstrating ringed sideroblasts on bone marrow aspirate. In the anemia of chronic renal insufficiency, caused by erythropoietin deficiency, the iron studies are normal and the red cells are normocytic.

302. The answer is c. Macrocytic anemia and indirect hyperbilirubinemia suggest hemolysis, which in this patient is likely due to IgM antibodies which may follow *Mycoplasma* infections and which cross-react with RBC surface molecules of the I/i system. These antibodies are termed cold-reacting antibodies because they react at temperatures less than 37°C (98°F). Examination of the peripheral blood smear is the first step in evaluation of hemolytic anemia. The young red cells (which would show up as reticulocytes when properly stained) are much larger than mature RBCs, accounting for the macrocytosis (the MCV can be as high as 140 with vigorous reticulocytosis). The presence of microspherocytes suggests immune-mediated hemolysis, while the presence of fragmented RBCs or schistocytes suggests a mechanical cause of hemolysis, as seen in the microangiopathic hemolytic anemias. Serum protein electrophoresis is useful to diagnose multiple myeloma, which is rarely associated with hemolysis, but this would not be the best initial test; the anemia in multiple myeloma is normocytic. Flow cytometry can detect surface proteins such as CD55, CD59 on granulocytes and red blood cells in paroxysmal nocturnal hemoglobinuria (a rare cause of hemolysis), but again is not the best first test. Glucose-6-PD levels might be useful once hemolytic anemia is established by a peripheral smear and negative Coombs test. Bone marrow biopsy would show erythroid hyperplasia, but is usually not required to diagnose hemolytic anemia.

303. The answer is c. Acute intermittent porphyria (AIP) is a disorder of heme biosynthetic pathway due to a deficiency in the enzyme porphobilinogen deaminase. Since the biosynthetic pathway cannot move forward due to defective enzyme activity, accumulation of the upstream substrates delta-aminolevulinic acid and porphobilinogen cause various clinical manifestations including abdominal pain, nausea, vomiting, peripheral neuropathy, neurogenic bladder, tachycardia, hypertension, and tremor during acute attack. Since the pain is neurogenic, and not due to infection or inflammation, rebound tenderness, leukocytosis, and fever are uncommon. Patients may have mild hepatic dysfunction with slight elevation of ALT and AST. Both serum and urine porphobilinogen and delta-aminolevulinic acid are elevated during an acute attack. Fecal porphyrins are normal. Many factors are known to cause acute exacerbation of AIP. Drugs such as phenytoin, barbiturates, alcohol, starvation or reduced carbohydrate intake, and stress can cause exacerbation.

Porphyria cutanea tarda is due to an acquired deficiency of hepatic enzyme uroporphyrinogen decarboxylase. A chronic blistering skin condition is highly characteristic of this porphyria. Urinary delta-aminolevulinic acid and porphobilinogen excretion may be normal or slightly elevated. Alcoholism and iron overload are frequently found to be exacerbating factors.

Variegate porphyria (VP) is due to the deficiency of protoporphyrinogen oxidase, which is a mitochondrial enzyme in heme biosynthetic pathway. Patients may present with symptoms of acute intermittent porphyria, cutaneous blistering porphyria, or both. Plasma and fecal total porphyrin determinations are most useful in distinguishing VP and AIP since they are elevated in VP but not in AIP.

Thalassemia syndromes constitute a heterogeneous group of genetic disorders, the clinical manifestations of which result from decreased or absent production of normal globin chains of hemoglobin. These abnormalities result in hypochromic, microcytic anemias of varying severity. Urine porphobilinogen and total porphyrin level are not elevated in any form of thalassemia. Autoimmune hepatitis could cause the transaminase elevation but would not account for the recurrent bouts of abdominal pain, the peripheral neuropathy, or the red urine.

304. The answer is d. This patient presents with the superior vena cava (SVC) syndrome. Such patients have jugular venous distension but no other signs of right-sided heart failure. They have prominent facial (especially periorbital) puffiness and may complain of headache, dizziness, or lethargy. SVC syndrome is caused by a malignant tumor 90% of the time. Lung cancer and lymphoma, both of which are often associated with bulky mediastinal lymphadenopathy, predominate. Gastric cancer often metastasizes to the supraclavicular nodes (most often on the left, the so-called Virchow node) but does not usually affect the mediastinal nodes to this degree. Prompt diagnosis is necessary to prevent CNS complications or laryngeal edema. Sensitive tumors (lymphoma, small cell lung cancer) may be treated with chemotherapy, while most other cell types are treated with radiation therapy. Hypertension, emphysema, and nephrotic syndrome do not cause SVC syndrome.

305. The answer is c. This patient has thrombotic thrombocytopenic purpura (TTP). TTP is an acute life-threatening disorder that is characterized by the pentad of microangiopathic hemolytic anemia, nonimmune thrombocytopenia, fever, renal insufficiency, and CNS involvement (confusion or multifocal encephalopathy). Not all patients have the full pentad; the essential features are the red blood cell fragmentation (schistocytes and helmet cells) and the thrombocytopenia. TTP may be triggered by endothelial damage and is associated with deficiency of a plasma protein (ADAMTS 13) that breaks down multimers of von Willebrand factor. Plasma exchange (with the infusion of fresh frozen plasma to provide the missing ADAMTS 13 protein) can be lifesaving. The hemolytic uremic syndrome (HUS), often associated with Shiga toxin-producing strains of *Escherichia coli* O157:H7, is similar but is usually not accompanied by CNS changes. Renal failure is usually more severe in HUS. Disseminated intravascular coagulation (DIC) associated with sepsis can resemble TTP, but the coagulation pathway is usually activated in DIC. In TTP the prothrombin time, PTT, and fibrinogen level are normal. Antiplatelet antibodies are associated with idiopathic thrombocytopenic purpura (ITP), but this patient has multiple abnormalities, not just thrombocytopenia. Hypersplenism can cause thrombocytopenia but rarely with a platelet count of below 50,000; it is not associated with red cell fragmentation.

306. The answer is b. This is a classic presentation of a patient with vitamin B_{12} deficiency. This is commonly seen in patients with gastric resection and malabsorption. Patients with gastric resection lose intrinsic factor production from parietal cells. Loss of intrinsic factor leads to decreased absorption of vitamin B_{12}. Megaloblastic anemia with hypersegmented neutrophils (as seen on this patient's peripheral blood smear) can be found in both folic acid and vitamin B_{12} deficiency. Folic acid deficiency does not produce peripheral neuropathy. B_{12} deficiency may cause bilateral peripheral neuropathy or degeneration (demyelination) of the posterior and pyramidal tracts of the spinal cord as well as cortical dysfunction leading to dementia. Iron deficiency anemia would show microcytic and hypochromic red blood cells on peripheral blood smear. Vitamin K deficiency results in a coagulopathy but does not cause neurologic symptoms or hypersegmented neutrophils on peripheral blood smear. Thiamine deficiency causes beriberi; this vitamin does not depend on gastric factors for absorption.

307. The answer is b. This patient has chronic myeloid leukemia (CML). Patients may be asymptomatic and diagnosed by abnormal CBC found incidentally, or patients may present with symptoms of fatigue, malaise, weight loss, early satiety, or left upper quadrant pain due to splenomegaly. Patients with CML typically have a normocytic anemia, leukocytosis with mature cells more than immature cells, and thrombocytosis. Diagnosis can be confirmed with bone marrow biopsy and cytogenetic analysis. The cytogenetic hallmark is reciprocal translocation between chromosome 9 (*Abl* gene) and 22 (*BCR* gene) - t(9;22)(q34;q11.2), known as the Philadelphia chromosome. This translocation results in an oncogene (*BCR-ABL* gene) that produces an abnormal fusion protein with tyrosine kinase activity. Treatment with the tyrosine kinase inhibitor imatinib is strikingly effective in this condition. The Philadelphia chromosome is not specific to CML. Some patients, with acute lymphocytic leukemia (ALL) also have the *BCR-ABL* gene, but these patients do not have thrombocytosis. Acute myeloid leukemia and the lymphocytic leukemias are not associated with this chromosomal abnormality. None of the other choices are associated with thrombocytosis and the cytogenetic pattern shown.

308. The answer is c. This woman's lifelong history of excessive bleeding suggests an inherited bleeding problem, as does the positive family history. The prolonged PTT indicates a deficiency of factors VIII, IX, XI, or XII, but the commonest of these deficiencies (classic hemophilia A and Christmas disease, or hemophilia B) are vanishingly rare in women. Furthermore, the continued oozing from dental sites and the absence of ecchymoses or hemarthroses suggest a platelet function disorder, as does the prolonged bleeding time. Von Willebrand disease is an autosomal dominant condition that leads to both platelet and factor VIII dysfunction and is the likeliest diagnosis in this patient. Although factor VIII concentrates can be used for life-threatening bleeding, most will respond to desmopressin, which raises the von Willebrand factor level in the most common form (the so-called type 1 form) of this disease. Mild von Willebrand disease is fairly common (1 in 250 individuals). Fresh frozen plasma and whole blood are much less effective ways to deliver factor VIII. Platelet transfusion would not be as effective as correction of the von Willebrand factor level.

309. The answer is c. Epstein-Barr virus is regarded as primary etiologic agent in the pathogenesis of nasopharyngeal carcinoma, particularly in the Chinese population. Pre- and post-treatment Epstein-Barr virus (EBV) DNA levels have significant prognostic value, with higher DNA copies indicating poor 5-year survival. Human papilloma virus is associated with a small subgroup of head and neck cancer, particularly arising from the base of the tongue and tonsillar fossa. Unlike EBV, HPV-positive head and neck cancer patients have a favorable prognosis. Cytomegalovirus does not have any prognostic relation with nasopharyngeal carcinoma. Every patient should get baseline liver and renal function test before onset of therapy, but these tests do not have prognostic implications.

310. The answer is c. This patient has an unexplained pancytopenia. If all three elements (red blood cells, white blood cells, and platelets) are affected, the cause is usually in the bone marrow (although peripheral destruction from hypersplenism can cause pancytopenia as well). In this patient without a history of liver disease or palpable splenomegaly on physical examination, a bone marrow production problem is the most likely culprit. Although B_{12} deficiency can cause pancytopenia, usually a macrocytic anemia is the most prominent feature; a serum B_{12} level would be reasonable, but the most productive approach would be to examine the bone marrow. Leukemia can present without leukocytosis (so-called aleukemic leukemia), but the most likely diagnosis would be aplastic anemia. In the elderly patient, myelodysplastic syndrome (MDS) may present with pancytopenia. Decreased levels of erythropoietin can cause decreased RBC production, but will not cause pancytopenia. A corticosteroid trial is not warranted until a diagnosis is established.

311. The answer is e. Although ovarian cancer is the leading cause of death from gynecologic malignancy in the United States, currently no screening test for early detection in the general population is recommended.

Screening with annual CA-125 levels, transvaginal ultrasonography, or pelvic CT scan has not shown reduction in mortality. *BRCA-1* and *BRCA-2* mutations are associated with familial breast-ovarian cancer syndrome, but screening of *BRCA-1* and *BRCA-2* are recommended for women with two or more relatives with breast or ovarian cancer.

312. The answer is a. This patient has likely developed hepatocellular carcinoma (HCC) as a complication of his macronodular cirrhosis. HCC is a feared complication of patients with cirrhosis resulting from hepatitis B, hepatitis C, or hemochromatosis (although it occurs with modestly increased frequency in patients with alcoholic cirrhosis as well). The incidence in high-risk patients is 3% per year. An α-fetoprotein (AFP) level greater than 500 μg/L is suggestive, and greater than 1000 μg/L virtually diagnostic, of this tumor. In patients with cirrhosis, elevated AFP, and tumors greater than 2 cm in size with typical CT appearance, diagnosis can be made without biopsy. Most patients will die within 6 months if untreated; resection of the tumor is often difficult due to the underlying liver disease. Liver transplantation can be curative in selected patients. If the α-fetoprotein is unexpectedly normal, CT-guided biopsy of the lesion would be more productive than a blind search (EGD, colonoscopy) for a primary tumor. PET scans are very expensive and would be unlikely to provide information that would change his management.

313. The answer is e. Renal cell carcinoma is twice as common in men as women and tends to occur in the 50- to 70-year age group. Many patients present with hematuria or flank pain, but the classic triad of hematuria, flank pain, and a palpable flank mass occurs in only 10% to 20% of patients. Paraneoplastic syndromes such as erythrocytosis, hypercalcemia, hepatic dysfunction, and fever of unknown origin are common. Surgery is the only potentially curable therapy; the results of treatment with chemotherapy or radiation therapy for nonresectable disease have been disappointing. Interferon-alpha and interleukin-2 produce responses (but no cures) in 10% to 20% of patients. Newer tyrosine kinase inhibitors (eg, sunitinib) are active against renal cell cancers and hold promise for more effective treatment. The prognosis for metastatic renal cell carcinoma is dismal. Pheochromocytoma can cause erythrocytosis and occasionally hypercalcemia but would not cause hematuria or an intrarenal mass. Polycystic kidney disease can cause erythrocytosis because of erythropoietin production by the cysts but would cause numerous bilateral cysts, not a solid mass.

Renal adenomyolipoma is a benign tumor that can present as a solitary renal mass on ultrasound. It has a characteristic CT appearance due to fat in the tumor. Neither renal adenomyolipoma nor adrenal carcinoma would cause erythrocytosis or hypercalcemia.

314. The answer is d. Spinal cord compression is an oncologic emergency. Major neurological deficit is often irreversible and severely compromises the patient's remaining quality of life. Vertebral and then epidural involvement precede the neurological findings; the thoracic cord is involved 70% of the time. The patient is often given high-dose dexamethasone before being sent for MRI. In the presence of neurological compromise, the definitive test, MRI scan, should be performed as quickly as possible. Multiple epidural metastases are noted in 25% of patients; their presence can affect treatment (eg, the extent of radiation therapy fields). If no neurological abnormalities are present, most experts recommend plain radiographs of the painful vertebra as the initial diagnostic test. A radionuclide bone scan would reveal the vertebral involvement but would not show the degree of spinal cord compromise. Electromyogram and nerve conduction studies would be normal in spinal cord disease. Bone scan and thoracic spine films are less specific than MRI. Hypercalcemia might cause confusion but not spinal cord signs.

315. The answer is a. The first step in evaluating a scrotal mass is to determine whether the mass is in the testis or outside it. Most solid masses arising from within the testis are malignant. Palpation of the scrotal mass and transillumination (holding a flashlight directly against the posterior wall of the scrotum) will distinguish testicular lesions from other masses within the scrotum, such as hydrocele. Ultrasonography will confirm a solid testicular mass. The tumor markers β-hCG and α-fetoprotein are not used in the initial evaluation of a scrotal mass, but will be important for staging if a solid mass suggestive of testicular carcinoma is found. Beta-hCG or AFP will be elevated in about 70% of patients with disseminated nonseminomatous testicular cancer. Seminomas are associated with normal tumor cell markers. The lymphatic drainage of the testis is into the periaortic nodes, not to the inguinal nodes. The periaortic nodes must be assessed radiographically, usually by CT scanning, if a testicular neoplasm is found. Orchiectomy is recommended if an intratesticular mass is confirmed but is not the best initial diagnostic step.

316. The answer is d. Unexplained gross hematuria requires evaluation. Patients who have gross hematuria in association with clear-cut urinary tract infection are usually treated and followed with a repeat urinalysis to confirm clearing of the RBCs, but this patient has no symptoms of urinary tract infection. Although benign causes (prostatitis, renal stones) are most common, as many as 15% of patients with gross hematuria will have bladder or ureteral cancer. Cigarette smoking increases the risk of bladder cancer two- to fourfold. Exposure to aniline dyes, chronic cyclophosphamide treatment, external beam radiation, and *Schistosoma* infection of the bladder are other risk factors. This patient should be referred to a urologist for cystoscopy to rule out transitional cell carcinoma of the bladder; the urologist will usually do a contrast retrograde pyelogram to assess for a ureteral cancer as well. If no lesion is found, CT scanning of the kidneys would be indicated despite the previous negative sonogram. Bladder scan is an ultrasonographic technique that assesses the volume of urine in the bladder. It does not visualize the bladder mucosa. Gross hematuria is uncommon in prostate cancer, which can be associated with an elevated PSA.

317. The answer is a. The long-term nature of these symptoms, the fact that the nodes are nontender, and their location (including scalene and supraclavicular) all suggest the likelihood of malignancy. Although infectious mononucleosis and toxoplasmosis can cause diffuse lymphadenopathy, these infections are usually associated with other evidence of infection such as pharyngitis, fever, and atypical lymphocytosis in the peripheral blood. It would be unusual for the lymphadenopathy associated with these infections to persist for 2 months. Serum angiotensin-converting enzyme level is a nonspecific test for sarcoidosis but is also elevated in other granulomatous diseases and is not sensitive or specific enough to be used as an initial diagnostic test. Lymphadenopathy associated with sarcoidosis requires a biopsy for diagnosis. In this patient, an excisional biopsy is necessary primarily to rule out malignancy, particularly lymphoma. Needle aspiration biopsy, useful for the diagnosis of metastatic carcinoma, is insufficient to diagnose suspected lymphoma, where assessment of the lymph node architecture is important.

318. The answer is e. The staging of Hodgkin disease is important so that proper treatment can be planned. Stage I (single lymph node bearing area) or stage II (more than one lymph node site on the same side of the diaphragm) patients with good prognostic features may be treated with radiation therapy. Those with stage III (affected lymph nodes on both sides of the diaphragm) or stage IV (extranodal disease) are treated with combination chemotherapy. CT or MRI of the abdomen and pelvis will show evidence of lymph node involvement below the diaphragm. Staging laparotomy with splenectomy, formerly done to provide pathology of the periaortic nodes and spleen, is rarely done today. Gallium scans can be useful in difficult cases. Bone marrow biopsy can later be performed to exclude bone marrow disease, which would imply stage IV, if less invasive studies have not clarified the proper stage. Liver biopsy is rarely indicated and the ESR is a nonspecific test.

319. The answer is a. Anorexia, weight loss, and back pain are common presenting symptoms of adenocarcinoma of the pancreas. Some patients present with new-onset diabetes. Although diabetes itself can cause weight loss, this would usually be associated with nocturia. Polyphagia rather than anorexia would characterize the weight loss of diabetes and malabsorption. In this patient, a CT scan would likely show a mass in the pancreas. Although cancer in the head of the pancreas can present with obstructive jaundice, cancer of the body or tail of the pancreas is usually associated with normal liver enzymes. This patient's symptoms are not suggestive of colon cancer, and the anemia associated with colon cancer is usually microcytic. Although PET scan may be used to stage certain cancers, it is rarely indicated as an initial test when cancer is suspected. Malabsorption is associated with diarrhea, not constipation. A glucose tolerance test will not add to the evaluation of this patient with known diabetes.

320. The answer is d. Patients with metastatic prostatic carcinoma are treated with endocrine therapy to shrink primary and secondary lesions by depriving prostatic tissue of circulating androgens. Estrogens are no longer recommended because of the high incidence of cardiovascular events. Most patients now receive a GnRH analogue or surgical castration. When GnRH analog drugs (leuprolide, goserelin) are used continuously, they suppress luteinizing hormone production via a negative feedback mechanism, resulting in reduced production of testicular androgen. At the beginning of treatment with GnRH agonists, there is a transient rise of the luteinizing hormone before the level falls. As a result, there may be a flare-up of symptoms which can be managed with antiandrogen medications (flutamide, bicalutamide). The bisphosphonate zoledronic acid can decrease pain and skeletal-related complications in patients with bony metastases and may be added to hormonal therapy. Radiotherapy is used for localized disease, but is less effective than hormonal therapy. The survival benefit of chemotherapy is small.

321. The answer is e. Heparin is the commonest cause of drug-induced thrombocytopenia. Between 10% and 15% of patients receiving unfractionated heparin develop thrombocytopenia. The drop in platelet count is attributed to the production of an antibody against a complex of heparin and platelet factor 4. Low-molecular-weight heparin can also cause thrombocytopenia, although less frequently than unfractionated heparin. It is important to remember the four Ts when suspecting HIT: (1) **T**hrombocytopenia, (2) **T**iming of platelet count fall, (3) **T**hrombosis, and (4) o**T**her causes of thrombocytopenia are excluded. Usually the platelet count drops 5 to 10 days after heparin is started. In this case, however, the patient likely had been exposed to heparin at the time of her CABG. With previous exposure, the thrombocytopenia can begin within hours of the reinstitution of any form of heparin.

Although low-molecular-weight heparin causes heparin-induced thrombocytopenia (HIT) less frequently than unfractionated heparin, all heparin products must be discontinued in the patient with HIT. In all patients with an active clot and those with heparin-induced thrombocytopenia with thrombosis (HITT), a direct thrombin inhibitor must be started and used as a bridge to full-potency warfarin therapy. The chief consequence of HIT is not bleeding but accelerated clotting resulting from the aggregation of platelet-heparin complexes in the circulation. HITT is a feared complication of HIT. Even with proper treatment, the amputation rate (owing to intra-arterial clotting) is as high as 40%, and the death rate as high as 25%.

322. The answer is c. Familial adenomatous polyposis (FAP) is characterized by the appearance of thousands of adenomatous polyps throughout the large bowel. It is transmitted as an autosomal dominant trait. It is associated with a deletion in the long arm of chromosome 5, which contains the *APC* gene. The colonic polyps are usually evident by age 25. If untreated, patients usually develop colon cancer by the age of 40. Once multiple polyps are detected, patients should undergo a total colectomy, which is the primary therapy to prevent colon cancer. Current guidelines recommend that patients with a family history of FAP should have screening with flexible sigmoidoscopy or colonoscopy beginning at the age of 25, followed by annual screening until age 35. An alternative method for identifying carriers is testing peripheral blood mononuclear cell DNA for the presence of a mutated *APC* gene. The detection of this mutation can lead to a definitive diagnosis before the development of polyps. The *MEN 1* gene is associated with multiple endocrine neoplasia type 1, which does not increase the risk of colon cancer. The *RET* gene is associated with multiple endocrine neoplasia type 2. The *MSH* gene is associated with hereditary nonpolyposis colon cancer (HNPCC), also known as Lynch syndrome. In contrast to FAP, patients with HNPCC or Lynch syndrome do not develop multiple polyps but instead develop only one or a few adenomas that rapidly progress to cancer. This condition is also strongly associated with ovarian and endometrial carcinoma. The *BRCA* gene is associated with familial breast and ovarian cancers.

323. The answer is c. Rifampin induces the cytochrome P450 system that metabolizes warfarin; higher doses of warfarin are required to overcome this effect. When rifampin is stopped, the dose of warfarin necessary to produce a therapeutic prothrombin time will decrease. Barbiturates and carbamazepine also accelerate the metabolism of warfarin. Most other drugs that interact with warfarin do so by blocking the microsomal enzymes that metabolize warfarin. These drugs therefore increase the prothrombin time and the therapeutic effect of warfarin. The dose of warfarin will need to be decreased when these drugs are started and increased when these drugs are discontinued. Drugs such as nonsteroidal anti-inflammatories can compete with warfarin for albumin-binding sites and will lead to an increased prothrombin time. The list of medications that can either increase or decrease the effect of warfarin is long; all patients given this drug should be advised to contact their physician before taking any new drug. They should also be counseled about over-the-counter drugs (aspirin and NSAIDs) and even health food supplements (such as ginkgo biloba) which can affect the prothrombin time in these patients. A stable intake of vitamin K-containing foods (ie, green leafy vegetables) is recommended.

324. The answer is b. Patients with hemochromatosis and cirrhosis have a very high incidence of hepatocellular carcinoma. The lifetime incidence of this complication is 30% and increases with age. Weight loss and abdominal pain suggest hepatocellular carcinoma in this patient. A CT scan or ultrasound and measurement of α-fetoprotein are indicated. The picture of right upper quadrant pain and elevated alkaline phosphatase would not suggest acute hepatitis (which causes an elevation of transaminases) or worsening of the cirrhosis caused by hemochromatosis. Primary biliary cirrhosis (associated with antimitochondrial antibodies) can cause obstructive biliary disease, but would be much less likely in this patient.

325. The answer is e. This woman is at high risk of recurrent breast cancer, an ultimately fatal event. Adjuvant therapy has been shown to decrease the chance of recurrence by 40%. This translates into a proven survival advantage for the woman; the advantages of treatment far outweigh the risk of side effects. Therefore, no therapy or only local therapy (eg, radiation therapy) would represent inadequate treatment.

Postmenopausal women who are ER or PR positive are generally treated with adjuvant hormonal therapy. Premenopausal women, or women whose tumor does not contain ER or PR, will usually need adjuvant chemotherapy. Both aromatase inhibitors (eg, letrozole, anastrozole) and tamoxifen (a selective estrogen receptor modulator) are effective in decreasing the rate of recurrence. Aromatase inhibitors are modestly more effective than tamoxifen and are the usual drugs chosen in a postmenopausal woman. Osteoporosis and musculoskeletal pains are common side effects of aromatase inhibitors. In a woman 5 or more years after menopause, the ovaries produce inconsequential amount of estrogens. Therefore oophorectomy, sometimes used in the premenopausal woman, is an inappropriate choice for this patient.

326. The answer is b. This patient's pancytopenia is likely caused by myelodysplastic syndrome (MDS), and the next best step for diagnosis will be a bone marrow biopsy. MDS is a hematopoietic stem cell disorder resulting in dysplastic and ineffective blood cell production. The disease is most evident in sixth or seventh decade of life and usually presents with variable decrease in blood cell lineage (anemia, leukopenia, and thrombocytopenia), high MCV, and dysplastic cells in peripheral smear. Many patients are asymptomatic. Some patients present with symptomatic anemia or infection, as in this case. There is a risk transformation to acute leukemia. Bone marrow biopsy usually reveals hypercellular marrow with dysplasia. The blast cells represent less than 20% of the total cells of the bone marrow aspirate. Hemoglobin electrophoresis is recommended for diagnosis of hemoglobinopathies such as thalassemia or sickle cell disease. *JAK2* mutation is considered for polycythemia vera and methylmalonic acid level for confirming vitamin B_{12} deficiency. Liver biopsy would be normal in MDS.

327. The answer is b. This patient has polycythemia vera, a clonal proliferative disorder of the bone marrow in which all three cell lines (red blood cells, platelets, and myelocytes) are overproduced. The other classic myeloproliferative disorders are chronic myeloid leukemia, essential thrombocythemia, and myelofibrosis. In polycythemia vera, nearly 98% patients are

JAK2 mutation positive. It is important to distinguish myeloproliferative syndromes (where one or more cell lines proliferate) from myelodysplastic syndromes (where one or more cell lines—usually red cells—are deficient). In myelodysplastic disorders, white blood cells and platelets are normal, at least initially. These patients present with anemia, often in association with mild macrocytosis and other features of altered marrow maturation (ringed sideroblasts, hypolobulated polys, etc). Splenomegaly and cellular overproduction are not features of the myelodysplastic syndromes. Cushing syndrome can cause facial plethora but would not account for the splenomegaly or hematological changes. Gaisböck syndrome causes erythrocytosis with a normal red cell mass (resulting from diminished plasma volume) but does not cause splenomegaly, leukocytosis, or thrombocytosis. Polycythemia vera does not occur as part of a paraneoplastic process.

328. The answer is c. Splenomegaly is not typical of sickle cell anemia. Recurrent splenic infarcts usually occur during childhood and lead to a small, infarcted spleen with functional asplenia. These patients often have Howell-Jolly bodies on peripheral blood smear (indicative of asplenia) and have an increased incidence of infection with encapsulated organisms. The presence of an enlarged spleen in a patient with sickled cells on peripheral blood smear is most often seen in hemoglobin SC disease. Any hemolytic anemia can result in an unconjugated hyperbilirubinemia and scleral icterus. Anemia results in a hyperdynamic circulation and a systolic ejection murmur. Ankle ulcers and other chronic skin ulcers may be persistent problems in patients with SS disease, particularly in those with severe anemia. Patients with sickle cell crisis often present with leukocytosis, related both to stress and to the asplenia.

329. The answer is e. This patient has developed a hemolytic anemia secondary to an antimalarial drug. Toxins or drugs such as primaquine, sulfamethoxazole, and nitrofurantoin cause hemolysis in patients with G6PD deficiency, which occurs most commonly in African-Americans. Since the *G6PD* gene is carried on the X chromosome, almost all affected patients are males. The drugs that cause hemolysis in G6PD deficiency are oxidizing agents. Oxidant stress on red blood cells is normally counteracted by reduced glutathione. NADPH (which is required to regenerate reduced glutathione after it has been oxidized) is produced by the hexose monophosphate shunt. G6PD is the first enzyme in this metabolic pathway. If this enzyme is less active, the cell cannot replace reduced glutathione and succumbs to oxidizing stress. Clinically this can range from mild to life-threatening hemolysis. It is usually necessary to wait several weeks or months after the hemolytic episode to measure G6PD levels. In mild cases, no treatment is necessary; once the offending drug is eliminated, the hemolysis resolves. Splenectomy is sometimes required in chronic hemolytic anemias such as hereditary spherocytosis or autoimmune hemolytic anemia, but not in G6PD deficiency. Methylene blue is used to treat methemoglobinemia. Vitamin E has no beneficial effect in G6PD deficiency.

330. The answer is c. This patient has testicular carcinoma. A solid mass arising from the testis (ie, not an extratesticular scrotal mass) is almost always malignant. Bulky retroperitoneal lymphadenopathy is characteristic of the metastatic pattern of testicular cancer. The evaluation first involves staging the tumor with CT rather than PET scanning. Stage I is confined to the testicle, stage II involves retroperitoneal or periaortic lymphadenopathy, and stage III implies distant spread to mediastinal or supraclavicular nodes, lung, or brain. The intensity of treatment is decided by placing the patient into good, intermediate, or poor prognostic groups. This is based on histological type (determined from the radical inguinal orchiectomy), stage, and tumor markers (AFP, β-hCG, and LDH). Diagnosis requires orchiectomy as needle biopsy or aspiration can spread the tumor. In general, favorable prognostic features include seminomatous histology, absent or (in the case of nonseminomatous tumors) low levels of serum tumor markers, absence of metastases beyond the retroperitoneal nodes, and testicular site of origin (extragonadal tumors carry a less favorable outlook). Favorable prognosis seminomas are often cured with orchiectomy and retroperitoneal radiation therapy. Chemotherapy is usually necessary to cure nonseminomatous tumors, but even intermediate prognosis nonseminomatous tumors can be cured 80% of the time. Other cancers may also be associated with tumor markers (CEA in colon cancer and α-fetoprotein in hepatocellular carcinoma).

331. The answer is c. Patients with acute myeloid leukemia (AML) usually present with nonspecific symptoms such as fever, bone pain, headache, night sweats, and fatigue. Bone pain is attributed to the expansion of the marrow by leukemic cells. Laboratory abnormalities include anemia and thrombocytopenia. Patients with French American British (FAB) classification M3 variety (acute promyelocytic leukemia) of AML can also present with symptoms of disseminated intravascular coagulation (DIC) or can develop it during treatment. Nearly 95% cases of acute promyelocytic leukemia have balanced translocation t(15;17) involving the retinoic acid receptor-alpha gene on chromosome 17 and the *PML* gene on chromosome 15. As a result, all-trans retinoic acid is used as a chemotherapeutic agent in cases of acute promyelocytic leukemia with good success. The blood smear in this patient shows a leukemic myeloblast containing an Auer rod. Auer rods are formed by fusion of lysosomal granules and appear as clumps of azurophilic, granular, needle-shaped material found in the cytoplasm of blast cells. Myelofibrosis would have a more insidious course and is usually associated with splenomegaly. Multiple myeloma can present with bone pain, but patients usually have chronic pain that is localized to the back or ribs. Acute lymphocytic leukemia (ALL) is less common in adults, and patients usually have generalized lymphadenopathy. Auer rods are found in myeloblasts but not in lymphoblasts of ALL. In ALL bone marrow biopsy would show a predominant lymphocytic pattern rather than myeloid predominance.

332. The answer is b. This patient with gram-negative bacteremia has developed disseminated intravascular coagulation (DIC), as evidenced by multiple-site bleeding, thrombocytopenia, fragmented red blood cells on peripheral smear, prolonged PT and PTT, and reduced fibrinogen levels from depletion of coagulation proteins. Initial treatment is directed at correcting the underlying disorder—in this case, infection. Although heparin was formerly recommended for the treatment of DIC, it is now used rarely and only in unusual circumstances (such as acute promyelocytic leukemia). For the patient who continues to bleed, supplementation of platelets and clotting factors (with fresh frozen plasma or cryoprecipitate) may help control life-threatening bleeding. Red cell fragmentation and low platelet count can be seen in microangiopathic disorders such as thrombotic thrombocytopenic purpura (TTP), but in these disorders the coagulation pathway is not activated. Therefore, in TTP the prothrombin time, partial thromboplastin time, and plasma fibrinogen levels will be normal. Plasmapheresis, vitamin K therapy, and RBC transfusion will not correct the underlying cause.

333. The answer is c. Propylthiouracil often causes a mild leukopenia that does not require discontinuation of the drug. Drug-induced agranulocytosis, however, is a life-threatening complication occurring in 0.1% to 0.2% of patients on antithyroid medications and requires immediate discontinuation of the drug. Agranulocytosis is an immune-mediated disorder; the absolute neutrophil count is often extremely depressed (usually <100). Generally the neutrophil count will recover 5 to 7 days after the offending drug has been discontinued. During this time the patient is at grave risk of septicemia. Although blood cultures and CXR may be indicated in this patient prior to the administration of antibiotics, the most important initial step is evaluating the white blood cell count. Evaluation of thyroid function (with TSH or T_3) will not diagnose the agranulocytosis.

334. The answer is c. This is a classic presentation of diffuse large cell lymphoma. These neoplasms usually present with a rapidly enlarging nodes and B symptoms (fever, night sweats, >10% weight loss). Extranodal disease (eg, gastric involvement) is occasionally seen, whereas extra-lymphatic disease is unusual in the more indolent small cell lymphomas. Although Hodgkin disease can also present in this fashion, the histological features are those of non-Hodgkin lymphoma.

Untreated large cell lymphomas are progressive and rapidly fatal. Usually, however, they respond to combination therapy (multidrug chemotherapy, often combined with the anti-CD 20 antibody rituximab). As opposed to indolent lymphomas, which respond but almost always relapse, most large cell lymphomas are cured with therapy. Exceptions are mantle cell lymphomas and primary central nervous system lymphomas, which are more refractory to therapy.

335. The answer is a. A breast mass, even in a young woman, requires definitive evaluation. Although most such masses are benign, breast cancer is still the most common cause of cancer death in this age group. Risk factor assessment cannot provide sufficient reassurance. A negative mammogram never rules out breast cancer. Either excisional biopsy or core needle biopsy under sonographic or stereotactic guidance will be needed to detect cases of breast cancer before metastases outside the breast have occurred. Reassurance and reevaluation in 6 months may lead to delay in diagnosis of breast cancer. Neither oral contraceptives nor tamoxifen are indicated prior to a definitive diagnosis.

336. The answer is e. Testing for thrombophilia is generally reserved for patients who develop unprovoked venous thromboses, especially when those events occur before age 40 in a patient with a positive family history of abnormal clotting. This patient should simply be treated with low-molecular-weight heparin followed by 3 to 6 months of warfarin in the standard fashion. If she develops recurrent DVT, thrombophilia testing would be considered.

The prothrombin gene mutation (*G20210A*) and factor V Leiden are the commonest genetic factors associated with DVT, but they cause only a modestly increased risk of DVT and their presence may not change the management of the patient. Patients with factor V Leiden who are taking oral contraceptives have a 35-fold increased risk of DVT, but OCPs should be avoided if possible in women with any history of DVT. Protein C, S, and AT III deficiencies confer a much greater risk, but are significantly less common. Their presence will usually be identified by the history including family history. Remember that these genetic conditions have been associated with an increased risk of venous, not arterial, thrombosis. Only the antiphospholipid antibody syndrome and elevated homocysteine levels have been associated with arterial thromboses.

337 to 339. The answers are 337-b, 338-g, 339-c. Malignancy is a recognized risk factor for venous thromboembolism (VTE), and VTE is the second leading cause of death in cancer patients. Procoagulant molecules expressed both by cancer cells and host tissue contribute to this condition. Low-molecular-weight heparin (LMWH) is the preferred anticoagulant for long-term treatment in patients with cancer. When compared with warfarin, LMWH reduces the rate of recurrent VTE without significant risk of bleeding. Newer anticoagulants such as rivaroxaban have not been adequately tested for cancer-induced VTE yet.

Young patients with unprovoked VTE, a history of unexplained VTE, or family history of VTE raise the suspicion of an inherited hypercoagulable disorder. The common inherited hypercoagulable disorders are Factor V Leiden mutation, prothrombin gene mutation, protein S deficiency, protein C deficiency, antithrombin III deficiency, dysfibrinogenemia, and antiphospholipid antibody syndrome. When inherited hypercoagulable disorders are strongly suspected, tests for above mentioned disorders can be ordered. In the event of an acute thrombosis, however, it is not recommended to test for protein C, protein S, and anti-thrombin III since active coagulation can reduce the plasma concentration of these proteins resulting in false-positive result. To avoid confusion, it is recommended to order only Factor V Leiden mutation, prothrombin gene mutation, and antiphospholipid antibody with acute VTE or when patients are on warfarin.

Warfarin-induced skin necrosis results from a transient hypercoagulable state. Warfarin initially affects all the vitamin K-dependent clotting proteins (Factors II, VII, IX, X, and proteins C and S). Since Protein C has a short half-life (8-12 hours), the serum protein C concentration drops quickly to 50% of normal in first 24 hours. Since circulating levels of other vitamin K-dependent proteins are still high, this gives rise to a hypercoagulable state which may cause microthrombi in the dermal and subcutaneous vessels, resulting in skin necrosis. The risk is particularly high in case of congenital protein C deficiency; nearly one-third cases of warfarin-induced skin necrosis are associated with congenital protein C deficiency.

340 to 342. The answers are 340-a, 341-d, 342-c. Multiple myeloma would best explain this patient's presentation. The onset of myeloma is often insidious. Pain caused by bone involvement, anemia, renal insufficiency, and bacterial pneumonia often follow. This patient presented with fatigue and bone pain, then developed bacterial pneumonia probably secondary to *Streptococcus pneumoniae,* an encapsulated organism for which antibody to the polysaccharide capsule is not adequately produced by the myeloma patient. There is also evidence for renal insufficiency. Hypercalcemia is frequently seen in patients with multiple myeloma and may be life-threatening. Definitive diagnosis of multiple myeloma is made by demonstrating greater than 30% plasma cells in the bone marrow. Seventy-five percent of patients with myeloma will have a monoclonal M spike on serum protein electrophoresis, but 25% will produce primarily Bence-Jones proteins, which, because of their small size, do not accumulate in the serum but are excreted in the urine. Urine protein electrophoresis will identify these patients. Approximately 1% of patients with myeloma will present with a nonsecretory myeloma. Patients with nonsecretory myeloma have no M-protein on serum/urine electrophoresis and immunofixation; the diagnosis can be made only with bone marrow biopsy. The bone scan in myeloma is usually negative. The radionuclide is taken up by osteoblasts, and myeloma is usually a purely osteolytic process. Renal biopsy might show monoclonal protein deposition in the kidney or intratubular casts but would not be the first diagnostic procedure. Rouleaux formation in peripheral smear is a characteristic finding of myeloma, although it is neither sensitive nor specific.

Waldenström macroglobulinemia may cause hyperviscosity syndrome with CNS manifestations including headache, blurring of vision, dizziness, nystagmus, ataxic gait, drowsiness, or even coma. Peripheral neuropathy, coagulopathy, lymphadenopathy, hepatosplenomegaly, and nonspecific constitutional symptoms are often present. An unusual gap between serum total protein and albumin indicates hyperglobulinemia, and a monoclonal IgM spike on serum protein electrophoresis helps establish an initial diagnosis. Bone marrow biopsy revealing more than 10% of lymphoid and plasmacytoid cells confirms the diagnosis. Unlike multiple myeloma, bony lesions are uncommon in Waldenström macroglobulinemia, whereas lymphadenopathy and organomegaly are uncommon in myeloma.

Monoclonal gammopathy of undetermined significance (MGUS) is a premalignant plasma cell disorder which is often suspected and detected incidentally from routine blood workup. The patients are asymptomatic with no end-organ damage such as renal failure, hypercalcemia, anemia, or lytic bone lesion. The serum electrophoresis reveals an M spike but the amount of M-protein on immunofixation is usually less than 3 gm/dL and bone marrow contains less than 10% of monoclonal plasma cells. Monitoring of patients is important since MGUS can progress to multiple myeloma over a period of time. It is recommended to get the first evaluation 6 months after initial diagnosis followed by annual or biannual checkup.

343 and 344. The answers are 343-c, 344-d. Syndrome of inappropriate of antidiuretic hormone (SIADH) is a disorder of impaired water excretion due to excessive secretion of ADH hormone, often by neoplastic cells. Antidiuretic hormone makes the urine concentrated, thereby preventing free water excretion. This leads to water retention and hyponatremia. As total body water increases, the serum osmolality decreases. In normal person, when serum osmolality decreases, the kidneys produce dilute urine to excrete excess water. In SIADH, however, continued ADH release from the tumor prevents urinary dilution, and urine osmolality remains inappropriately high. Urine osmolality more than 100 mOsm/kg in face of hyponatremia is highly suspicious of SIADH. Urine Na value is also higher than 40 mEq/L in SIADH. It is most commonly seen in small cell cancer of the lung.

Tumor lysis syndrome (TLS) is an oncologic emergency resulting from breakdown of tumor cells with subsequent release of potassium, phosphate, and uric acid into the circulation. It is most commonly seen in hematologic malignancy such as non-Hodgkin lymphoma or Burkitt lymphoma. Diagnostic criteria (the Cairo-Bishop criteria) for TLS include both laboratory and clinical features. Laboratory TLS includes two or more of the following values: uric acid $\geq$ 8 mg/dL, calcium $\leq$ 7 mg/dL, potassium $\geq$6 mEq/L, and phosphorus $\geq$ 6.5 mg/dL for children or 4.5 mg/dL for adults. Clinical TLS is laboratory TLS plus one of the following: increased serum creatinine concentration (≥1.5 times the upper limit of normal, cardiac arrhythmia, sudden death, or seizure).

The classic Trousseau syndrome consists of migratory superficial thrombophlebitis. A single episode of tenderness and inflammation in a superficial vein is common and usually benign, but recurrent unprovoked episodes should prompt a search for an underlying neoplasm. Cancer of the pancreas is the most common tumor, but any mucin-producing carcinoma can produce this syndrome. Sézary syndrome is skin infiltration by malignant T-cells in cutaneous T-cell lymphoma. Lambert-Eaton myasthenic syndrome is a disorder of the neuromuscular junction due to antibodies directed against the voltage-gated calcium channel. The antibody prevents normal calcium flux required for the release of acetylcholine, resulting in neuromuscular weakness. It is often a paraneoplastic syndrome associated with small cell carcinoma of the lung

345 to 347. The answers are 345-d, 346-b, 347-e. Chronic lymphocytic leukemia is monoclonal proliferation of mature lymphocytes, often found incidentally during routine checkup. Some patients may have constitutional symptoms such as weight loss, fever, night sweats, and fatigue. Painless lymphadenopathy is the most common physical finding. Hepatosplenomegaly can occur as well. Lymphocytosis is the most striking feature, and peripheral smear usually contains numerous mature lymphocytes. Bone marrow usually contains lymphocytes accounting for >30% of all nucleated cells.

Immune thrombocytopenic purpura is a common cause of thrombocytopenia in otherwise normal individual; it is caused by immune-mediated destruction of platelets by antibodies against platelet antigens. Other causes of thrombocytopenia including sepsis, viral and other infections, drugs, pregnancy, liver disease, and hypersplenism should be ruled out. Patients may present with petechiae, purpura, epistaxis, or severe hemorrhage. Glucocorticoids and intravenous immune globulin (IVIG) are usually the first choice to treat this condition. Anti-D (RhoGAM) can be used instead of IVIG in patients with Rh-positive blood. Thrombotic thrombocytopenic purpura (TTP) usually presents with microangiopathic hemolytic anemia, nonimmune thrombocytopenia, fever, renal insufficiency, and CNS involvement. The peripheral smear in TTP contains schistocytes and decreased number of platelets.

Hemophilia is an X-linked recessive disorder resulting is Factor VIII or Factor IX deficiency. It mainly manifests as bleeding in joints, muscles, subcutaneous tissue, and from the gastrointestinal tract; the bleeding may be spontaneous or trauma-related, depending on the severity of deficiency. A normal platelet count and prothrombin time but prolonged activated partial thromboplastin time (aPTT) are suggestive of hemophilia. Mild cases may escape detection until adulthood. Obtaining a detailed family history is very important. Specific assays for Factor VIII and Factor IX will confirm the diagnosis.

Acute lymphoblastic leukemia is primarily a malignancy of childhood and young adulthood, and presents commonly with bone pain and lymph-adenopathy. The peripheral smear and bone marrow usually contain a large number of lymphoblasts. Leukemoid reaction is a reactive leukocytosis with increased number of myelocytes, metamyelocytes, and bands in the peripheral circulation.

Suggested Readings

1. Kasper DL, Fauci AS, Hauser SL, Longo DL, Jameson JL, Loscalzo J. *Harrison's Principles of Internal Medicine*. 19th ed. New York: McGraw-Hill; 2015. Chapters 77, 78, 79, 107, 108, 109, 110, 112, 114, 115, 116, 126, 128, 130, 131, 132, 133, 134, 136, 140, 141.
2. NCCN Clinical Practice Guidelines in Oncology (NCCN Guidelines®), available at: http://www.nccn.org/
3. American Society of Clinical Oncology (ASCO) Clinical Practice Guideline, available at: http://www.asco.org/quality-guidelines
4. Schulman S, Crowther MA. How I treat with anticoagulants in 2012: New and old anticoagulants, and when and how to switch. *Blood*. 2012;119:3016-3023.
5. Palumbo A, Anderson K. Multiple myeloma. *N Engl J Med*. 2011;364: 1046-1060.
6. George JN. Clinical practice. Thrombotic thrombocytopenic purpura. *N Engl J Med*. 2006;354:1927-1935.

Neurology

Questions

348. A 30-year-old man complains of unilateral headaches. He was diagnosed with migraine headaches at age 24. The headaches did not respond to triptan therapy at that time, but after 6 weeks the headaches resolved. He has had three or four spells of severe headaches since then. Currently his headaches have been present for the past 2 weeks. The headaches start with a stabbing pain just below the right eye. Usually the affected eye feels "irritated" (reddened with increased lacrimation). He saw an optometrist during one of the episodes and a miotic pupil was noted. Each pain lasts from 60 to 90 minutes, but he may have several discrete episodes each day. The neurological examination, including cranial nerve examination, is now normal. What is your best approach to treatment at this time?

a. Prescribe oral sumatriptan for use at the onset of headache
b. Prednisone 60 mg daily for 2 to 4 weeks
c. Obtain MRI scan of the head with gadolinium contrast
d. Begin propranolol 20 mg bid
e. Refer for neuropsychiatric testing

349. A 47-year-old dentist consults you because of tremor, which is interfering with his work. The tremor has come on gradually over the past several years and seems more prominent after the ingestion of caffeine; he notices that, in the evening after work, an alcoholic beverage will decrease the tremor. No one in his family has a similar tremor. He is otherwise healthy and takes no medications. On examination his vital signs are normal. Except for the tremor, his neurological examination is normal; in particular there is no focal weakness, rigidity, or bradykinesia. When he holds out his arms and extends his fingers, you detect a rapid fine tremor of both hands; the tremor goes away when he rests his arms at his side. What is the best next step in the management of this patient?

a. MRI scan to visualize the basal ganglia
b. Electromyogram and nerve conduction studies to more fully characterize the tremor
c. Therapeutic trial of propranolol
d. Therapeutic trial of primidone
e. Neurology referral to rule out motor neuron disease

350. A 35-year-old previously healthy woman suddenly develops a severe headache while lifting weights. A minute later she has transient loss of consciousness. She awakes with vomiting and a continued headache. She describes the headache as "the worst headache of my life." She appears uncomfortable and vomits during the physical examination. Blood pressure is 140/85, pulse rate is 100/min, respirations are 18/min, and temperature is 36.8°C (98.2°F). There is neck stiffness. Physical examination, including careful cranial nerve and deep tendon reflex testing, is otherwise normal. Which of the following is the best next step in evaluation?

a. CT scan without contrast
b. CT scan with contrast
c. Cerebral angiogram
d. Holter monitor
e. Lumbar puncture

351. A 64-year-old man is evaluated because of weakness and difficulty in weaning from mechanical ventilation. The patient had been admitted to the intensive care unit 2 weeks ago because of septic shock related to alcoholism, pneumonia, and *Klebsiella* bacteremia. He had developed respiratory failure requiring intubation and mechanical ventilation as well as acute kidney injury. His pulmonary infiltrates had responded to appropriate intravenous antibiotics and his hypotension had responded to intravenous norepinephrine. Now the patient is alert and responsive to verbal commands, is afebrile with blood pressure of 114/74 but has not tolerated several trials of weaning from the ventilator. On physical examination, the patient is cooperative. Cranial nerves are normal. Muscle strength is poor, especially in distal musculature, where he displays only 2/5 strength in the hands and feet. Proximal strength is 3/5. Ankle and knee reflexes are unobtainable. Sensory examination is difficult because of problems communicating with the patient but suggests distal sensory loss in the lower extremities. Laboratory studies show that his creatinine level has spontaneously improved to 2.4 mg/dL. Electrolytes are normal, and the patient has a mild normochromic normocytic anemia with resolving leukocytosis. Serum creatine kinase is 78 units/L (normal <140). What is the most likely cause of his weakness?

a. Muscle degeneration with loss of myosin in myocytes
b. Persistent neuromuscular blockade due to aminoglycoside use
c. Thiamine depletion from intravenous glucose administration
d. Axonal degeneration of peripheral nerves with denervation potentials in myocytes
e. Demyelination of peripheral nerves from unrecognized Guillain-Barré syndrome (GBS)

352. An 82-year-old woman is evaluated for progressive dementia. She is on no medications; the family has not noticed urinary incontinence or seizure activity. Her mini-mental state examination (MMSE) score is 21 out of 30; she has no focal weakness or reflex asymmetry on physical examination. MR scan shows a 2.4-cm partly calcified, densely enhancing mass near the falx (shown in the following figure). There is no surrounding edema or mass effect. What is the best approach to the management of this patient's intracranial mass?

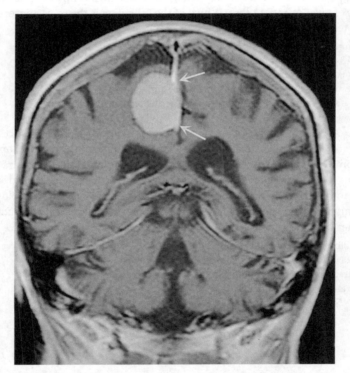

Reproduced, with permission, from Fauci A, et al. *Harrison's Principles of Internal Medicine*. 17th ed. New York, NY: McGraw-Hill Education, 2008:2606.

a. Neurosurgical resection of the mass
b. Radiation therapy to the mass
c. Serial CT scans and cholinergic treatment for the dementia if indicated
d. Ventriculoperitoneal shunting
e. Phenytoin and watchful waiting

353. A 30-year-old man complains of bilateral leg weakness and clumsiness of fine movements of the right hand. Five years ago he had an episode of transient visual loss. On physical examination, there is hyperreflexia with Babinski sign in the lower extremities and cerebellar dysmetria with poor finger-to-nose movement on the right. When the patient is asked to look to the right, the left eye does not move normally past the midline. Nystagmus is noted in the abducting eye. A more detailed history suggests the patient has had several episodes of gait difficulty that have resolved spontaneously. He appears to be stable between these episodes. He has no systemic symptoms of fever or weight loss. Which of the following is the most appropriate next test to order?

a. Lumbar puncture
b. MR scan with gadolinium contrast
c. Quantitative cerebrospinal fluid (CSF) IgG levels
d. Testing for oligoclonal bands in cerebrospinal fluid
e. CT scan of the head with intravenous-iodinated contrast

354. A 76-year-old woman consults you because of leg discomfort. Her legs are comfortable during the day, but in the evening she develops an uncomfortable creepy-crawly sensation that keeps her awake for hours. The feeling is temporarily relieved by movement; she will awaken, pace around, and sometimes run water on her legs to achieve relief. Her neurological examination is normal. Which of the following is the best initial treatment for her condition?

a. Zolpidem 5 mg po at bedtime
b. Trazodone 50 mg po at bedtime
c. Stretching exercises of the legs
d. Pramipexole 0.125 mg po in the evening
e. Cyclobenzaprine 10 mg po at bedtime

355. A 50-year-old man complains of slowly progressive weakness over several months. Walking has become more difficult, as has using his hands. There are no sensory, bowel, or bladder complaints; he denies problems with thinking, speech, or vision. Examination shows distal muscle weakness with muscle wasting and fasciculations. There are also upper motor neuron signs, including extensor plantar reflexes and hyperreflexia in wasted muscle groups. The remainder of the neurological examination is unremarkable. Which of the following tests is most likely to be abnormal in this patient?

a. Cerebrospinal fluid white blood cell count
b. Sensory nerve conduction studies
c. CT scan of the brain
d. Electromyography
e. Thyroid studies and vitamin B_{12} level

356. A 22-year-old woman seeks advice for the treatment of headaches. The first of these headaches began at age 16, but their frequency has increased to two to three per month over the past year. The headaches are not preceded by an aura. The headaches are usually bilateral, are throbbing, and are so intense that she has to go home from work. Loud noise and physical activity make the pain more severe. Each headache lasts until the evening; she will awaken the next morning without pain or nausea, and will be able to return to work. She takes acetaminophen at the onset of the headache without benefit. She is on no other medications including oral contraceptives. Neurological examination is normal. What is the best step in the management of these headaches?

a. Topiramate starting at a dose of 25 mg twice daily
b. An oral triptan such as sumatriptan at the onset of pain
c. Combination acetaminophen/hydrocodone at the onset of pain
d. Long-acting propranolol 40 mg daily, increasing until the headaches are completely prevented
e. Gabapentin 300 mg daily at bedtime, increasing until the headaches are controlled

357. A 20-year-old woman complains of weakness that is worse in the afternoon, worse during prolonged activity, and improved by rest. When fatigued, the patient is unable to hold her head up or chew her food. She often notes diplopia when driving home from work. On physical examination, she has no loss of reflexes, sensation, or coordination. Which of the following is the likely pathogenesis of this disease?

a. Autoantibodies directed against the postsynaptic acetylcholine receptor causing neuromuscular transmission failure
b. Destruction of anterior horn cells by virus
c. Progressive muscular atrophy caused by spinal degeneration
d. Demyelinating disease
e. Defect in muscle glycogen breakdown

358. A 65-year-old man presents with right-sided weakness and expressive aphasia that began suddenly 2 hours ago. He has a history of osteoarthritis, gout, and hypertension. He has no history of recent head trauma or surgery. Medications include lisinopril, allopurinol, and acetaminophen. On physical examination the patient is alert. His blood pressure is 164/90 and his pulse rate is 66. He has a dense right hemiparesis and is not able to speak. Complete blood count, platelet count, prothrombin time, glucose, and ECG are normal. CT of the head without IV contrast is normal. What is the next best step?

a. Urgent carotid ultrasonography
b. Anticoagulation with heparin
c. Discuss with patient and his family the risks and benefits of intravenous recombinant tissue-type plasminogen activator
d. Aspirin 81 mg orally now
e. MRI scan of the brain

359. Three weeks after an upper respiratory illness, a 25-year-old man develops weakness of his legs, which progresses over several days. On physical examination he has 4/5 strength in his arms but only 2/5 in the legs bilaterally. There is no sensory deficit, but knee and ankle reflexes cannot be elicited. During a 2-day observation period the weakness ascends, and he begins to notice increasing weakness of the hands. He notices mild tingling, but the sensory examination continues to be normal. The workup of this patient is most likely to show which of the following?

a. Acellular spinal fluid with high protein
b. Abnormal electromyogram/nerve conduction velocity (EMG/NCV) showing axonal degeneration
c. Positive edrophonium (Tensilon) test
d. Elevated creatine kinase (CK)
e. Respiratory alkalosis on arterial blood gas measurement

360. A 32-year-old woman presents to you for evaluation of headache. The headaches began at age 18, were initially unilateral and worse around the time of her menses. Initially the use of triptans two or three times a month would provide complete relief. Over the past several years, however, the headaches have become more frequent and severe. Triptans provide only partial relief; the patient requires a combination of acetaminophen, caffeine, and butalbital to achieve some improvement. Prophylactic medications including beta-blockers, tricyclics, and topiramate have been unsuccessful in preventing the headaches, and she has been to the emergency room three times over the past 2 weeks for a "pain shot." The general physical examination is unremarkable. Her funduscopic examination shows no evidence of papilledema, and a careful neurological examination is likewise normal. What is the most likely explanation for her headache syndrome?

a. Status migrainosus
b. Medication overuse headache
c. Space-occupying intracerebral lesion
d. CNS vasculitis
e. Pseudotumor cerebri

361. A 76-year-old woman presents with numbness and mild weakness in the legs. She has noticed mild numbness in the fingertips bilaterally. The symptoms have been slowly progressive over the past year. She rarely goes to the doctor and takes no medications. Neurological examination shows sensory loss to light touch distal to the knees and wrists in a symmetric pattern. Joint position and vibratory sensation are normal. Ankle reflexes are absent, and she has mild distal weakness. Which of the following is the most likely abnormality on laboratory testing?

a. Hyperglycemia
b. Macrocytic anemia with a low vitamin B_{12} level
c. Oligoclonal bands on CSF analysis
d. Low T_4, elevated TSH
e. Positive acetylcholine receptor antibody titers

362. A 68-year-old man with a history of hypertension and coronary artery disease presents with right-sided weakness, sensory loss, and an expressive aphasia. Symptoms began 6 hours prior to arrival in the ED. Neuroimaging studies are shown in the following figure. In the emergency department the patient's blood pressure is persistently 180/95. Which of the following is the best next step in management of this patient's blood pressure?

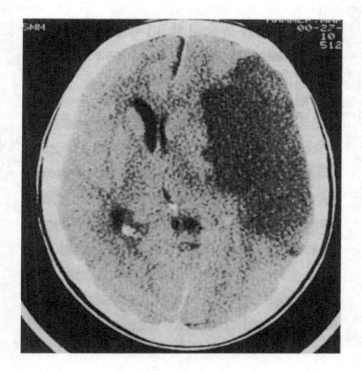

a. Administer IV nitroprusside
b. Administer clonidine 0.1 mg po until the blood pressure drops below 140/90
c. Observe the blood pressure
d. Administer IV mannitol
e. Administer IV labetalol

363. A 45-year-old woman presents to her physician with a 6-week history of gradually increasing limb weakness. She first noticed difficulty climbing stairs, then problems rising from a chair, and, finally, lifting her arms above shoulder level. Aside from some difficulty swallowing, she has no ocular, bulbar, or sphincter problems and no sensory complaints. Family history is negative for neurological disease. Examination reveals significant proximal limb and neck muscle weakness with minimal atrophy, normal sensory findings, and normal deep tendon reflexes. Affected muscles are slightly tender; there is no skin rash. What is the likely pathogenesis of her condition?

a. B- and T-cell mediated attack against muscle autoantigens
b. Anterior horn cell degeneration in the spinal cord
c. Antibodies to the acetylcholine receptor at the neuromuscular junction
d. Vasculitis with focal nerve and muscle necrosis
e. Abnormal trinucleotide repeat in the *DMPK* gene

364. A 55-year-old diabetic woman suddenly develops weakness of the left side of her face as well as of her right arm and leg. She also has diplopia on left lateral gaze. Where is the responsible lesion?

a. Right cerebral hemisphere
b. Left cerebral hemisphere
c. Right side of the brainstem
d. Left side of the brainstem
e. Right median longitudinal fasciculus

365. A 26-year-old woman presents for follow-up of her multiple sclerosis (MS). She has had two separate episodes of optic neuritis and has noticed stutteringly progressive weakness in her lower extremities. She has a mild neurogenic bladder. Her symptoms have been stable over the past 4 months. MRI scanning reveals several plaques in the periventricular white matter (MR scan shown in the following figure) and several other plaques in the brainstem. What is the best next step in her management?

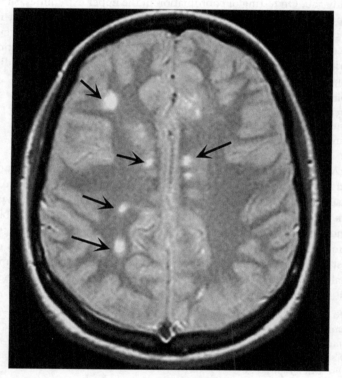

Reproduced, with permission, from Fauci A, et al. *Harrison's Principles of Internal Medicine.* 17th ed. New York, NY: McGraw-Hill Education, 2008:2615.

a. Intravenous methylprednisolone 1 g daily for 3 days
b. Oral cyclophosphamide
c. Oral anticholinergics for the urinary incontinence and observation of the demyelinating process
d. Interferon-beta
e. Intravenous mitoxantrone every 3 months

366. A 58-year-old woman has a history of alcohol abuse, coronary artery disease, and atrial fibrillation. Her medications include metoprolol, lisinopril, simvastatin, and warfarin. She develops urinary urgency and frequency and is treated with oxycodone and ciprofloxacin. Three days later she develops a headache, dizziness, vomiting, and has difficulty walking. On neurological examination her strength, sensation (including vibratory sensation), and reflexes are normal. She walks with an uncoordinated, unsteady gait. On testing of coordination in the upper extremities, she displays past-pointing and poor rapid alternating movements with her right upper extremity. In the lower extremities, her heel-shin testing also reveals poor coordination on the right. INR is 6.5 (normal <1, therapeutic for warfarin 2.0-3.0). What is the most likely cause of her neurologic findings?

a. Right cerebellar hemorrhage
b. Multiple small infarcts in the basal ganglia
c. Cerebellar degeneration due to chronic alcohol abuse
d. Posterior column degeneration as a result of vitamin deficiency
e. Combined effects of oxycodone and ethanol

367. A 68-year-old man is seen in the emergency room after an unwitnessed syncopal episode. His wife heard a strange noise and found him confused and on the floor of the living room where he had been watching television. His wife tells you that he has no ongoing medical problems, does not take any medications, and does not use alcohol or illicit drugs. On examination the patient is drowsy, has a tongue laceration, and his pants are wet with urine. Serum electrolytes (including sodium and calcium) are normal and urine drug screen is negative. Which of the following is the best next step in evaluation?

a. MRI scan of brain
b. Lumbar puncture
c. Holter monitor
d. CT scan of head
e. Echocardiography

368. A 74-year-woman consults you because of tremor and difficulty completing her daily tasks on time. She has hypertension and takes hydrochlorothiazide 25 mg every morning. She does not smoke and uses alcohol infrequently. On examination, her BP is 126/84; her vital signs are otherwise unremarkable. Eye movements are normal as are her reflexes and motor strength. She moves slowly; her timed up-and-go (TUG) test takes 24 seconds (normal 10 seconds). She has a slow resting tremor with a frequency of about 3 per second; the tremor is more prominent on the right than the left. The tremor decreases with intentional movement. Her handwriting has deteriorated and is small and crabbed. Which therapy is most likely to improve her functional disabilities?

a. Switching her antihypertensive to propranolol 20 mg po bid
b. Benztropine mesylate 0.5 mg po tid
c. Lorazepam 0.5 mg po tid
d. Ropinirole beginning at a dose of 0.25 mg tid
e. Carbidopa/levodopa beginning at a dose of one-half of a 25 mg/100 mg tablet tid

369. A 72-year-old woman is found unconscious at home by her daughter. The daughter last spoke to her mother 1 day ago, at which time her mother seemed fine. The patient has diabetes, hypertension, atrial fibrillation, and chronic back pain. Her medications include metformin, lisinopril, warfarin, and oxycodone. On examination her blood pressure is 167/70, pulse 48 beats/min, respiratory rate 12 breaths/min and irregular, and temperature 37.2°C (98.9°F). There are no signs of trauma. Neck is supple. The patient does not respond to verbal stimuli. Pupils are equally reactive to light. The oculocephalic reflex (doll's eye maneuver) is normal. On applying firm pressure to the orbital rim, the patient flexes her right arm, but does not move her left arm. Which of the following is the most likely cause of her condition?

a. Hypoglycemia
b. Narcotic overdose
c. Lacunar infarct in the right internal capsule
d. Acute subdural hematoma
e. Anterior cerebral artery embolism

370. A 37-year-old factory worker develops increasing weakness in the legs; coworkers have noted episodes of transient confusion. The patient has bilateral foot drop and atrophy; mild wrist weakness is also present. Deep tendon reflexes are absent in the lower extremities. His CBC shows an anemia with hemoglobin of 9.6 g/dL; examination of the peripheral blood smear shows basophilic stippling. Which of the following is the most likely cause of this patient's symptoms?

a. Amyotrophic lateral sclerosis
b. Lead poisoning
c. Overuse syndrome
d. Myasthenia gravis
e. Alcoholism

371. A 73-year-old woman presents with increasing weakness, most noticeable in the legs. She has noticed some cramping and weakness in the upper extremities as well. She has more difficulty removing the lids from jars than before. She has noticed some stiffness in the neck but denies back pain or injury. There is no bowel or bladder incontinence. She takes naproxen for osteoarthritis and is on alendronate for osteoporosis. She smokes one pack of cigarettes daily. The general physical examination reveals decreased range of motion in the cervical spine. On neurological examination, the patient has 4/5 strength in the hands with mild atrophy of the interosseous muscles. She also has 4/5 strength in the feet; the weakness is more prominent in the distal musculature. She has difficulty with both heel walking and toe walking. Reflexes are hyperactive in the lower extremities. Sustained clonus is demonstrated at the ankles. What is the best next step in her management?

a. Obtain MRI scan of the head
b. Begin riluzole
c. Obtain MRI scan of the cervical spine
d. Check muscle enzymes including creatine kinase and aldolase
e. Refer for physical therapy and gait training exercises

372. A 73-year-old man has had three episodes of visual loss in the right eye. The episodes last 20 to 30 minutes and resolve completely. He describes the sensation as like a window shade being pulled down in front of the eye. He has a history of hypertension and tobacco use. He denies dyspnea, chest pain, palpitations, or unilateral weakness or numbness. On examination the patient appears healthy; his vital signs are normal and the neurological examination is unremarkable. An ECG shows normal sinus rhythm without evidence of ischemia or hypertrophy. Initial laboratory studies are normal. Both noncontrast CT scan of the head and MR scan of the brain are normal. What is the best next step in this patient's management?

a. Admit the patient to the hospital for intravenous unfractionated heparin.
b. Obtain an echocardiogram.
c. Check for antiphospholipid antibodies and homocysteine levels.
d. Order a carotid duplex ultrasonogram and begin antiplatelet therapy.
e. Begin lamotrigine for probable nonconvulsive seizure.

Questions 373 and 374

Match the clinical description with the most likely mechanism of disease. Each lettered option may be used once, more than once, or not at all.

a. Large-vessel stroke due to cardiogenic embolism
b. Large-vessel stroke due to atherosclerotic middle cerebral artery (MCA) occlusion
c. CNS vasculitis due to giant cell arteritis
d. Small vessel (lacunar) stroke
e. Stroke due to carotid artery dissection
f. Hemorrhagic stroke due to uncontrolled hypertension

373. A 73-year-old woman presents with sudden-onset right-sided weakness. She has a 18-year history of type 2 diabetes mellitus which has been treated with metformin 1000 mg bid; a recent hemoglobin A1C level was 7.8. She also has hypertension and osteoarthritis. On physical examination, she is alert and oriented. BP is 172/88 and she is afebrile. Speech and mentation are normal. She has a right facial droop with sparing of the forehead. Right arm and right leg strength are 3/5; the right Babinski response is equivocal while the left is clearly downgoing. Sensory examination (including tests for stereognosis and graphesthesia) is normal bilaterally.

374. A 52-year-old Hispanic man presents with left-sided weakness and difficulty with speech. He takes no medications but has noticed mild exertional dyspnea for the past 2 to 3 months. His neurological symptoms came on suddenly and without warning, like a "bolt out of the blue." He denies previous weakness or visual loss. On examination BP is 136/74 and pulse is irregular at 92/min. Cardiac examination shows an irregular rhythm and a soft diastolic rumble at the apex. He has moderate right facial weakness and pronator drift of the right hand and arm. Strength of the right leg and the left side of his body are normal. Heat-cold discrimination and light touch to microfilament testing are diminished in the right face and arm. The patient's speech is halting and nonfluent. He is unable to name simple objects such as "watch" and "pencil."

Questions 375 to 377

For each of the clinical descriptions, select the most likely diagnosis. Each lettered option may be used once, more than once, or not at all.

a. Senile dementia of Alzheimer type
b. Creutzfeldt-Jacob disease
c. Vascular (multi-infarct) dementia
d. Vitamin B_{12} deficiency
e. Tertiary syphilis
f.   Dementia with Lewy bodies
g. Normal-pressure hydrocephalus

375. An 80-year-old woman has developed gradually progressive memory loss; she is aware of her deficit, which is frustrating to her. Over the past month or two, she has had difficulty controlling her voiding to the point that she is now using adult diapers. Her gait has become unsteady, with a shuffling lurching quality and frequent falls. MRI shows dilated ventricles bilaterally, normal sulci, and no mass lesion.

376. A 70-year-old man with history of hypertension and diabetes presents with a stepwise loss of intellectual function. Earlier episodes have been associated with unilateral weakness and difficulty swallowing. A unilateral Babinski sign is found on neurological examination.

377. A 52-year-old man presents with emotional lability, weight loss, and hallucinations. Over several months he has developed a rapidly progressive dementia associated with quick jerks of his arms and legs that are precipitated by movement. An electroencephalogram is abnormal with diffuse slowing and periodic sharp waves. Cerebrospinal fluid analysis shows normal cell count, glucose, and protein.

Questions 378 and 379

Match each clinical description with the correct diagnosis. Each lettered option may be used once, more than once, or not at all.

a. Pneumococcal meningitis
b. Cryptococcal meningitis
c. Coxsackievirus (aseptic) meningitis
d. Pyogenic brain abscess
e. *Listeria monocytogenes* meningitis
f. Herpes simplex encephalitis
g. Cerebral cysticercosis

378. A 52-year-old previously healthy woman presents with behavioral abnormalities and aphasia. Her husband reports that her symptoms began 3 days ago with fever and headache. On examination, she has a temperature of 38.4°C (101°F), mild nuchal rigidity, and agitation. When questioned, she repeats the question or responds with nonsense words. CT scan shows mild temporal hypodensity on the right; CSF examination shows 354 WBC with 75% lymphocytes. The CSF protein is elevated at 167 mg/dL, but the CSF glucose is normal at 112 (simultaneous peripheral glucose 142).

379. A 28-year-old alcoholic has recently been treated for lung abscess. Three days before this admission, the patient develops headache, fever, and mild right-sided weakness. His MRI scan is shown in the following figure.

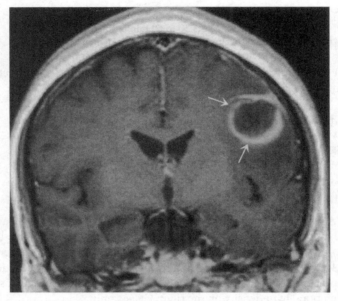

Reproduced, with permission, from Fauci A, et al. *Harrison's Principles of Internal Medicine*. 17th ed. New York, NY: McGraw-Hill Education, 2008.

380. A 62-year-old man presents with several weeks of excruciating stabbing pain in his right cheek. This pain occurs several times a day, lasts for a few seconds, and is so intense that he often winces or cries out. Episodes of pain can sometimes be caused by touching the face, or by air blowing on his face. What is the most likely diagnosis?

a. Carotid artery aneurysm
b. Migraine
c. Trigeminal neuralgia
d. Glossopharyngeal neuralgia
e. Brain tumor

381. A 72-year-old man complains of memory difficulties. He is worried that he has Alzheimer disease. He has trouble recalling the names of friends, and last month forgot his son's birthday, which had never happened before. On two occasions he became lost driving to a familiar department store. He is now afraid to make trips away from home. His children tell him that he has forgotten things they have discussed even 1 day previously. He lives independently and has not had any difficulty preparing meals, paying bills, using the telephone, or taking his medications. He takes lisinopril and hydrochlorothiazide for hypertension. He does not use alcohol. Folstein MMSE score is 27/30 and Montreal Cognitive Assessment (MoCA) score is 26/30. Neurologic examination is normal. Which of the following is most appropriate?

a. Inform the patient that his symptoms are a normal consequence of aging and that his risk of Alzheimer disease is no higher than average
b. Tell the patient that he has dementia and must stop driving
c. Perform screening tests for vitamin deficiency and psychiatric disease
d. Begin donepezil
e. Order a Holter monitor

Questions 382 and 383

Match each scenario with the appropriate antiepileptic drug treatment. Each lettered option may be used once, more than once, or not at all.
a. Intravenous lorazepam, 0.1 mg/kg
b. Intravenous fosphenytoin, 20 phenytoin equivalents/kg
c. Carbamazepine, 200 mg po bid
d. Phenytoin, 100 mg po tid
e. Levetiracetam 500 mg po bid
f. No treatment

382. A 67-year-old woman is admitted because of a witnessed generalized seizure associated with urinary and fecal incontinence and followed by postictal confusion. She has recently been started on hydrochlorothiazide for essential hypertension and is found to have a serum sodium level of 114 mEq/L. The neurological examination is nonfocal, and neuroimaging studies are normal. A second seizure occurs just as the infusion of 3% hypertonic saline is begun, but the patient has no further neurologic events after the serum sodium concentration is corrected. She is now ready for discharge and has a serum sodium level of 136 mEq/L. Her hypertension has responded to an angiotensin-converting enzyme inhibitor. What antiepileptic drug regimen should be started?

383. A 20-year-old woman presents to the emergency department after a witnessed seizure. She is a college student and had been awake most of the previous night studying for her final examinations. On the morning of admission she suffered a generalized seizure in the college cafeteria. There was no warning aura and no evidence of focal weakness when she was evaluated by the EMTs. The patient denies a history of seizures and denies recreational drug or alcohol use. Her father, however, has been on an unknown antiepileptic drug for many years. The patient does note that she often has muscle twitches in the morning so severe that she has dropped objects. Neurological examination and an MRI scan are both normal. Complete blood count and electrolytes are normal. What antiepileptic drug regimen should be recommended?

384. A 57-year-old banker complains of 2 days of severe dizziness. When she sits up or rolls over in bed, she has a spinning sensation that lasts for a few seconds and is followed by nausea. These episodes have occurred many times a day and prevent her from working. She denies fever or upper respiratory symptoms and takes no medications. When moved quickly from a sitting to a lying position with her head turned and hanging below the horizontal plane, she complains of dizziness, and horizontal nystagmus is noted. The most likely diagnosis is

a. Orthostatic hypotension
b. Meniere disease
c. Acoustic neuroma
d. Benign paroxysmal positional vertigo (BPPV)
e. Ischemic infarct in the lateral medulla (Wallenberg syndrome)

385. A 42-year-old woman presents with several weeks of increasingly severe morning headaches and mild right arm weakness. Contrast-enhanced CT scan of the brain reveals a 3×4 cm lesion in the left parietal lobe. Which of the following statements is true?

a. Cerebrospinal fluid analysis is often helpful in establishing the cell type of brain tumors
b. If glioblastoma multiforme is identified, her life expectancy is about 1 year
c. In patients with metastatic brain lesions, the primary site can almost always be identified
d. Most meningiomas are aggressive and have a poor prognosis
e. Central nervous system lymphomas occur almost exclusively in patients with AIDS

Neurology

Answers

348. The answer is b. The history is classic for cluster headache, an often debilitating periodic pain syndrome. The typical cluster lasts for weeks and then remits. Like classic migraines, cluster headaches are unilateral and can be associated with autonomic symptoms (including Horner syndrome) on the symptomatic side. The following table helps you to distinguish cluster headache from migraine:

	Cluster Headache	Migraine Headache
Aura	No	Sometimes
Duration of pain	30 min-3 h	4-72 h
Gender	Male	Female
Activity	Pt paces in agitation	Pt prefers to lie quietly in the dark
Eyes	Unilateral lacrimation and rhinorrhea	Photophobia, otherwise normal

Treatment of cluster headache involves three principles: (1) relieving the acute headache, (2) aborting or shortening the cluster, and (3) preventive (or prophylactic) therapy. It is harder to relieve the individual headache in cluster disorder than in migraine because each episode of pain is of shorter duration. High-flow oxygen (7-10 L/min via face mask) is most effective, but subcutaneous sumatriptan may also be tried. This patient is not having an acute headache; so acute treatment is not necessary. This patient needs prednisone to abort the cluster; 40 to 60 mg/d is given for weeks and then tapered over a month or two. Verapamil (often at high dose) is used for prophylaxis if the clusters occur frequently or are not relieved by steroids. Propranolol and tricyclic antidepressants (which are given for migraine prevention) are much less helpful in the patient with cluster headache. The pain in cluster headache is very severe, and suicides have occurred when the patient enters another stereotypical cluster. Proper diagnosis and treatment are therefore crucial. Neuroimaging studies might be indicated in headaches of recent onset or with focal neurological findings, but treatment should take precedence. Neuropsychiatric testing is expensive and would not be indicated in this patient with classic cluster headache.

349. The answer is c. This patient's action tremor (ie, brought out by sustained motor activity) and otherwise normal neurological examination are diagnostic of essential tremor. Fifty percent of patients will have a positive family history (benign familial tremor). The tremor is termed "benign" to separate it from Parkinson disease and other progressive neurological diseases and because it does not affect other areas of function; however, about 15% of patients (especially those in professions that require fine motor control) will be functionally impaired. An identical rapid fine action tremor can be seen in normal persons after strenuous motor activity or with anxiety. Hyperthyroidism, caffeine overuse, alcohol withdrawal, and use of sympathomimetic drugs (such as cocaine and amphetamines) can cause an identical tremor and can exacerbate the tremor in familial cases.

Neurological imaging is normal in patients with essential tremor. The EMG is nonspecific. This patient has no features (eg, weakness, fasciculations) to suggest motor neuron disease. Patients with essential tremor are managed with medications, especially beta-blockers, to decrease the severity of the tremor. Most neurologists feel that nonselective beta-blockers (blocking both beta-1 and beta-2 receptors) are most effective. They can be used on an "as needed" basis (ie, before performance of fine tasks) if the patient is not troubled by the tremor at other times. Primidone is also effective but is associated with more side effects, especially at higher doses.

350. The answer is a. An excruciating headache with syncope requires evaluation for subarachnoid hemorrhage (SAH). This occurs with leakage or rupture of an intracranial aneurysm, usually located at an arterial bifurcation in the anterior cerebral circulation. Rupture may occur spontaneously or at times of exercise. About 2% of persons have "berry" aneurysms. Fortunately only a small percentage of these persons ever experience rupture, which may be fatal. The headache that precedes or accompanies SAH is severe and often described as a "thunderclap" headache, meaning that it reaches its maximum intensity in seconds. Migraine may also cause severe headache, but usually reaches maximum intensity in 5 to 30 minutes. Syncope occurs in about one-half of patients with SAH and is thought to be due to accompanying cerebral artery spasm. Blood in the cerebrospinal fluid irritates the meninges and may cause neck stiffness. Suspected subarachnoid hemorrhage mandates CT scanning as the initial test. In about 90% of patients, there will be enough blood to be visualized on a noncontrast CT scan. A contrast CT scan sometimes obscures the diagnosis because, in an enhanced scan, normal arteries may be mistaken for subarachnoid blood. If the CT scan is normal, a lumbar puncture will establish the diagnosis by demonstrating blood in the cerebrospinal fluid (CSF). As opposed to CSF blood from a traumatic lumbar puncture, the CSF blood does not clear with continued collection of fluid. Cerebral angiography is necessary to assess the need for surgery and to detect other aneurysms, but it is usually delayed because angiography may precipitate spasm, especially if performed immediately after the acute rupture. Holter monitor might be helpful in unexplained syncope but would not address the severe headache. Electroencephalography is sometimes used to diagnose seizures in a patient with unwitnessed and unexplained syncope, but would not be appropriate until subarachnoid hemorrhage has been excluded.

351. The answer is d. This patient suffers from critical care polyneuropathy, which affects 25% to 50% of ICU patients who have suffered multiorgan failure or who have required long-term mechanical ventilation. It typically presents with motor weakness and difficulty in weaning the patient from the ventilator. Cranial nerves are spared. Distal reflex loss, sensory changes in neuropathic distribution, and normal CK help distinguish it from critical care myopathy. Both conditions can coexist in the same patient and distinction between the two conditions may not be important, as treatment of both conditions is supportive. Patients usually improve slowly with time, but prolonged dependence on the ventilator as well as weakness and sensory loss lasting months or years often occur. The cause of critical care polyneuropathy is unknown, but axonal degeneration on nerve conduction studies is characteristic.

Loss of myosin characterizes the closely related condition of critical care myopathy, but sensory changes and reflex loss would not be anticipated in a myopathic process. Neuromuscular blockade again would not cause sensory and reflex changes. Thiamine deficiency can be provoked in a malnourished patient (such as one suffering from chronic alcoholism) but would be associated with nystagmus, ataxia, and mental status changes rather than distal weakness and neuropathy. Demyelination (rather than axonal degeneration) is associated with Guillain-Barré syndrome, but this condition would be very unlikely in this ICU patient without antecedent viral or *Campylobacter* infection.

352. The answer is c. This patient has an asymptomatic meningioma, a common CNS tumor. The radiographic picture of a densely enhancing tumor near the surface of the brain, often with the so-called "dural tail," is essentially diagnostic, and biopsy is not necessary. An occasional patient will have bony overgrowth of the skull as a result of the hypervascular tumor; such a patient may notice a change in the contour of the skull. Almost all meningiomas are benign and grow slowly. Many are discovered incidentally during CNS imaging for other problems. While large or symptomatic meningiomas may require surgical resection, this patient's tumor should be followed at 3 to 6 month intervals with serial CT scans. Radiation therapy is unnecessary. Ventriculoperitoneal shunting is indicated only if neuroimaging studies show hydrocephalus. Phenytoin is used if seizures occur; seizures are less common in meningioma than in glial tumors that arise within the brain parenchyma. This patient's tumor would not account for her intellectual decline (bilateral cortical disease is necessary to affect higher intellectual function), and craniotomy with resection in the very elderly often causes more problems that it treats.

353. The answer is b. This patient's symptoms and signs are worrisome for a demyelinating process such as multiple sclerosis. The episode of transient blindness was likely a result of optic neuritis, which occurs in 25% to 40% of multiple sclerosis patients (a similar presentation can occur in systemic lupus erythematosus [SLE], sarcoidosis, or syphilis). In addition, the patient gives a history of a relapsing-remitting process. There are abnormal signs of cerebellar and upper motor neuron disease; the eye movement abnormalities indicate intranuclear ophthalmoplegia. Signs and symptoms therefore suggest multiple lesions in space and time, making multiple sclerosis the most likely diagnosis. All patients with suspected multiple sclerosis should have MR imaging of the brain. MRI is sensitive in defining demyelinating lesions in the brain and spinal cord; gadolinium infusion is necessary to demonstrate active demyelination. Disease-related changes on MRI are found in more than 95% of patients who have definite evidence for MS. Most patients do not need spinal fluid analysis for diagnosis. Although 70% will have elevated IgG levels and 85% will have oligoclonal bands on CSF analysis, lumbar puncture is reserved for cases where the diagnosis is uncertain. Finding pleocytosis of greater than 75 cells per microliter or any polymorphonuclear leukocytes in the CSF makes the diagnosis of MS unlikely. In some cases, chronic infection with syphilis or HIV may mimic MS. CT scanning is much less sensitive than MRI in detecting demyelinating lesions, especially in the posterior fossa and cervical cord.

354. The answer is d. This woman has restless leg syndrome (RLS), a common sensory complaint in the elderly. It is characterized by ill-defined leg discomfort that occurs in the evening when the patient is reclining or at night when the patient is trying to sleep. The uncomfortable sensation is relieved by movement. Examination is normal or shows at most mild distal sensory loss. There are no motor or reflex changes. Although most often idiopathic, RLS can be associated with iron-deficiency or renal insufficiency; iron studies (serum iron, total iron-binding capacity [TIBC], and/or ferritin levels) and serum creatinine should be measured. Although several agents (benzodiazepines, opioids) can provide symptomatic relief, dopamine-enhancing drugs are most effective. Levodopa-carbidopa is effective but may lead to rebound effects, so direct dopamine agonists (pramipexole, ropinirole) are now preferred. Soporifics such as zolpidem or trazodone are usually ineffective. RLS is a sensory, not a motor, syndrome, so muscle stretching exercises or muscle relaxants rarely provide symptom relief.

355. The answer is d. This patient's findings are worrisome for the progressive motor neuron disease amyotrophic lateral sclerosis (ALS). Amyotrophic lateral sclerosis affects both upper and lower motor neurons but spares the sensory and autonomic systems. Upper motor neuron signs include an extensor plantar response and an increased tendon reflex in a weakened muscle. Lower motor neuron signs include focal weakness, focal wasting, and fasciculations. Muscular dystrophy, polymyositis, and the neuromuscular junction disorder myasthenia gravis cause (usually proximal) muscle weakness but not the atrophy, fasciculations, and upper motor neuron signs seen in this patient. EMG in the patient with ALS shows widespread denervation and fibrillation potentials with preserved nerve conduction velocities. Sensory testing is normal. There is no inflammatory reaction in the CSF. CT or MRI of the brain and cervical spine may be necessary to rule out a mass in the region of the foramen magnum or cervical cord compression as can be seen in cervical spine stenosis, but would not be the first test chosen. Thyroid studies and vitamin B_{12} levels may be useful in peripheral neuropathy but not in motor neuron disease.

356. The answer is b. Although the classic migraine is unilateral and is preceded by an aura, many patients experience migraines without aura (formerly termed "common" migraines). This patient's female gender, the onset of the headaches in adolescence, the severity of the pain, and the worsening with light, noise, or activity are all suggestive of migraine. Muscle contraction headaches are often bilateral but occur more frequently (often every afternoon), are less intense (rarely debilitating), and are usually relieved by simple analgesics. Medication overuse headaches are often bilateral but occur more frequently (usually daily); this patient's occasional use of acetaminophen is insufficient to cause medication overuse headache. Space-occupying lesions can cause bilateral headaches, but the headaches occur more frequently, at increasing severity (as the lesion expands), often worsen at night or with Valsalva maneuver, and are usually associated with (sometimes subtle) focal abnormalities on neurological examination.

Triptans are very effective medications to abort migraines and are usually the first agents tried in patients either with or without aura. Parenteral or nasal triptans are favored if the patient needs rapid relief or if vomiting precludes the use of oral medications. It is often necessary to try two or three different agents to find the one that works best for the individual patient. If the headaches occur frequently (more than twice weekly) or are debilitating despite triptan treatment, prophylactic medications are called for. These medications are administered daily in order to prevent the migraines from occurring; they are ineffective if used at the onset of the headache. Beta-blockers, tricyclic antidepressants, and certain anticonvulsants (topiramate, divalproex) are the usual prophylactic agents that are tried. Gabapentin is less effective. Narcotics such as hydrocodone are often less effective than triptans and carry the risk of habituation if used frequently.

357. The answer is a. The disease process described is myasthenia gravis (MG), a neuromuscular disease marked by muscle weakness and fatigability. Myasthenia gravis results from a reduction in the number of junctional acetylcholine receptors as a result of autoantibodies. Antibodies cross-link these receptors, causing increased endocytosis and degradation in lysosomes. A decreased number of available acetylcholine receptors results in decreased efficiency of neuromuscular transmission. MG patients also have autoantibodies against muscle-specific tyrosine kinase (MuSK) receptors. MG presents with weakness and fatigability, particularly of cranial muscles, causing diplopia, ptosis, nasal speech, and dysarthria. Proximal limb weakness also occurs. Diseases of the central nervous system (poliomyelitis, Friedreich ataxia, or multiple sclerosis, as in answers b, c, and d) cause changes in reflexes, sensation, or coordination. ALS, a pure motor disorder, causes fasciculations and muscle atrophy as a result of lower motor neuron involvement. McArdle disease, a glycogen storage disease, causes muscle cramping and occasionally rhabdomyolysis with heavy exertion but only very rarely with usual daily activities.

Ten percent of myasthenia patients have thymic tumors. Surgical removal of a thymoma is necessary because of local tumor spread. Even in the absence of tumor, 85% of patients clinically improve after thymectomy. It is common practice to perform thymectomy in most patients with generalized MG who are between puberty and age 55.

358. The answer is c. This patient presents with a major left middle cerebral artery territory stroke. Patients who present within 3 to $4^1/_2$ hours of onset of symptoms of ischemic stroke are candidates for thrombolysis, which has been shown to improve disability and decrease long-term neurologic deficit. In one study, 50% of patients treated with recombinant tissue-type plasminogen activator (rtPA) had little or no neurologic deficit 6 months after the stroke, compared to 35% of controls. rtPA is contraindicated in hemorrhagic strokes. Thus all patients who are candidates should have CT imaging to exclude a hemorrhagic stroke. CT scanning in acute ischemic stroke is frequently normal (as in this patient) and thus the diagnosis of stroke is made on clinical grounds. rtPA use in acute ischemic stroke is associated with a 6% risk of intracranial hemorrhage, which is fatal in 50% of these patients; thus patients and/or their families should be carefully informed of the relative risks and benefits. Patients with intracranial hemorrhage on imaging, recent head trauma (within the past 90 days), surgery within the past 2 weeks, uncontrolled hypertension, coagulopathy, or who present with seizures are not candidates for rtPA. Aspirin and heparin are to be avoided for 24 hours in patients who are given tPA. Extracranial cerebrovascular disease can be diagnosed with carotid ultrasonography, but carotid artery surgery is done to prevent a subsequent stroke and thus carotid ultrasonography can be done nonurgently. MRI scanning is more sensitive for diagnosing acute stroke, but does not need to be done to confirm a stroke in this patient who has clear-cut ischemic findings. MRI scanning is more time-consuming than CT and might put this patient outside the time window for benefit from rtPA.

359. The answer is a. This patient presents with an acute symmetrical polyneuropathy characteristic of Guillain-Barré syndrome. This demyelinating process is often preceded by a viral illness or infection with *Campylobacter jejuni*. Characteristically, there is little sensory involvement; about 30% of patients require ventilatory assistance. Loss of deep tendon reflexes, especially in the lower extremities, is an important clue to the lower motor neuron involvement that characterizes GBS. Guillain-Barré syndrome is characterized by an elevated CSF protein with few, if any, white blood cells. EMG usually shows a demyelinating (not an axonal) process with nonuniform slowing and conduction block. A positive edrophonium test is characteristic of myasthenia gravis, but this patient's loss of tendon reflexes would not occur in MG. CK levels are normal, as there is no damage to muscle in this disease process. Arterial blood gases in Guillain-Barré syndrome might show a respiratory acidosis (not respiratory alkalosis) secondary to hypoventilation.

360. The answer is b. Patients who use medications for headache more than twice weekly are at risk of medication overuse headache. Any analgesic, including triptans themselves, can contribute, but opiates and barbiturates are the main culprits. In this setting, the migraine may "transform" into a chronic daily headache. Medication overuse headaches usually start in the morning and improve but do not completely resolve with analgesic therapy. The patient must completely discontinue the offending drug for 2 to 12 weeks for the headaches to resolve. Treating headaches during the period of abstinence can be very difficult. The physician should be vigilant about the development of another cause of headache (mass lesion, inflammatory disorder) in a patient with transformed migraines. CNS imaging and laboratory workup, not generally recommended in the patient with typical migraine, are sometimes indicated. In this patient without focal neurological findings, however, the most likely diagnosis is still medication overuse headache. Status migrainosus (continuous migraine) and CNS vasculitis are much less common than medication overuse headache. Pseudotumor cerebri usually causes papilledema.

361. The answer is a. The insidious onset of a distal and progressive sensory loss is characteristic of diabetic neuropathy. In many metabolic neuropathies, the longest nerve fibers are affected first, leading to the stocking-glove pattern of sensory loss. Autonomic changes can accompany the sensory loss. Some diabetics will have vascular changes in the vasa nervorum that can lead to asymmetric peripheral or cranial neuropathies; these are often reversible, while the distal neuropathy is usually progressive. It is not rare for neuropathy to be a presenting symptom of type-2 diabetes, particularly if the patient has not had prior glucose testing. Other conditions associated with peripheral neuropathy include medication side effect, toxins, uremia, neoplasm, vitamin deficiency, and amyloidosis. EMG with nerve conduction velocity testing will categorize neuropathy into axonal and demyelinating varieties and will often provide important diagnostic information. In vitamin B_{12} deficiency, posterior column function (eg, vibratory sensation) would be affected out of proportion to small pain and temperature fibers. Multiple sclerosis (which can cause oligoclonal bands) is an upper motor neuron disease that would not cause distal weakness or hyporeflexia. Symptomatic hypothyroidism (detected by low T_4 and elevated TSH levels) often causes delayed relaxation phase of muscle stretch reflexes; although fatigue and paresthesias are common symptoms of hypothyroidism, an overt peripheral neuropathy is uncommon. Myasthenia gravis (usually associated with antibodies against the Ach receptor) does not affect sensation or reflexes.

362. The answer is c. Although hypertension is an important cause of stroke, it should not be aggressively treated in the setting of acute cerebral ischemia. Since cerebral autoregulation is disrupted in acute stroke, a drop in blood pressure can decrease perfusion and worsen the so-called ischemic penumbra. Generally, blood pressure elevation up to 220/120 is tolerated. If the patient were a candidate for thrombolytic therapy, it would be acceptable to lower the BP to less than 185/110 with labetalol or nicardipine. Since this patient's symptoms began 6 hours ago, however, he is not a candidate for rtPA. Some stroke specialists recommend more aggressive blood pressure control in acute intracranial hemorrhage, but this patient has an ischemic (not hemorrhagic) stroke. Mannitol is of minimal benefit in cerebral edema associated with acute stroke.

363. The answer is a. Polymyositis is an acquired myopathy characterized by subacute symmetrical weakness of proximal limb and trunk muscles that progresses over several weeks or months. When a characteristic skin rash occurs, the disease is known as dermatomyositis. Both of these disorders are felt to have an autoimmune pathogenesis. Autoantibodies (including antinuclear antibodies and antibodies to the Jo-1 antigen) are common, and up to 50% of cases will have additional features of connective tissue diseases (rheumatoid arthritis, lupus erythematosus, scleroderma, Sjögren syndrome). Laboratory findings in polymyositis include an elevated serum CK level, an EMG showing myopathic potentials with fibrillations, and a muscle biopsy showing necrotic muscle fibers and inflammatory infiltrates. Anterior horn cell degeneration of unknown cause characterizes amyotrophic lateral sclerosis (ALS), but evidence of denervation (such as muscle fasciculations) and upper motor neuron involvement (hyperreflexia) would be expected. ALS is often asymmetric at onset. Antibodies to the acetylcholine receptor (AchR) are seen in myasthenia gravis (MG), but other autoantibodies and in particular evidence of direct immunological attack against muscle fibers do not occur. The weakness in MG is episodic and usually brought on by prolonged exertion; ptosis and diplopia (indicative of involvement of the bulbar musculature) are common in MG but rare in polymyositis. Vasculitis (for instance, polyarteritis nodosum) typically affects nerves more than muscles, usually causing an asymmetric mononeuritis multiplex. Systemic involvement such as fever, necrotic skin lesions, and renal involvement would be expected in a vasculitic process. Muscular dystrophies cause insidious onset of muscle weakness and wasting and will present with pure motor weakness without other evidence of neurological abnormality. Muscular dystrophy, however, would be uncommon at this age in a patient with negative family history. Myotonic muscular dystrophy is associated with abnormal CTG trinucleotide repeat in the *DMPK* gene and can present in adulthood, but would be expected to cause myotonia, cardiac dysfunction, and distal muscle weakness.

364. The answer is d. This patient has weakness of the left face and the contralateral (right) arm and leg, commonly called a *crossed hemiplegia*. Such crossed syndromes are characteristic of brainstem lesions. In this case, the lesion is an infarct localized to the left inferior pons caused by occlusion of a branch of the basilar artery. The infarct has damaged the left sixth and seventh cranial nerves or nuclei in the left pons with resultant diplopia on left lateral gaze and left facial weakness. Also damaged is the left descending corticospinal tract, proximal to its decussation in the medulla; this damage causes weakness in the right arm and leg. This classic presentation is called the Millard-Gubler syndrome. Hemispheric lesions cause motor and sensory loss all on the same side (contralateral to the lesion). A lesion in the median longitudinal fasciculus causes third and sixth cranial nerve dysfunction but not motor deficit of the face or body.

365. The answer is d. Interferon-beta is a standard therapy used to prevent progressive disease in relapsing-remitting multiple sclerosis. Both interferon-beta 1b and several forms of interferon-beta 1a are available and are similarly effective. Glatiramer acetate (Copaxone) is also approved for MS. While patients who receive any one of these treatments have 30% fewer exacerbations, fewer new MRI lesions and less long-term disability, the treatments do not cure the disease. Interferon-beta can cause side effects, particularly a flulike syndrome that usually resolves within several months. Acute exacerbations of MS are treated with high-dose methylprednisolone followed by tapering oral prednisone. This treatment improves symptoms during a relapse but does not affect the long-term course of the disease. This patient, however, is not having an acute exacerbation of her disease. Steadily progressive MS, especially primary progressive disease, when the disease never remits but worsens inexorably, is a difficult management problem. Immunosuppressives such as cyclophosphamide and mitoxantrone are often tried. Such patients often progress to debility and mortality from urinary infection, aspiration pneumonia, or infected pressure ulcers. Providing this patient with stutteringly progressive disease with symptomatic treatment alone would be inappropriate.

366. The answer is a. This patient has evidence of cerebellar dysfunction, most likely due to cerebellar hemorrhage. Many drugs (including ciprofloxacin) interact with warfarin, excessively prolong anticoagulation, and may result in spontaneous hemorrhage. Cerebellar lesions are typically associated with ataxia and dizziness. This patient's bleeding can be localized to the right cerebellar hemisphere since a focal lesion in one lobe of the cerebellum (eg, a cerebellar tumor, hemorrhage or infarct) causes dyscoordination on the same side of the body (ipsilateral) as the lesion. Infarcts in the basal ganglia would cause extrapyramidal signs with rigidity and uncontrolled movements in addition to discoordination. Midline cerebellar lesions (most commonly alcoholic cerebellar degeneration) cause midline signs (especially gait ataxia) out of proportion to the findings in the extremities. Posterior column disease would cause sensory abnormalities (especially, loss of proprioception and vibratory sensation) rather than problems with coordination. Acute alcohol ingestion and narcotic overdose can cause dizziness and ataxia, often with nystagmus, but would not be expected to cause unilateral dysmetria.

367. The answer is a. Though syncope is often due to a cardiovascular cause, the presence of a tongue laceration and urinary incontinence suggest syncope due to a seizure. Furthermore, patients with syncope due to cardiac causes usually recover normal mentation within a few minutes. Prolonged drowsiness is a common postictal phenomenon that can follow a generalized seizure. These findings all point to the likelihood of an unwitnessed seizure in this patient. New-onset seizure in a young person is often idiopathic or related to substance abuse (amphetamine or cocaine), but seizures that begin in older adults are worrisome for structural brain disease. The evaluation of a new seizure in an older adult includes an electroencephalogram (EEG) to confirm the diagnosis, even though the EEG will be nondiagnostic in about one-half of patients. An MRI is the best test to look for structural brain disease, such as a brain tumor, old stroke, brain abscess, or vascular malformation. Even small lesions can provide the trigger for a seizure, so the more sensitive MRI is preferred to CT scanning in this circumstance. Though often performed, routine blood tests are rarely helpful in the evaluation of seizures. Lumbar puncture is performed only if meningitis or encephalitis is suspected. Holter monitoring is used to detect rhythm disturbances that can be associated with syncope, but cardiac syncope is rarely associated with seizures. Another cause of cardiac syncope is aortic stenosis that could be detected by echocardiography, but syncope associated with aortic stenosis is almost never associated with seizures.

368. The answer is e. Parkinson disease (PD) is marked by depletion of dopamine-rich cells in the substantia nigra. The resulting decrease in striatal dopamine is the basis for the classic symptoms of rigidity, bradykinesia, tremor, and postural instability. Many experts consider bradykinesia to be the fundamental feature of PD. Although tremor is often the first manifestation, about 20% of patients do not have a tremor. When present, the tremor occurs at rest, is slower than most other tremors, and decreases with intentional activity (so that a watch repairman with PD is often able to function normally).

The most effective treatment for PD is levodopa. Levodopa is converted to dopamine in the substantia nigra and then transported to the striatum, where it stimulates dopamine receptors. This is the basis for the drug's clinical effect on PD. Levodopa is usually administered with carbidopa (a dopa decarboxylase inhibitor) in one pill. Carbidopa prevents levodopa's metabolism in the peripheral circulation and central nervous system, and thus allows it to be given at a lower dose less likely to cause nausea and vomiting. The major problems with levodopa have been (1) limb and facial dyskinesias, (2) motor fluctuations ("off-on" effects), and (3) the fact that levodopa treats PD only symptomatically while neuronal loss in the substantia nigra continues despite drug treatment. Direct dopamine agonists (such as ropinirole or pramipexole), although less potent than dopamine itself, are often used as the first drug in younger patients. Side effects (in particular, motor fluctuations) are often less troublesome. Anticholinergic agents, such as benztropine mesylate, work by restoring the balance between striatal dopamine and acetylcholine; they are particularly effective in decreasing the degree of tremor. In the elderly, however, they often cause

CNS side effects (especially confusion) and would not be a good choice in this elderly woman. Propranolol would help essential tremor but has no benefit in Parkinson disease. Chronic benzodiazepine use should be avoided because of the risk of habituation as well as confusion and falls in the elderly. Benzodiazepines do not improve the symptoms of PD.

369. The answer is d. This woman presents with coma and requires rapid and careful evaluation. The most common causes of coma are central nervous system infections (meningitis and encephalitis), structural central nervous system lesions, which produce compression of the brainstem, metabolic abnormalities, and drug overdose. The neurologic examination is very helpful in the evaluation of comatose patients, and should focus on specific maneuvers: (1) testing for nuchal rigidity, (2) pupillary response to light, (3) response to painful stimulus (typically by applying firm pressure to the sternum or orbital rim), and (4) the oculocephalic reflex (doll's eye maneuver). Neck stiffness and fever in the comatose patient would suggest meningitis or subarachnoid hemorrhage. Pupillary response to light is preserved in metabolic derangements, drug overdose, and early in space-occupying lesions. Preserved pupillary light reflex in the absence of an oculocephalic reflex is seen almost exclusively in drug overdose. In space-occupying lesions with early brainstem compression (the so-called diencephalic stage) the pupillary response to light and the oculocephalic reflex are preserved. As brainstem compression progresses to midbrain and then pons compression, pupillary response to light and the oculocephalic reflex are lost. When unilateral arm flexion with painful stimulation occurs in the comatose patient, this suggests a hemispheric mass with mild brainstem compression. As brainstem compression progresses to involve the midbrain, the comatose patient will respond to painful stimulation with arm flexion and leg extension (decorticate posturing). When brainstem compression progresses further to involve the pons, painful stimulation results in extension of both arms and legs (decerebrate posturing).

This comatose patient has preserved pupillary and oculocephalic reflexes, and right arm flexion with painful stimulation. This suggests a left hemispheric space-occupying lesion with early brainstem compression. The widened pulse pressure, bradycardia, and irregular breathing (Cushing reflex) also suggest increased intracranial pressure. In this patient on warfarin, these findings are likely due to an acute subdural hematoma, which may occur spontaneously or with trauma (such as falling). Emergency non-contrast CT of the head will almost always show the hematoma.

Hypoglycemia is uncommon with metformin. Neither hypoglycemia nor drug overdose would cause unilateral arm flexion with painful stimulation. In the absence of fever and neck stiffness, meningitis is unlikely. A lacunar infarct will cause focal findings (such as pure motor or pure sensory stroke) but not global brain dysfunction (coma). Anterior cerebral artery occlusion causes motor and sensory deficits of the contralateral leg and foot but does not impair consciousness.

370. The answer is b. Lead poisoning often causes a peripheral neuropathy with primary motor involvement. It can superficially resemble ALS, but upper motor neuron signs (such as hyperreflexia) are not seen in lead poisoning. In addition, the cognitive changes of lead encephalopathy are not seen in early ALS, in peripheral nerve injuries (eg, carpal or tarsal tunnel syndromes), or in myasthenia. Alcoholism can cause peripheral neuropathy but would not cause this patient's prominent motor weakness or the basophilic stippling. The presence of any anemia in a patient with peripheral neuropathy should prompt the clinician to think of a single disease entity (such as heavy metal poisoning) that can cause both entities. Lead lines may be seen at the gingiva-tooth border. Laboratory testing focuses on protoporphyrin levels (free erythrocyte or zinc) and blood lead levels. Industries often associated with lead exposure include battery and ceramic manufacturing, the demolition of lead-painted houses and bridges, plumbing, soldering, and, occasionally, exposure to the combustion of leaded fuels.

371. The answer is c. Cervical spondylosis (arthritis) or midline disc protrusion can cause cervical myelopathy, which can mimic amyotrophic lateral sclerosis. The neck pain and stiffness can be mild. The patient can have both lower motor neuron signs such as atrophy, reflex loss, and even fasciculations in the arms and upper motor neuron signs such as hyperreflexia and clonus (from cord compression) in the legs. Therefore, the diagnosis of ALS is never made without imaging studies of the cervical cord, as compressive cervical myelopathy is a remediable condition. Starting riluzole to slow the progression of ALS would, therefore, be inappropriate at this point. Disease in the cortex would never cause this combination of bilateral upper and lower neuron disease, so an MRI scan of the brain would be superfluous. Myopathies such as polymyositis or metabolic myopathy cause more proximal than distal weakness and would not be associated with hyperreflexia. You should think of disease of the neuromuscular junction (eg, myasthenia gravis) or muscle when the neurological examination is normal except for weakness.

Simply referring the patient for physical or occupational therapy would leave her potentially treatable cervical spine disease undiagnosed. Decompressive surgery can improve symptoms and halt progressive loss of function in cervical myelopathy.

372. The answer is d. This patient has suffered several transient ischemic attacks with the classic description of amaurosis fugax. Although the traditional symptom duration of less than 24 hours is often cited, most TIAs last less than 1 hour, usually 15 or 20 minutes. Many patients whose symptoms last for several hours are found to have ischemic strokes on MRI imaging. TIAs carry a high risk of neurological morbidity and should be promptly evaluated and treated. Five percent of patients will have a full-blown stroke within the next 2 weeks.

Assessing the extracranial carotid arteries for evidence of atherosclerosis is crucial in patients with anterior circulation TIAs. If a common or internal carotid stenosis of 70% or greater is found, carotid endarterectomy has been proven to decrease the risk of subsequent stroke. Carotid angioplasty with stenting is used in some centers, but has not been studied as rigorously as carotid endarterectomy. Lesions of the external carotid artery do not cause CNS symptoms.

The reason to acutely admit a patient with TIA to the hospital is to obtain rapid carotid evaluation and to evaluate for cardiac emboli. The ABCD2 system is used to stratify patients for hospital admission. Patients are given 2 points each for focal weakness (as opposed to speech or visual symptoms only) and duration of symptoms greater than 1 hour. Patients are given 1 point for age >60 years, BP above 140/90, speech impairment without weakness, duration of symptoms 10 to 59 minutes, and diabetes. Patients with an ABCD2 score of 3 or more are usually admitted for prompt evaluation. The use of anticoagulants in acute stroke has diminished greatly and is primarily used in cases of demonstrated cardiogenic emboli. For the typical atherosclerotic process, antiplatelet therapy is preferred. Cardiogenic sources of clots (ie, atrial fibrillation, mitral valve disease, intracardiac tumors) usually cause large vessel ischemic strokes rather than TIAs, so echocardiography would be less important in this patient. In addition, the normal cardiac exam and ECG make a cardiogenic source unlikely. Testing for thrombophilia is rarely helpful in patients with TIA. These tests may be helpful in patients with a large-vessel stroke and no identifiable source of the stroke. Amaurosis fugax would not be a manifestation of seizure disorder.

373 and 374.   The answers are 373-d, 374-a. Sudden onset of focal neurological deficit strongly suggests stroke. The time course and anatomic extent of involvement are important clues to the pathogenesis of the stroke, which can provide important therapeutic information. A focused history and physical examination (especially neurological examination) is the most important first step. Emergent CT scanning without IV contrast will reveal a hemorrhagic process but will initially be normal in cases of cerebral ischemia.

The patient in question 373 has a lacunar (small-vessel) stroke in the internal capsule on the left. Lacunar strokes are due to occlusion of the small penetrating vessels that supply blood to subcortical white matter and brainstem; the size of the infarct will be less than 1 cm. Since the descending motor and ascending sensory fibers in the internal capsule are separate, the deficit is usually confined to one or the other. "Pure motor stroke" is the commonest lacunar syndrome. Pure sensory stroke, clumsy hand-dysarthria syndrome, and various well-localized brainstem defects are frequently seen. Cortical deficits (aphasia, seizure, cortical blindness) should not occur. Diabetes and hypertension are the usual underlying substrates for lacunar stroke.

The patient in question 374 has evidence of large vessel occlusion of the left middle cerebral artery. The middle cerebral artery supplies both the motor and sensory strips of the cortex; since Broca's area is just in front of the motor cortex, an expressive aphasia is common with dominant hemisphere MCA stroke. The paramedian cortex (which controls the lower extremity) is supplied by the anterior cerebral artery; so the leg and foot are often spared in an MCA stroke. Equal involvement of face, arm, and leg suggests internal carotid occlusion (lacunar pure motor stroke also affects all three areas). Although CT or MR angiography would be necessary to distinguish embolic occlusion from atherothrombotic disease, this patient's irregular heart rhythm and murmur of mitral stenosis suggest atrial fibrillation, the commonest cause of cardiogenic embolism. Patients with stroke due to cardiogenic embolism require long-term anticoagulation; atherothrombotic and lacunar strokes are usually treated with antiplatelet drugs.

Giant cell (temporal) arteritis can cause headache, fever, weight loss, and sudden visual loss due to ophthalmic artery occlusion but does not cause intracranial occlusion or stroke. Carotid artery dissection can cause stroke due to distal embolization from the intimal flap but would be associated with neck pain (usually severe); Doppler ultrasound will often show the intimal flap. Severe headache and progressive neurological deficit usually accompany hemorrhagic stroke. Hypertension is usually marked and subcortical structures (ie, thalamus, basal ganglia, cerebellum, pons) are most often affected. Obtundation suggests mass effect with brainstem compression; uncomplicated ischemic cortical strokes do not cause alterations of level of consciousness such as drowsiness or coma.

375 to 377. The answers are 375-g, 376-c, 377-b. The development of a dementing illness is a catastrophe for patient and family alike. Once it is clear that multiple domains (not just memory) are affected, and that the defect is interfering with daily function, evaluation for "treatable" causes of dementia is indicated. The triad of cognitive decline, recent onset of urinary incontinence, and apraxia of gait should suggest normal pressure hydrocephalus (NPH). The gait disturbance resembles parkinsonism, but leg function will usually be near-normal in the supine position. CNS imaging (either CT or MRI) will reveal enlargement of ventricles out of proportion to cortical atrophy. Some of these patients will improve or stabilize in response to CSF shunting (usually into the peritoneum); deciding which patients are candidates for a shunt procedure is complicated and is often guided by the patient's response to a temporary CSF drainage procedure.

The 70-year-old with hypertension and previous focal deficits is most likely to have vascular dementia. This is associated with progressive stepwise deterioration, usually the result of recurrent bilateral cortical or subcortical (lacunar) infarcts. Focal findings, including hemiparesis, extensor plantar responses, and pseudobulbar palsy, are common.

Creutzfeldt-Jacob disease is a rare form of dementia that is distinguished from other dementias by early personality change, a rapidly progressive course, the presence of myoclonus (90% of patients), and distinctive EEG abnormalities (periodic sharp waves). In these patients the cerebrospinal fluid cell count, glucose, and protein levels are normal, but the 14-3-3 protein is often present. The causative agent is a prion or transmissible protein. The disease usually occurs sporadically though familial cases have been reported. Transmission has also occurred by consumption of contaminated beef as well as by transplantation of affected tissue such as dura mater, cornea, or pituitary gland. Creutzfeldt-Jacob disease is rapidly fatal with death occurring in most cases within a year of symptom onset.

Alzheimer disease (AD), the commonest cause of dementia, is steadily and inexorably progressive. Insight and judgment often deteriorate along with memory; so the patient is not usually aware of the deficit. Dementia with Lewy bodies (DLB) causes dementia with bradykinesia, visual hallucinations, and sensitivity to the side effects of anticholinergic medications.

Although both AD and DLB may show temporary response to cholinergic medications, the underlying process is inexorably progressive. Vitamin B_{12} deficiency can cause a dementing illness, often but not always in association with a macrocytic anemia and decrease in proprioception and vibratory sensation. Tertiary syphilis can cause parenchymal destruction and dementia, but is much less common than in previous eras. Often there is a compatible history or evidence of tabes dorsalis (severe neuropathy). Evaluation for treatable causes of dementia include medication history, thyroid studies, B_{12} (or methylmalonic acid) level, chemistry panel (to exclude renal failure or electrolyte imbalance), and CNS imaging. Further evaluations such as RPR, lumbar puncture, or specialized testing, are reserved for those with atypical feature (such as rapid progression) or a compatible history.

378 and 379. The answers are **378-f, 379-d.** CSF infections can present with meningeal inflammation, parenchymal involvement, or both. The patient in question 378 has both meningitis (fever, nuchal rigidity, CSF pleocytosis) and focal brain involvement (temporal lobe signs). The combination of high lymphocyte count in the CSF with cortical brain dysfunction indicates encephalitis. The most common cause of sporadic (ie, nonepidemic) encephalitis is herpes simplex encephalitis; prompt diagnosis and treatment with intravenous acyclovir can decrease permanent brain damage and improve survival. The commonest cause of seasonal encephalitis in the United States is now West Nile virus infection. Viral (aseptic) meningitis causes a similar lymphocytic pleocytosis with normal CSF glucose level but is not associated with brain dysfunction such as confusion, aphasia, ataxia, or focal weakness.

The patient in question 379 with focal findings and a history of pyogenic lung infection has a brain abscess. Organisms can gain access to the pulmonary veins and then be spread hematogenously to various organs of the body, bypassing the normal sieving effect of the pulmonary capillaries. Lumbar puncture is contraindicated in the presence of mass effect, but would usually show only a small number of white blood cells, a high protein, and elevated CSF pressure.

Bacterial meningitis (due to the pneumococcus or *Listeria monocytogenes*, for instance) almost always causes a neutrophilic pleocytosis and low CSF glucose due to phagocytosis of the proliferating organisms by polymorphonuclear leukocytes. CSF glucose will also be low (<2/3 of simultaneous blood glucose) in fungal, tuberculous, and carcinomatous meningitis, but these conditions can easily be separated from bacterial meningitis by their subacute to chronic onset and the predominance of lymphocytes (rather than neutrophils) in the CSF. Cryptococcal meningitis, fungal meningitis seen in patients with T-cell dysfunction such as AIDS, presents with chronic to subacute symptoms and a very high CSF protein level; India ink stain and elevated cryptococcal antigen levels will be diagnostic.

Cerebral cysticercosis (due to *Taenia solium* infection) is often associated with calcified or multiple small cystic lesions, which serve as a seizure focus, although hydrocephalus and chronic meningitis can occasionally occur. Almost all patients acquire the tapeworm infection in emerging nations, where meat inspection and sanitation practices are less well developed. History and CNS imaging will usually distinguish pyogenic brain abscess from cysticercosis.

380. The correct answer is c. Facial or head pain that is repetitive, severe, stabbing, and lasts just a few seconds is characteristic of the cranial neuralgias: trigeminal, glossopharyngeal, and occipital neuralgia. Of the cranial neuralgias, trigeminal neuralgia (tic douloureux) is the most common and typically occurs in middle-aged patients. Earlier onset can indicate underlying multiple sclerosis. The pain usually occurs unilaterally in the second or third division of the trigeminal nerve, and is classically precipitated by light touch of the face. The first-line treatment is carbamazepine, but about one-third of patients do not respond to medical treatment and require invasive management such as microvascular decompression of the trigeminal nerve. Glossopharyngeal neuralgia is much less common, is felt in the throat, and is precipitated by swallowing or yawning. In occipital neuralgia the episodes of pain originate from the base of the skull. Headaches associated with migraine tend to be throbbing and last for hours at a time. Headaches associated with brain tumors are steadily progressive and are often made worse by Valsalva maneuver and by recumbency (ie, typically worse at night). Carotid artery aneurysms may cause stroke or facial swelling but rarely cause headache.

381. The answer is c. Difficulty recalling names and temporarily misplacing objects are commonly seen with advancing age, but becoming lost and having trouble recalling recent conversations are more worrisome symptoms of significant cognitive impairment. This patient does not have dementia, which requires impairment in memory and one other cognitive domain (language, spatial orientation, or executive function). The Folstein mini-mental state examination (MMSE) and the Montreal Cognitive

Assessment (MoCA) are screening tests for Alzheimer disease. Most authorities use MMSE and MoCA scores of less than 26 as a positive screen. This patient is on the borderline of a positive screen. Patients with isolated but significant cognitive impairment, but who do not meet the diagnostic criteria for dementia, are often classified as having mild cognitive impairment (MCI). MCI is often accompanied by depression, and can be due to vitamin B_{12} deficiency, for which the patient should be screened. Patients with mild cognitive impairment are at higher risk for progression to frank dementia (12% per year in some series), but some of these patients will never develop progressive memory loss. Randomized trials of the acetylcholinesterase inhibitors donepezil and galantamine have failed to establish efficacy of either of these drugs in patients with MCI. Holter monitoring is used to detect cardiac arrhythmias, which can be associated with syncope but not selective memory impairment.

382 and 383. The answers are 382-f, 383-e. The evaluation of a first seizure should focus on (1) excluding seizure mimics such as convulsive syncope or nonconvulsive seizures (formerly termed pseudoseizures), (2) determining if the seizure is focal or primary generalized seizure, and (3) assessing the patient for secondary seizures (such as seizures caused by metabolic derangements or a structural brain abnormality such as tumor or previous stroke). Patients with a remediable cause of the seizure (as in question 382) do not need to be placed on antiepileptic drugs (AEDs). Most patients with a single unprovoked and unexplained seizure are not given AEDs, but those with high risk features for recurrence (age >65, focal findings on clinical examination, MRI, or EEG) are often offered AEDs. AEDs decrease the risk of recurrent seizures by about 50%.

The patient in question 383 has juvenile myoclonic epilepsy, an idiopathic generalized epilepsy disorder that may present in adulthood. The positive family history and the morning myoclonic jerks (sometimes dismissed by the patient "jitteriness" or ascribed to alcohol withdrawal) are characteristic. These patients require lifelong AED therapy. While most AEDs are beneficial in focal (partial) epilepsy, drugs such as phenytoin and carbamazepine may actually worsen primary generalized seizures and should not be used in this patient. Levetiracetam, lamotrigine, topiramate, and valproic acid are better agents for primary generalized seizures. Intravenous medications such as lorazepam (the drug of first choice) and phenytoin or fosphenytoin are used in status epilepticus but would not be appropriate in either of these cases. Although status epilepticus is classically defined as continuous or repetitive seizure activity lasting longer than 30 minutes, treatment should be considered if an individual seizure lasts more than 5 minutes.

384. The answer is d. Dizziness is a nonspecific symptom that may refer to several different sensations, including impending faint, spinning sensation, or impaired balance. A sensation of spinning or rotation is referred to as vertigo, and may be due to central or peripheral causes. Peripheral causes of vertigo are usually associated with nystagmus and more troublesome to the patient but are not due to life-threatening disease. The commonest cause of peripheral vertigo is benign paroxysmal positional vertigo (BPPV), which characteristically begins in middle-age persons, occurs with sudden changes of position, and is thought to be due to cellular debris in the semicircular canals. The diagnosis is supported by the Dix-Hallpike maneuver, where the patient is moved quickly from a sitting to a lying position with head turned and hanging below the horizontal plane. The occurrence of dizziness and horizontal nystagmus after a few second latency period constitutes a positive test. This patient's symptoms are not brought on by standing; so orthostatic hypotension is unlikely. Meniere disease is a chronic disease of both the labyrinth and the cochlea; so progressive unilateral hearing loss and tinnitus are usually present. Acoustic neuroma is also a chronic (rather than episodic) condition associated with hearing loss, unsteadiness of gait, and loss of corneal reflex on the affected side. Central causes of vertigo (vertebrobasilar stroke, cerebellar hemorrhage) cause constant (rather than intermittent) symptoms and are associated with ataxia and focal CNS signs. The Dix-Hallpike test in brainstem disorders causes immediate vertigo (ie, no latent period) and often vertical or rotatory nystagmus.

385. The answer is b. Headache is a common symptom in patients with brain tumors. The headache is often worse in the morning and increases in intensity with time. Seizures, change in personality, and motor weakness are other common symptoms that occur in patients with brain tumors. CSF examination is rarely helpful in delineating cell type, and lumbar puncture can be dangerous in the presence of a space-occupying lesion. Certain tumor types have typical radiographic appearance, but this is almost never definitive enough to be confident of cell type without a biopsy, except in the case of a meningioma. Brain tumors may be primary or metastatic. Glioblastoma multiforme (GBM) is the commonest primary glial tumor; it can usually be distinguished from meningioma and schwannoma by its intraparenchymal location. GBM is an aggressive high-grade tumor that is usually resistant to therapy, and carries a poor prognosis. Most patients with this tumor die within 1 year of diagnosis.

Metastatic brain tumors are most commonly from lung, breast, or melanoma, but the primary site is unidentified in about one-fifth of patients even after careful study. In the vast majority of cases, meningiomas grow slowly, and are histologically benign. CNS lymphomas are B-cell tumors; although most common in immunocompromised patients, they may occur in immunocompetent patients as well. CNS lymphomas usually arise from the subcortical white matter and may spread across the midline, which is uncommon in glial tumors such as GBM, astrocytoma, or oligodendroglioma.

Suggested Readings

1. Kasper DL, Fauci AS, Hauser SL, Longo DL, Jameson JL, Loscalzo J. *Harrison's Principles of Internal Medicine.* 19th edition. New York: McGraw-Hill; 2015. Chapters 30, 31, 32, 36, 437, 445, 446, 447, 455, 458, 459, 461.
2. Guidelines for Diagnosis and Management of Neurological Conditions, available at: www.aan.com/guidelines
3. Chou KL. In the clinic. Parkinson disease. *Ann Intern Med.* 2012;157:ITC5 1-16.
4. Grotta JC. Clinical practice. Carotid stenosis. *JAMA.* 2013;369:1143-1150.
5. MacGregor EA. In the clinic. Migraine. *Ann Intern Med.* 2013;159:ITC1 1-15.
6. Rabins PV, Blass DM. In the clinic. Dementia. *Ann Intern Med.* 2014;161: ITC1 1-15.

Dermatology

Questions

386. A 25-year-old woman consults you for management of acne. Her acne began at puberty. Initially it was controlled with topical benzoyl peroxide, topical clindamycin, and oral contraceptives. Recently, however, she and her husband have decided to start a family, and she has discontinued the oral contraceptives. Her acne has flared despite continuing the topical clindamycin. Her menses have resumed with a normal pattern. Physical examination shows comedones, some inflammatory pustules, and one or two mild cystic lesions. She does not have hirsutism or evidence of virilization. What is the best next step in her management?

a. Start oral spironolactone.
b. Start oral erythromycin.
c. Start oral tetracycline.
d. She should resume secure contraception and take oral isotretinoin.
e. Check serum DHEA-S and testosterone levels.

387. A 22-year-old man presents with a 6-month history of a red, non-pruritic rash over the trunk, scalp, elbows, and knees. These eruptions are more likely to occur during stressful periods and have occurred at sites of skin injury. The patient has tried topical hydrocortisone without benefit. On examination, sharply demarcated plaques are seen with a thick scale. Pitting of the fingernails is present. There is no evidence of synovitis. What is the best first step in the therapy of this patient's skin disease?

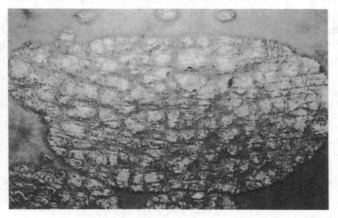

Reproduced, with permission, from Fauci A, et al. *Harrison's Principles of Internal Medicine.* 17th ed. New York, NY: McGraw-Hill Education, 2008:311.

a. Photochemotherapy (PUVA)
b. Oral methotrexate
c. Topical tacrolimus
d. Oral cyclosporine
e. Topical betamethasone valerate ointment (high-potency)

388. A 25-year-old man complains of fever, nausea, and myalgias for 5 days, and now has developed a macular rash over his wrists, palms, ankles, and soles with some petechial lesions. The rash recently ascended to his arms and legs. The patient recently returned from a summer camping trip in Tennessee. On examination, he has fever to 38.5°C (101°F) and appears moderately toxic. Which of the following is the most likely cause of the rash?

a. Contact dermatitis
b. Sexual exposure
c. Tick exposure
d. Contaminated water
e. Undercooked pork

389. A 42-year-old woman presents with pruritus primarily affecting the wrists, finger webs, and periumbilical area. Her children have similar symptoms. Examination reveals excoriations in the symptomatic areas. On the volar aspect of the right wrist, you find a single 2-mm long serpiginous lesion. What is the likely pathogenesis of her symptoms?

a. Immunoglobulin A deposition in the papillary dermis
b. Xerotic desiccation of the stratum corneum
c. Infection with a highly communicable DNA virus
d. Heavy metal poisoning from lead-based paint
e. Infestation with an arthropod

390. A 35-year-old asthmatic woman develops an itchy rash over her back, legs, and trunk a few minutes after taking amoxicillin-clavulanate for a urinary tract infection. Erythematous, edematous blanchable plaques are noted. The wheals vary in size. There are no mucosal lesions and no swelling of the lips or shortness of breath. What is the best first step in management of her symptomatic rash?

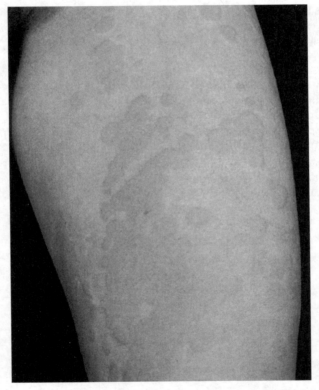

Reproduced, with permission, from Wolff K, et al. *Fitzpatrick's Color Atlas & Synopsis of Clinical Dermatology*. 6th ed. New York: McGraw-Hill Education, 2009. Figure 14.9.

a. Intravenous glucocorticoids
b. Subcutaneous epinephrine
c. Oral antihistamines (H_1 blockers)
d. Aspirin
e. Oral doxepin

391. A 64-year-old woman presents with diffuse hair loss. She says that her hair is "coming out by the handfuls" after shampooing. She was treated for severe community-acquired pneumonia 2 months ago but has regained her strength and is exercising regularly. She is taking no medications. Examination reveals diffuse hair loss. Several hair can be removed by gentle tugging. The scalp is normal without scale or erythema. Her general examination is unremarkable; in particular, her vital signs are normal, she has no pallor or inflammatory synovitis, and her reflexes are normal with a normal relaxation phase. What is the best next step in her management?

a. Reassurance
b. Measurement of serum testosterone and DHEA-S levels
c. Topical minoxidil
d. Topical corticosteroids
e. CBC and antinuclear antibodies

392. A 30-year-old African-American woman has a 2-month history of nonproductive cough and painful skin lesions in the lower extremities. She denies fever or weight loss. Physical examination shows several nontender raised plaques around the nares and scattered similar plaques around the base of the neck. In the lower extremities she has several erythematous tender nonulcerated nodules, measuring up to 4 cm in diameter. Chest x-ray reveals bilateral hilar adenopathy and a streaky interstitial density in the right upper lobe. What is the best way to establish a diagnosis?

a. Punch biopsy of one of the plaques on the neck
b. Incisional biopsy of one of the lower extremity nodules
c. Sputum studies for acid-fast bacilli (AFB) and fungi
d. Mediastinoscopy and biopsy of a hilar or mediastinal nodes
e. Serum angiotensin-converting enzyme assay

393. A 72-year-old woman presents with pruritus for the past 6 weeks. She is careful to moisturize her skin after her daily shower and uses soap sparingly. The itching is diffuse and keeps her awake at night. Over this time she has lost 15 lb of weight and has noticed diminished appetite. She has previously been healthy and takes no medications. Physical examination shows no evidence of rash; a few excoriations are present. She appears fatigued with mild temporal muscle wasting. The general examination is otherwise unremarkable. What is the best next step in her management?

a. Topical corticosteroids
b. Oral antihistamines
c. Psychiatric referral for management of depression
d. Skin biopsy at the edge of one of the excoriations
e. Laboratory testing including CBC, comprehensive metabolic panel, and thyroid studies

394. A 53-year-old woman presents to the clinic with an erythematous lesion on the dorsum of her left hand. The lesion has been present for the past 7 months and has not responded to topical corticosteroid treatment. She is concerned because the lesion occasionally bleeds and has grown in size during the past few months. On physical examination you notice an 11-mm erythematous plaque with a small central ulceration. The skin is indurated with mild crusting on the surface. Which of the following describes this process?

a. It is a malignant neoplasm of the keratinocytes with the potential to metastasize.
b. This lesion is unrelated to actinic keratosis.
c. It is a chronic inflammatory condition, which can be complicated by arthritis of small- and medium-sized joints.
d. It is a malignant neoplasm of the melanocytes with the potential to metastasize.
e. It is the most common skin cancer.

395. A 50-year-old woman develops pink macules and papules on her hands and forearms in association with a sore throat. The lesions are target-like, with the centers a dusky violet. What are the most likely causes of this patient's rash?

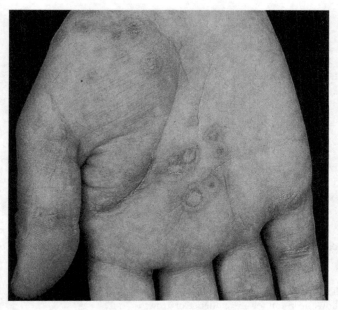

Reproduced, with permission, from Wolff K, et al. *Fitzpatrick's Color Atlas & Synopsis of Clinical Dermatology.* 5th ed. New York, NY: McGraw-Hill Education, 2005:141.

a. Tampons and superficial skin infections
b. Drugs and herpesvirus infections
c. Rickettsial and fungal infections
d. Anxiety and emotional stress
e. Harsh soaps and drying agents

396. A 25-year-old woman with blonde hair and fair complexion complains of a mole on her upper back. The lesion is 8 mm in diameter, darkly pigmented, and asymmetric, with an irregular border (shown in the following figure). Which of the following is the best next step in the management?

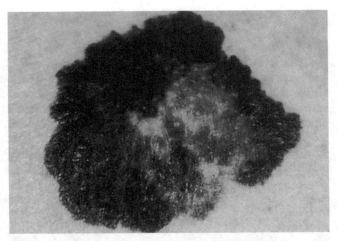

Reproduced, with permission, from Fauci A, et al. *Harrison's Principles of Internal Medicine.* 17th ed. New York, NY: McGraw-Hill, 2008:308.

a. Tell the patient to avoid sunlight
b. Follow the lesion for any evidence of growth
c. Obtain metastatic workup
d. Obtain full-thickness excisional biopsy
e. Obtain superficial shave biopsy

397. A 39-year-old man with a history of myocardial infarction complains of yellow bumps on his elbows and buttocks. Yellow-colored cutaneous plaques are noted in those areas. The lesions occur in crops and have a surrounding reddish halo. Which of the following is the best next step in evaluation of this patient?

a. Biopsy of skin lesions
b. Lipid profile
c. Uric acid level
d. Chest x-ray
e. Liver enzymes

398. A 45-year-old man presents with fever, generalized weakness, and a skin rash. He was healthy until 1 month before admission, when he was found to have a low-grade astrocytoma in the right parietal lobe. The tumor was successfully resected, and the patient was started on phenytoin for seizure prevention. Five days ago he noticed low-grade fever and malaise. Two days thereafter, painful reddish macules developed, began to coalesce, and then became fluid-filled vesicles. He has noticed pain and irritation of the mouth and eyes. Examination shows that 40% of his body and most mucosal surfaces are affected by a desquamating rash. Nikolsky sign is present (the skin shears off when lateral pressure is applied). What is the best next step in this patient's management?

a. Discontinue phenytoin and prescribe prednisone 60 mg daily by mouth.
b. Discontinue phenytoin, prescribe topical emollients, and see the patient back in the office the next day.
c. Discontinue phenytoin, admit the patient to a general medicine ward, and begin plasma exchange.
d. Discontinue phenytoin, admit the patient to a burn unit, and monitor for electrolyte disturbance and infection.
e. Discontinue phenytoin, begin empiric ciprofloxacin and hydrocodone for the pain, and see the patient back in 1 week.

399. A 17-year-old adolescent girl noted a 2-cm annular pink, scaly lesion on her back. Over the next 2 weeks she develops several smaller oval pink lesions with a fine collarette of scale. They seem to run in the body folds and mainly involve the trunk, although a few occur on the upper arms and thighs. There is no lymphadenopathy and no oral lesions. Which of the following is the most likely diagnosis?

a. Tinea versicolor
b. Psoriasis
c. Lichen planus
d. Pityriasis rosea
e. Secondary syphilis

400. A 67-year-old man with Parkinson disease has macular areas of erythema with a greasy scale behind the ears and on the scalp, eyebrows, glabella, nasolabial folds, and central chest. Which of the following is true?

a. A high-dose topical steroid is the best long-term treatment.
b. Oral fluconazole is usually necessary to eradicate the problem.
c. This condition flares with sun exposure.
d. Topical ketoconazole or 1% hydrocortisone cream (low potency) is good initial therapy.
e. This patient is likely to have destructive arthritis of the distal interphalangeal joints.

401. A 45-year-old woman presents with the complaint that her toenails are thick and yellow. She is otherwise healthy and takes no medications. On examination, two toenails on the right foot and the great toenail on her left foot are affected. There is no periungual erythema, and her peripheral pulses are good. What is the best advice for this patient?

a. This nail disease will spontaneously remit.
b. CBC, comprehensive metabolic profile, chest x-ray, and abdominal CT scan should be ordered to look for underlying malignancy.
c. Oral therapies will need to be used for months until the nails have grown out.
d. Sampling the nail is unnecessary for definitive diagnosis.
e. Topical therapies are as effective as oral agents.

402. A 33-year-old fair-skinned woman has telangiectasias of the cheeks and nose along with red papules and occasional pustules. She also appears to have conjunctivitis with dilated scleral vessels. She reports frequent flushing and blushing. Drinking red wine produces a severe flushing of the face. There is a family history of this condition. Which of the following is the most likely diagnosis?

a. Carcinoid syndrome
b. Porphyria cutanea tarda
c. Systemic lupus erythematosus
d. Rosacea
e. Seborrheic dermatitis

403. A 46-year-old construction worker is brought to the clinic by his wife because she has noticed an unusual growth on his left ear for the past 8 months (shown in the following figure). The patient explains that, except for occasional itching, the lesion does not bother him. On physical examination, you notice an 8-mm pearly papule with central ulceration and a few small dilated blood vessels on the border. What is the natural course of this lesion if left untreated?

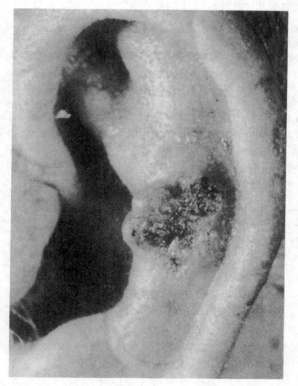

Reproduced, with permission, from Fauci A, et al. *Harrison's Principles of Internal Medicine.* 17th ed. New York, NY: McGraw-Hill Education, 2008:499.

a. This is a benign lesion and will not change
b. Local invasion of surrounding tissue
c. Regression over time
d. Metastasis via lymphatic spread
e. Disseminated infection resulting in septicemia

404. A 25-year-old postal worker presents with a pruritic, nonpainful skin lesion on the dorsum of his hand. It began like an insect bite but expanded over several days. On examination, the lesion has a black, necrotic center associated with severe local swelling. The patient does not appear to be systemically ill, and vital signs are normal. Which of the following is correct?

a. The lesion is ecthyma gangrenosum, and blood cultures will be positive for *Pseudomonas aeruginosa*.
b. A skin biopsy should be performed and Gram stain examined for gram-positive rods.
c. The patient has been bitten by *Loxosceles reclusa*, the brown recluse spider.
d. The patient has bubonic plague.
e. The patient has necrotizing fasciitis and needs immediate surgical debridement.

405. A 25-year-old man who has been living in Washington, DC, presents with a diffuse vesicular rash over his face and trunk. He also has fever. He has no history of chickenpox and has not received the varicella vaccine. Which of the following information obtained from history and physical examination suggests that the patient has chickenpox and not smallpox from a bioterrorism attack?

a. Vesicular lesions on the palms and soles
b. Vesicular lesions concentrated on the trunk
c. Rash most prominent over the face
d. All lesions at the same stage of development
e. High fever several days prior to the rash

406. A 68-year-old man complains of several blisters arising over the back and trunk for the preceding 2 weeks. He takes no medications and has not noted systemic symptoms such as fever, sore throat, weight loss, or fatigue. The general physical examination is normal. The oral mucosa and the lips are normal. Several 2- to 3-cm bullae are present over the trunk and back. A few excoriations where the blisters have ruptured are present. The remainder of the skin is normal, without erythema or scale. What is the best diagnostic approach at this time?

a. Culture of vesicular fluid for herpes viruses
b. Trial of corticosteroids
c. Biopsy of the edge of a bulla with some surrounding intact skin
d. CT scan of the chest and abdomen looking for occult malignancy
e. Combination of oral H_1 and H_2 antihistamines

407. A 42-year-old woman has had a recurrent pruritic rash since childhood. The volar aspects of the wrists and antecubital fossae have generally been most affected, but recently the rash has spread to her face, including perioral areas. She has responded to topical corticosteroids in the past but has run out of her prescription. Her husband has psoriasis, and she has recently been using his topical clobetasol propionate 0.05% with good effect. She requests her own supply of clobetasol. The patient has mild asthma controlled with as-needed inhaled beta-agonist but is otherwise healthy. What is the best recommendation for the management of her facial dermatitis?

a. Continue the superpotent topical clobetasol 0.05%.
b. Switch from the superpotent clobetasol to a high-potency topical corticosteroid such as fluocinonide 0.05%.
c. Switch from clobetasol to a low-potency topical corticosteroid such as 1% hydrocortisone cream.
d. Switch the patient to an oral antihistamine such as loratadine 10 mg daily.
e. Add oral prednisone 10 mg daily and taper to as low a dose as will control her symptoms.

408. A 65-year-old man presents with nail discoloration as shown. He has no skin rash or systemic symptoms; other nails are normal. The nail changes have been present for several months. What is the likely pathogenesis of this lesion?

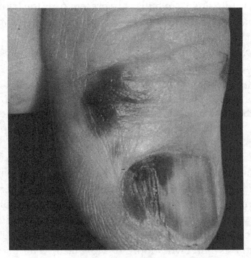

Reproduced, with permission, from Wolff K, et al. *Fitzpatrick's Color Atlas & Synopsis of Clinical Dermatology*. 6th ed. New York: McGraw-Hill Education, 2009. Figure 33.14.

a. Postinflammatory hyperpigmentation
b. Previous trauma to the nail bed with disruption of the growth plate
c. Malignant transformation of melanocytes in the nail bed
d. Involvement of the growth plate in the cellular proliferation of psoriasis
e. Lead poisoning with deposition of heavy metal in the growth plate

409. A 34-year-old homosexual man with a history of HIV presents to the clinic complaining of wheezing and multiple violaceous plaques and nodules on his trunk and extremities. Physical examination of the oral mucosa reveals similar findings on his palate, gingiva, and tongue. Chest x-ray is also significant for pulmonary infiltrates. What is the most likely pathogenesis of this process?

a. Proliferation of neoplastic T cells
b. Infection with human herpesvirus 6
c. Infection with *Mycobacterium avium* due to decreasing CD4 count
d. Angioproliferative disease caused by infection with human herpesvirus 8
e. Disseminated herpes simplex infection

Dermatology

Answers

386. The answer is b. Intensity of acne treatment is determined by the severity of the disease. Mild (comedonal) acne is managed with topical agents—typically topical benzoyl peroxide and topical antibiotics (clindamycin, erythromycin), often supplemented by a topical retinoid in the evening. Moderate acne is associated with papules and pustules; oral antibiotics are often added at this stage. More potent topicals such as azelaic acid may be tried for moderate acne. Severe acne is defined by nodules and cysts. Long-term oral antibiotics are the cornerstones of treatment at this stage. Because of numerous side effects including severe teratogenicity, hypertriglyceridemia, and depression, isotretinoin (the most effective single agent) is reserved for refractory cases. Therefore, this woman, even if she were to practice double contraception and to sign up for the iPLEDGE program, would not be a candidate for isotretinoin.

Since women of reproductive age often suffer from acne, it is important to know which agents are safe for planned conception and pregnancy. Of the agents listed, oral erythromycin is pregnancy category B. Tetracyclines and spironolactone are category D. Although androgen excess can contribute to acne in women, in absence of hirsutism or menstrual irregularity, androgen testing is not indicated. Androgens are often measured in cases of acne that are refractory to treatment, but this woman has responded well to previously prescribed treatment.

387. The answer is e. The rash described is classic for psoriasis, a common chronic inflammatory skin disorder. Its characteristic features include sharply bordered papules or plaques with thick "micaceous" scale, usually located on the knees, elbows, and scalp. Stress, certain medications such as lithium, and skin injury commonly exacerbate the disease. The distribution of the described rash would make contact dermatitis unlikely. In the differential of psoriasis are lichen planus (polygonal pruritic purple papules with lacy mucous membrane lesions), cutaneous lupus (often in a "cape" distribution), and dermatophytes (usually spreading, fewer discrete lesions, with fine peripheral scale and central clearing).

Topical corticosteroids of moderate or high potency are the first agents to try in psoriasis without joint involvement. Topical vitamin D analogues such as calcipotriene or calcitriol may be combined with topical steroids, but they are much more expensive than topical steroids. Topical calcineurin antagonists are used in atopic dermatitis, not in psoriasis. Psoralens with UVA phototherapy (PUVA) are reserved for moderate to severe widespread cases because of an increased risk of squamous cell carcinoma of the skin. Methotrexate, oral cyclosporine, and immune response modifiers such as etanercept are useful in extensive disease (>10% body surface area) or if joint involvement is present. Systemic treatments carry higher risk of side effects.

388. The answer is c. The rash described is most consistent with Rocky Mountain spotted fever, for which a tick is the intermediate vector. Secondary syphilis could present with a macular rash in the same distribution, but does not cause an acute febrile syndrome with myalgia. Always think of these two diagnoses when a rash begins on the palms and soles. Contact dermatitis does not cause petechial lesions. The skin lesions in disseminated gonococcal infection can be distal, but are usually few in number and are grayish to pustular. Giardiasis is acquired from contaminated water but does not cause fever or a rash. Trichinosis, acquired from the ingestion of contaminated pork, can cause myalgias and a maculopapular rash, but rarely shows the distal involvement seen in this patient. Trichinosis causes prominent periorbital edema and eosinophilia.

389. The answer is e. Intense pruritus is a cardinal symptom of scabies, infestation with the mite *Sarcoptes scabiei*. Family members are often affected. If a tiny serpiginous burrow can be identified, potassium hydroxide (KOH) preparation of scrapings from the burrow often reveals the mite or its eggs. The whole family needs to be treated with 5% permethrin; retreatment is often necessary. The pruritus may take several weeks to resolve. Bedbugs can leave linear bites which do not hurt but are pruritic. Bedbugs don't actively infest the skin, so specific treatment of the bites is not necessary. Dermatitis herpetiformis (DH) is an intensely pruritic disease associated with IgA deposition in the dermis, but the skin eruption is vesicular at outset and usually affects the elbows, knees, and buttocks. DH is not contagious. Xerotic eczema is a common cause of pruritus, especially in winter months. Skin is dry with a fine scale; linear burrows are not found. Xerotic eczema responds to skin hydration, especially after bath or shower. Parvovirus B19 is a contagious DNA virus that may cause family outbreaks, but it causes fever, blanchable erythema ("slapped-cheek" rash is more common in children) and minimal pruritus. Lead ingestion is a risk for children in substandard housing; it causes intellectual decline, peripheral neuropathy, and anemia with basophilic stippling but not pruritus or skin rash.

390. The answer is c. Urticaria, or hives, is a common dermatologic problem characterized by pruritic, edematous papules and plaques that vary in size and come and go, often within minutes or hours. In cholinergic urticaria, mast cells may be stimulated by heat, cold, pressure, water, stress, or exercise. Immunologic mechanisms can also cause mast cell degranulation. Patients with atopic conditions, such as asthma or eczema, are more likely to suffer from cholinergic urticaria.

Avoidance of the offending agent, when it is identifiable, is most important in management of urticaria. Nonspecific stimuli that promote mast cell degranulation (ie, exercise, temperature extremes, vibration) should be limited until the urticaria resolves. Oral nonsedating antihistamines provide symptomatic relief but may need to be continued for several weeks after the inciting event. Some experts add histamine H2 blockers if H1 monotherapy is unsuccessful. Glucocorticoids play a minimal role in management of urticaria unless the process is severe and unremitting. Epinephrine plays no role unless there is concomitant angioedema or anaphylaxis. Agents such as aspirin or alcohol, which aggravate cutaneous vasodilation, should be avoided. Doxepin is used in chronic urticaria unresponsive to histamine blockade but would not be the first agent chosen.

391. The answer is a. This patient's diffuse hair loss after a severe illness is caused by telogen effluvium. Normal hair follicles go through a life cycle. Approximately 5% are in the death (telogen) phase where the hair shaft is released. In telogen effluvium, the hair follicles are "shocked" by the systemic stress, and many enter the telogen phase at the same time. The diagnosis is made by careful history and physical examination. CBC, ANA, and hormonal levels will be normal. Topical treatments are ineffective. The patient will recover fully in a month or two, although a wig may be necessary to hide cosmetically troubling alopecia in the meantime.

Diffuse hair loss may be seen with many drugs or with systemic illnesses such as hypothyroidism, systemic lupus, syphilis, or iron deficiency, but there is no evidence of any of these illnesses in this patient. Male pattern baldness (androgen-dependent alopecia) is seen in normal men, in some older women, and in women with androgen excess, but the hair loss affects the crown and frontal region rather than the scalp diffusely. The dramatic and acute hair loss of telogen effluvium does not occur in male pattern baldness.

392. The answer is a. This patient's ethnicity, her skin lesions, her hilar lymphadenopathy, and the streaky lung infiltrates suggest the diagnosis of sarcoidosis. The painful nodules on the legs represent erythema nodosum, a hypersensitivity reaction associated with several inflammatory conditions. Erythema nodosum can be seen with sarcoidosis, TB, inflammatory bowel disease, several other infectious processes, or can be idiopathic. Biopsy of one of the tender nodules would reveal a nonspecific panniculitis (inflammation of the subcutaneous fat) and would not be helpful diagnostically. Biopsy of one of the plaques, however, could reveal noncaseating granulomas characteristic of sarcoidosis and would be helpful in ruling out the less likely infectious pathogens. Skin biopsy is safer and less expensive than an invasive procedure such as mediastinoscopy. In the absence of sputum production, fever, or weight loss, AFB and fungal studies are unlikely to be productive. The serum ACE assay is nonspecifically elevated in many systemic granulomatous diseases and plays a minor role in the assessment and management of a patient with sarcoidosis.

393. The answer is e. In 20% of cases, diffuse itching is a manifestation of systemic illness. Renal insufficiency, obstructive liver disease (especially primary biliary cirrhosis), hematological conditions (such as polycythemia vera or lymphoma), and thyroid disorders can all present in this fashion. Although most patients with pruritus will have dry skin (xerosis) or dermatitis (usually the primary dermatitis is apparent from the examination), this patient's weight loss and anorexia should prompt a search for an underlying disorder. Topical agents, oral antihistamines, or doxepin (a tricyclic antidepressant with potent H_1 and H_2 blocking effects) can be used for symptomatic purposes but should not replace a search for an underlying cause in this elderly patient with new onset of symptoms. Depression can cause weight loss, but severe pruritus would be an unlikely presenting symptom. Excoriations are nonspecific manifestations of scratching; unless a specific primary lesion (eg, papule, vesicle) is found, skin biopsy will rarely be helpful in the evaluation of pruritus.

394. The answer is a. Cutaneous squamous cell carcinoma (SCC) is a malignant neoplasm of the keratinocytes; it can grow rapidly and may metastasize (1%-3% of cases). Actinic keratosis is considered a precancerous lesion.

Clinically, SCC commonly presents as an ulcerated erythematous nodule or superficial erosion on the skin. SCC can occur anywhere on the body but is most common on areas of sun-damaged skin, including the lower lip. Nodular lesions should be excised. Psoriasis is a chronic inflammatory disease characterized by well-marginated erythematous papules and plaques covered by a silvery scale. A complication of this disease is asymmetric arthritis of the distal and proximal interphalangeal joints. Ulceration is not seen in psoriatic plaques. Melanomas are malignant neoplasms of the melanocytes with metastatic potential. Metastasis and prognosis are related to depth of invasion. Melanomas, however, usually have areas of definite hyperpigmentation. Basal cell carcinoma (BCC) is the most common skin cancer, accounting for 70% to 80% of nonmelanoma skin cancers. It usually has a characteristic rolled or undermined border with telangiectasias around the lesion. Local invasion can be a serious problem, but BCCs almost never metastasize.

395. The answer is b. Target lesions, especially with nonblanching violet or petechial centers, are classic manifestations of erythema multiforme. Blanchable lesions and blisters may be found as well. Common causes of erythema multiforme include drugs and herpesvirus infections (especially herpes simplex or Epstein-Barr virus). It is most important to identify the offending agent, as continuation of a causative drug can lead to oral involvement, systemic illness, and the full-blown Stevens-Johnson syndrome (SJS). The rash may take 4 to 6 weeks to resolve. Readministration of the causative agent should be scrupulously avoided. Phenytoin, sulfa drugs, barbiturates, and penicillin are common causes. The rash, with its target lesions, should not be confused with toxic shock syndrome, which causes a blanchable erythema followed by desquamation of palms and soles. Rocky Mountain spotted fever causes a distal petechial rash as a result of endothelial damage. Neurodermatitis (associated with anxiety) and xerotic eczema (associated with drying agents) would not cause target lesions.

396. The answer is d. The lesion has characteristics of melanoma (remember ABCDE: *a*symmetry, irregular or ill-defined *b*order, dark black or variegated *c*olor, *d*iameter >6 mm, and *e*nlargement over time). A full-thickness excisional biopsy is required for diagnosis and should not be delayed. Shave biopsy of a suspected melanoma makes the assessment of depth of invasion difficult. Diagnosis is urgent; the lesion cannot be observed over time. After the diagnosis of melanoma is made, the tumor must then be staged to determine prognosis and treatment.

397. The answer is b. The description and location of these lesions are suggestive of eruptive xanthomas. Eruptive xanthomas occur primarily on buttocks or extensor surfaces and are associated with elevated triglycerides. Tophaceous gout can result in deposits of monosodium urate, usually in the skin around joints of the hands and feet. Tophi are usually white and may discharge a chalky material. Skin biopsy is not usually necessary to distinguish these lesions. The cutaneous lesions of sarcoidosis (which would usually show disease on CXR) are reddish-brown waxy papules, usually on the face. Obstructive liver disease can occasionally cause palmar xanthomas, which are seen as yellow plaques along the palmar creases.

Xanthomas can be important cutaneous clues for underlying lipid disorders. Xanthelasmas, yellowish plaques on the inner aspect of the upper eyelids, are nonspecific but are associated with hyperlipidemia 50% of the time. Tendon xanthomas are important clues for familial hypercholesterolemia. Tuberous xanthomas, which often present as plaques or even polypoid nodules over pressure points, usually signify hypercholesterolemia. Eruptive xanthomas, again, are associated with triglyceride levels above 1000 mg/dL. Treatment of the hypertriglyceridemia usually results in resolution of lesions. Biopsy of a xanthoma would show lipid-containing macrophages, but is usually not necessary for diagnosis.

398. The answer is d. Although most drug-induced rashes are self-limited and benign, this patient has developed skin necrosis as a consequence of phenytoin treatment and must be hospitalized in a burn unit. Even with modern supportive care, mortality is at least 25%. Treatment is largely supportive; steroids are controversial. Antibiotics are withheld unless the patient develops evidence of infection, but electrolyte disturbances are common and should be anticipated. The name given to this condition varies with severity. If target lesions and mucosal involvement are not accompanied by skin necrosis, the patient is said to have erythema multiforme. Stevens-Johnson syndrome (SJS) implies approximately 10% body surface area involvement, while toxic epidermal necrolysis (TEN) indicates >30% BSA necrosis. Most cases of TEN are caused by medications, especially antiepileptic drugs, antibiotics, and allopurinol. Outpatient management and even general ward admission do not give proper consideration to the considerable mortality and morbidity of SJS and TEN.

399. The answer is d. The description of this papulosquamous disease is classic for pityriasis rosea. This disease occurs at some time in about 10%

of the population, usually in young adults. Pityriasis rosea primarily affects the trunk and proximal extremities; it is usually asymptomatic, although some patients have an early, mild viral prodrome (malaise and low-grade fever), and itching may be significant. Drug eruptions, fungal infections, and secondary syphilis may mimic this disease, but the lesions of pityriasis rosea are usually centripetal (redder in the middle) while most tinea lesions are centrifugal (redder on the edges). Fungal infections (tinea) are rarely as widespread and sudden in onset; potassium hydroxide (KOH) preparation will be positive. Psoriasis, with its thick, scaly plaques on extensor surfaces, should not cause confusion. A rare condition called guttate parapsoriasis should be suspected if the rash lasts more than 2 months, since pityriasis rosea usually clears spontaneously in 6 weeks. Lichen planus is a papulo-squamous disorder, but it causes intensely pruritic polygonal plaques, often with intraoral involvement. It would not cause a "Christmas tree" pattern on the back as seen in this patient. Secondary syphilis is characterized by lymphadenopathy, oral patches, and lesions on the palms and soles (a VDRL test will be strongly positive at this stage).

400. The answer is d. The patient has the typical areas of involvement of seborrheic dermatitis. This common dermatitis appears to be worse in many neurological diseases. It is also very common and severe in patients with AIDS. In general, symptoms are worse in the winter. UV radiation improves the condition. *Pityrosporum ovale* appears to play a role in sebor-rheic dermatitis and dandruff, and the symptoms improve with the use of certain antifungal preparations (eg, ketoconazole) that decrease this yeast. Mild topical steroids also produce an excellent clinical response. High-dose topical steroids are rarely necessary; when used on the face for long peri-ods of time, they can cause irreversible atrophy and thinning of the skin. Oral fluconazole is used in refractory *Candida* infections, which usually affect the oral mucosa (thrush), the vaginal mucosa or moist intertriginous areas. Psoriasis (which can cause destructive arthritis) should be easily dis-tinguishable by the pattern of involvement (psoriasis does not usually affect the face) and by its characteristic thick micaceous scale.

401. The answer is c. This woman has onychomycosis, which often affects the toenails in an asymmetric pattern. Onychomycosis does not usually resolve spontaneously and is more difficult to eradicate than is tinea pedis (athlete's foot). The etiologic agents include several species of yeast, mold, and dermatophytes, therefore, direct microscopy and/or fungal culture may be necessary for definitive therapy. The condition is often asymptomatic and may not require treatment. Topical therapies are effective, but require daily application for many months. They have the advantage of safety. Oral treatment with terbinafine or itraconazole is more effective than topical treatment but must also be continued up to 6 months; oral antifungals carry the risk of hepatotoxicity. Yellow nail syndrome should be considered in the differential for widespread yellow nail changes and is associated with pulmonary disease and cancers. Yellow nail syndrome affects all 20 nails; a workup for systemic disease is unnecessary in the usual patient with onychomycosis.

402. The answer is d. Rosacea is a common problem in middle-aged, fair-skinned people. Sun damage appears to play an important role. Stress, alcohol, and heat contribute to the flushing. Men may develop rhinophyma (connective tissue overgrowth, particularly of the nose). Low-dose oral tetracycline, erythromycin, and metronidazole control the symptoms. Topical metronidazole, azelaic acid, and sodium sulfacetamide also work well. The carcinoid syndrome causes flushing but not papules and pustules and is usually associated with gastrointestinal symptoms; it is quite rare. Porphyria cutanea tarda can cause telangiectasias and can be associated with alcohol consumption, but patients with this disease usually have increased facial hair growth and fragile skin in sun-exposed areas as well. The butterfly-shaped macular rash of lupus does not cause pustules; usually the patient has other evidence of active disease, especially synovitis. Seborrheic dermatitis affects the eyebrows and nasolabial folds more prominently than the cheeks and nose.

403. The answer is b. This is a classic description of basal cell carcinoma. Basal cell carcinoma is a malignant neoplasm of the epidermal basal cells that clinically presents as a pearly papule or nodule with a central ulceration, raised borders, and telangiectasias. Basal cell carcinomas are locally invasive and rarely metastasize; distant spread is reported in fewer than 0.1% of these cancers. Invasion of surrounding tissue and metastasis are more frequently seen in squamous cell carcinoma. Squamous cell carcinoma is a malignant neoplasm of the keratinocytes; it is much more aggressive than basal cell carcinoma, grows rapidly, and may metastasize via lymphatic spread. Bacterial infections such as meningococcemia and necrotizing fasciitis could result in septicemia without appropriate treatment but are acute, not chronic, conditions.

404. The answer is b. The possibility of cutaneous anthrax in this postal worker is the most important consideration in the era of bioterrorism concern. The lesion described would be characteristic of cutaneous anthrax—beginning as a small papule that is painless and progressing to a black, necrotic lesion over several days. A skin biopsy would show the very characteristic gram-positive rods of anthrax. Cutaneous anthrax has occurred in postal workers who have handled letters containing anthrax spores, but can also occur in those who handle infected animals or their wool or hides. Unlike inhalational anthrax, these patients do not appear severely ill at the outset of the infection. Ecthyma gangrenosum also produces a black, necrotic skin lesion. These lesions occur in patients who are bacteremic and systemically ill from *P aeruginosa*. Ecthyma gangrenosum lesions are smaller and more widely disseminated (due to the bacteremia) than this patient's lesion. The brown recluse spider's bite can also produce a black necrotic ulcer. The bite is painful and usually spreads rapidly; systemic symptoms such as nausea, vomiting, myalgias and fever often accompany the bite. The bubo of plague produces a tender lymphadenitis. The patient with plague or necrotizing fasciitis is acutely ill with fever and other signs of systemic inflammatory response syndrome.

405. The answer is b. Although there have been no cases of smallpox in the world since 1977, the threat of bioterrorism has forced physicians to be vigilant about the disease's reemergence. It will be important for students and physicians to recognize the distinguishing characteristics of chickenpox versus smallpox. In chickenpox, lesions are more concentrated on the trunk. In smallpox, lesions are more likely to occur on face, palms, and soles. In chickenpox, lesions are more superficial, come out in crops, and are in many different stages of development. In smallpox, lesions are characteristically in the same stage of development. In chickenpox, fever usually occurs at the time of the appearance of the rash. In smallpox, fever and prostration precede the rash by several days; patients appear severely ill.

406. The answer is c. Blistering diseases are potentially serious conditions. Blisters that are smaller than 0.5 cm are termed vesicles; larger lesions are called bullae. The proper diagnosis and treatment of bullous disorders are paramount in order to prevent disability and even death from burn-like denudation of the skin and associated infection. Although many skin diseases such as allergic contact dermatitis, erythema multiforme, and bullous impetigo can cause blisters, this patient is more likely to have bullous pemphigoid or pemphigus. These are immunologically mediated disorders. Skin biopsy with immunofluorescence staining will reveal antibodies at the basal layer of the epidermis (bullous pemphigoid) or within the epidermis (pemphigus). Mucosal, especially oral, involvement is characteristic of pemphigus. Immunosuppressive agents including systemic corticosteroids are often necessary to treat these conditions. Antihistamines, sometimes helpful if itching is prominent, will not treat the underlying condition. It is no longer felt that bullous dermatoses are indicative of underlying malignancy, so a "shotgun" search for occult malignancy is not recommended. Dermatitis herpetiformis and porphyria cutanea tarda are other skin diseases that can be associated with blisters.

407. The answer is c. Topical steroids are widely used in dermatology, but their potency varies widely (1000-fold difference between 1% hydrocortisone cream and ultra-high potency clobetasol). Chronic use of high-potency topical steroids on the face often leads to permanent telangiectasias and atrophy of the skin ("cigarette-paper" skin") and should be avoided. The lowest-potency preparation that is effective should be employed. Use of ultrapotent preparations in occluded areas such as axillae can even cause systemic absorption and hypothalamic-pituitary-adrenal axis suppression and cataracts; children are particularly susceptible to side effects of absorbed corticosteroids.

This woman has a classic history for atopic dermatitis, a condition that often pursues a relapsing-remitting course; it may be associated with asthma and eosinophilia. Antihistamines, although effective as antipruritics, have little effect on the rash. Systemic steroids should be avoided in all but the most refractory cases. Skin moisturization, avoidance of triggers such as heat or stress, and topical calcineurin inhibitors (tacrolimus, pimecrolimus) are other potentially effective treatments.

408. The answer is c. Trauma, onychomycosis, and medication effect are common causes of dark nail pigmentation, but this patient's linear pigmentation and the hyperpigmentation of the nail fold (Hutchinson sign) are worrisome features for an acral subungual melanoma. This patient should be referred to a dermatologist or surgeon for biopsy.

Traumatic subungual hematoma often affects the toenails after vigorous exercise such as marathon running, when the nail may be pulled up off the nail bed. The patient will usually recall the event, and a linear pattern would be unusual. Papulosquamous disorders such as psoriasis and lichen planus often affect the nails, but they usually cause pitting or a roughened thickening of the nail surface. Numerous nails (both fingernails and toe-nails) are usually affected in psoriasis. Inspection of the nails can indicate underlying systemic disorders such as hypoalbuminemia (Beau lines) and lead poisoning, but these conditions do not cause nail hyperpigmentation.

409. The answer is d. This patient has Kaposi sarcoma (KS). In HIV-infected individuals, KS is associated with human herpesvirus 8 (HHV-8). KS lesions are derived from the proliferation of endothelial cells in blood/lymphatic microvasculature. They present as violaceous patches, plaques, and/or nodules on the skin, mucosa, and/or viscera. The pulmonary infiltrates observed on the chest x-ray of this patient are the result of visceral KS affecting the lungs. KS has become uncommon in the era of highly active antiretroviral therapy (HAART). Proliferation of neoplastic T cells is seen in cutaneous T-cell lymphomas such as mycosis fungoides. Human herpesvirus 6 (HHV-6) is the cause of exanthema subitum (roseola) in children. It consists of 2- to 3-mm pink macules and papules on the trunk following a fever. *Mycobacterium avium* causes fever and weight loss in HIV patients with a CD4 count less than 50/μL but would not cause skin and oral plaques as seen in this patient. Immunodeficient patients or patients with HIV who are infected with HSV can present with the disseminated form of the disease. However, these lesions consist of a vesicular rash that is different from the violaceous plaques observed in KS.

Suggested Readings

1. Kasper DL, Fauci AS, Hauser SL, Longo DL, Jameson LJ, Loscalzo J. *Harrison's Principles of Internal Medicine.* 19th ed. New York: McGraw-Hill; 2015. Chapters 70, 71, 72, 74.
2. Wolff K, Johnson RA, Saavedra AP. *Fitzpatrick's Color Atlas and Synopsis of Clinical Dermatology.* 7th ed. New York: McGraw-Hill Education; 2013.
3. Dermatology Practice and Management Guidelines, available at: http://www.aad.org.
4. Patel RV, Lebwohl M. In the clinic. Psoriasis. *Ann Intern Med.* 2011;155: ITC2 1-15.
5. Stern RS. Clinical practice. Exanthematous drug eruptions. *JAMA.* 2012;366:2492-2501.
6. YosipovitchG, Bernhard JD. Clinical practice. Chronic pruritus. *JAMA.* 2013;368:1625-34.

General Medicine and Prevention

Questions

410. A 53-year-old woman with type 2 diabetes mellitus is found to have a blood pressure of 152/98. She has never had any ophthalmologic, cardiovascular, or renal complications of diabetes or hypertension (HTN). Based on recent recommendations of the JNC 8 (The Eighth Report of the Joint National Committee on Prevention, Detection, Evaluation, and Treatment of High Blood Pressure), which of the following is the currently recommended goal for blood pressure control in this case?

a. Less than 160/90
b. Less than 145/95
c. Less than 140/90
d. Less than 130/80
e. Less than 120/70

411. A 60-year-old man has just moved to town and needs to establish care. He had a "heart attack" last year. Preferring a "natural" approach, he has been very conscientious about low-fat, low-cholesterol eating habits and a significant exercise program. He has gradually eliminated a number of prescription medications (he does not recall their names) that he was on at the time of hospital discharge. His medical history is negative for hypertension, diabetes, or smoking. His lipid profile shows the following:

Total cholesterol: 194 mg/dL
Triglycerides: 140 mg/dL
HDL: 42 mg/dL
LDL (calculated): 124 mg/dL
ECG shows Q waves in leads II, II, and aVF consistent with an old inferior MI

Based on the 2013 Guidelines for the American College of Cardiology/American Heart Association (ACC/AHA) which of the following recommendations would you make for treatment of his lipid disorder?

a. Continue current dietary efforts and exercise.
b. Add a high intensity statin (atorvastatin or rosuvastatin).
c. Add a fibric acid derivative such as gemfibrozil or fenofibrate.
d. Review previous medications and resume an angiotensin-converting enzyme (ACE) inhibitor.
e. Have the patient buy over-the-counter fish oil tablets and take 2 g in the morning and 2 g in the evening.

412. A 60-year-old man had an anterior myocardial infarction 3 months ago. He currently is asymptomatic and has normal vital signs and a normal physical examination. His echocardiogram shows a mildly depressed ejection fraction of 40%. He is on an antiplatelet agent, statin, and an ACE inhibitor. What other category of medication would typically be prescribed for secondary prevention of myocardial infarction?

a. Alpha-blocker
b. Beta-blocker
c. Calcium-channel blocker
d. Nitrates
e. Naproxen sodium

Questions 413 to 415 relate to the following abstract.

Title: What factors predict bicyclists colliding with motor vehicles?

Background: We wished to identify risk factors for bicyclists colliding with a motor vehicle (bicycle-MVC).

Methods: We reviewed emergency department records from 2000 to 2010 and identified 214 bicyclists presenting with an injury related to a bicycle-MVC. These bicyclists were compared to a control group of bicyclists (matched for age and gender) seen in the emergency department over the same time period for injuries not related to a MVC.

Results: In multivariate logistic regression, odd ratios for suffering a bicycle-MVC are included in the following table:

Characteristic	N	Odds Ratio	95% Confidence Limits
Injury occurring before dawn or after dark	106	2.0	1.2-4.5
Age of bicyclist > 50 years	130	3.1	1.9-5.0
Bicyclist riding against traffic	32	1.9	0.8-7.6

Conclusions: Bicycling after age 50 and bicycling before dawn or after dark puts bicyclers at risk for an injury-producing collision with a motor vehicle.

413. The epidemiologic type of study described in this abstract is best characterized as:

a. A randomized controlled trial
b. A case-control study
c. A cohort study
d. A cross-sectional study
e. A meta-analysis

414. A major advantage of the type of epidemiologic study described in this abstract is:

a. It is the best type of study to test for cause-and-effect.
b. It is the best type of study for determining disease incidence.
c. It is an easy way to determine disease prevalence at one point in time.
d. It is often the only practical way to study a rare disease or occurrence.
e. It combines data from several studies to improve statistical power.

415. What is the reason that the abstract authors did not include "bicyclist riding against traffic" as a characteristic associated with an injury-producing collision with a motor vehicle?

a. Statistical significance is defined as an odds ratio of 2.0 or greater.
b. The odds ratios of the other characteristics were higher.
c. The lower limit of the 95% confidence level is <1.
d. Statistical significance is not necessarily clinically relevant.
e. The number of patients in this category is too few.

416. You are the primary care physician for a 78-year-old man with severe dementia, coronary artery disease, chronic obstructive pulmonary disease (COPD), hyperlipidemia, and HTN. He takes hydrochlorothiazide, lisinopril, metoprolol, aspirin, simvastatin, and tiotropium as well as oxygen at 2 L/min. The patient no longer recognizes his wife or other family members and requires total care at a nursing home facility. The wife approaches you stating that her husband never wanted to live like this and instructs you to stop all of his medications including the oxygen and to enroll him in hospice for comfort care. The patient's living will states that his wife is to make decisions if he becomes incapacitated. The patient's two grown children object to this plan and ask you to continue all current medications. What is the appropriate next step?

a. Hold a family conference and explain that you would prefer that the family come to consensus, but if not you will need to follow the wife's expressed wishes as she legally has the power of attorney.
b. Continue all medications and follow the wishes of the children while explaining to the wife that a majority of the family desires this course of action.
c. Request an ethics consult to make the decision.
d. Attempt to negotiate separately with the wife and children for a middle ground course of action such as stopping all medications except the oxygen.
e. Advise the family that if they cannot come to an agreement they will need to find a new physician.

417. A 42-year-old banker sees you as a new patient. He states that he is healthy and takes no regular medications. His examination is normal except for a blood pressure of 150/94. When questioning him about alcohol use, he admits that he goes out drinking with friends several nights each week to relieve stress. At these times he will often have 8 to 10 mixed alcohol drinks. He and his wife have recently had several arguments about this habit, and she has threatened to divorce him if he doesn't change his ways. Despite this, he has been unable to change. On one occasion he was arrested for driving while intoxicated. Nonetheless, he has continued to be successfully employed, has never been hospitalized for an alcohol-related problem, and has never had symptoms of alcohol withdrawal. Which of the following statements regarding treatment of this patient is true?

a. Advice from a physician to reduce his alcohol consumption is likely to be successful.
b. Treatment of his alcohol use disorder should include complete abstinence from alcohol and participation in a mutual aid group.
c. Abstinence from alcohol may necessitate treatment of his blood pressure because he is currently using alcohol to treat stress.
d. Medications for alcohol dependence are not usually helpful.
e. The fact that this patient has had no symptoms of alcohol dependence demonstrates that he does not misuse alcohol.

418. A 26-year-old stockbroker sees you because she has felt anxious almost every day for the past 9 months. She feels "keyed up" at work. At times she has difficulty concentrating and has made several minor errors in clients' accounts. For the past year she has frequently had trouble falling asleep at night despite the fact that she always feels tired. She does not fall asleep during the day at inopportune times. She denies substance or alcohol abuse. Her vital signs and physical examination are normal. CBC, TSH, and chemistry panel are normal. What is the most appropriate initial treatment alternative?

a. Long-acting benzodiazepine such as clonazepam on a regularly scheduled basis
b. Selective serotonin reuptake inhibitor (SSRI) such as citalopram
c. Tricyclic antidepressant such as amitriptyline
d. Atypical antipsychotic such as olanzapine
e. Centrally acting antihypertensive such as clonidine

419. A 25-year-old PhD candidate recently traveled to Central America for 1 month to gain information regarding the socioeconomics of that region. While there, he took ciprofloxacin twice a day for 5 days for diarrhea. However, over the 2 to 3 weeks since coming home, he has continued to have occasional loose stools plus vague abdominal discomfort and bloating. His symptoms are more severe after a fatty meal, and he has lost 5 lb since his return. He denies rectal bleeding, fever, or chills. Which of the following therapies is most likely to relieve this traveler's diarrhea?

a. Another course of ciprofloxacin
b. Doxycycline
c. Metronidazole
d. Trimethoprim-sulfamethoxazole
e. Oral glucose-electrolyte solution

420. A 42-year-old pediatric nurse practitioner seeks your advice regarding his immunization needs. He is healthy and takes no regular medications. He had well-documented chickenpox as a child. He received a tetanus-diphtheria booster 5 years ago and influenza vaccine 2 months ago. Influenza A activity has been reported in your community in the past 2 weeks. Which of the following immunizations would you recommend for this patient at this time?

a. An influenza booster
b. Tetanus-diphtheria-acellular pertussis (Tdap)
c. Pneumococcal vaccine
d. Herpes zoster vaccine
e. Meningococcal vaccine

421. You see a debilitated 80-year-old woman who is being admitted to a nursing home in June. She has had no immunizations for many years except for a "tetanus" booster 15 years ago and a 23-valent pneumococcal polysaccharide vaccine (PPSV23) 3 years ago when discharged from the hospital after a stay for pneumonia. Which of the following immunizations should be given at this time?

a. Influenza vaccine
b. *Haemophilus influenzae* B immunization
c. Hepatitis B immunization series
d. Revaccination with PPSV23
e. Tetanus-diphtheria-acellular pertussis (Tdap)

422. A 52-year-old woman with a history of hypertension and diabetes comes to the office for review of preventive medicine recommendations. She had a mammogram at age 50 but has had no other preventive medicine tests or advice that she can recall. She does not smoke cigarettes, does not drink alcohol, and is overweight (BMI = 29). Her mother developed breast cancer at age 75 and her father had colon cancer detected at age 65. According to the U.S. Preventive Services Task Force, which combination of screening tests should you recommend?

a. Screening mammography, a chest x-ray, colonoscopy, a screening aortic sonogram, and a bone density scan
b. Screening mammography, Pap smear, and colonoscopy
c. Screening mammography, a chest CT scan, colonoscopy, and a bone density scan
d. Screening mammography, a CA-125 blood test, Pap smear, and a bone density scan
e. Screening mammography, colonoscopy, and a bone density scan

423. A 26-year-old medical student plans a 3-week mission trip to Mexico. She will be staying with local villagers and working indoors in a rural area 30 minutes from Mexico City. She has previously been vaccinated for hepatitis B. Of the following choices, which vaccination is most important?

a. Inactivated poliovirus vaccine (IPV) booster
b. Hepatitis A vaccine
c. Rabies vaccine
d. Meningococcal vaccine
e. Dengue vaccine

424. A 28-year-old laborer sees you because of low back pain. Ten days ago he strained his back while moving a refrigerator. Despite taking acetaminophen, his pain has worsened. He has difficulty sleeping because of the pain and for the past 3 days he has spent most of the day in bed. He has not had fever, leg numbness or weakness, or bladder or bowel problems. He takes no regular prescription medications. On examination he has difficulty getting on and off the examination table because of back pain. He has normal vital signs including a normal temperature. There is evidence of bilateral paraspinous muscle spasm. The patient is able to walk on his heels and toes and has negative straight leg raising test bilaterally. What is the best next step in the management of this patient?

a. Two-view lumbar spine x-ray
b. MRI of the lumbar spine
c. Continued bed rest
d. A nonsteroidal anti-inflammatory drug (NSAID) and physical therapy
e. Epidural steroid injection

Question 425 pertains to the following pharmaceutical advertisement.

Malignant melanoma is now the seventh most common cancer in the United States. The lifetime risk of melanoma in certain fair-skinned people is one in 75. SONPROTECTA is a new drug approved by the FDA for the prevention of melanoma in fair-skinned people.

Indications: SONPROTECTA is indicated for the prevention of melanoma in fair-skinned persons age 35 to 55 with a history of severe sunburn as a child.

Important Safety Information: SONPROTECTA can result in worsening seizures in patients who have an underlying seizure disorder and is contraindicated in such patients.

Adverse Reactions: The most common adverse reactions (SONPROTECTA incidence ≥ 5% more than placebo) include dry mouth (9% vs 2%), flatus (33% vs 25%), and brittle hair (7% vs 2%).

Efficacy: In a recent large multicenter prospective, randomized, double-blind, placebo-controlled trial, SONPROTECTA resulted in a 91% reduction in melanoma occurrence when administered over a 5-year period. Over 20,000 adults with Fitzpatrick I skin type were enrolled at multiple medical centers in the United States and Australia and were randomized to receive SONPROTECTA or placebo for 5 years (see the following Table). They were followed in a blinded fashion every 6 months by dermatologists who biopsied all suspicious lesions.

	SONPROTECTA (*n* = 10,000)	Placebo (*n* = 10,000)	Percent reduction	*p*-value
Persons developing melanoma	5	55	91%	<0.001

425. How many fair-skinned persons would need to take SONPROTECTA for 5 years to prevent one of them from developing melanoma?

a. 9
b. 50
c. 91
d. 200
e. Cannot be determined from the information provided

426. A 22-year-old man is persuaded by his wife to come to you for a general checkup. She hints of concern about alcohol use. He admits to drinking on average three to four beers every night with more on the weekends. He used alcohol rarely until 2 years ago when his brother died. He has never had withdrawal symptoms after several days of abstinence. What would be a practical next step to take that might help you further evaluate the physical consequences of this patient's drinking?

a. Order ultrasound of the liver
b. Order CT scan of the abdomen
c. Order liver function tests including aspartate transaminase (AST), alanine transaminase (ALT), gamma-glutamyl transpeptidase (GGT), and a complete blood count (CBC)
d. Order esophagogastroduodenoscopy (EGD) to look for silent esophageal varices
e. Order α-fetoprotein level and a CA-19-9 level

427. A 55-year-old woman comes to the clinic with insomnia, fatigue, 10-lb weight loss over the past month, loss of interest in most activities, and diminished ability to concentrate. She was widowed 2 years ago and lives alone. She denies delusions, hallucinations, and suicidal ideation. Physical examination is normal and basic laboratory workup is negative, including a normal TSH and CBC. You diagnose her with depression. Which of the following statements is true?

a. There is no advantage to initiating combination of pharmacotherapy and psychotherapy over prescribing either alone.
b. She should be admitted to a psychiatric facility.
c. Levels of neurotransmitters such as norepinephrine and serotonin are often low or effects are underactive in these patients.
d. The initial pharmacologic agent of choice is a tricyclic antidepressant such as amitriptyline.
e. Electroconvulsive therapy is recommended for most initial episodes.

428. A 65-year-old woman was hospitalized for pulmonary embolus and eventually discharged on warfarin (Coumadin) with a therapeutic INR. During the next 2 weeks as an outpatient, she is started back on her previously prescribed ACE inhibitor, given temazepam for insomnia, treated with ciprofloxacin for a urinary tract infection, started on over-the-counter famotidine for reflux symptoms, and told to stop the naproxen she was taking for osteoarthritis. A subsequent INR is 5.0. Which of the following drugs most likely potentiated the effects of warfarin and led to the high INR?

a. ACE inhibitor
b. Temazepam
c. Ciprofloxacin
d. Famotidine
e. Naproxen discontinuation

429. A 20-year-old college basketball player is brought to the university urgent care clinic after developing chest pain and palpitations during practice. There is no dyspnea or tachypnea. He denies family history of cardiac disease, and social history is negative for alcohol or drug use. Cardiac auscultation is unremarkable, and ECG shows frequent premature ventricular contractions (PVCs). Which of the following is the most appropriate next step in evaluation and/or management?

a. Obtain urine drug screen
b. Arrange treadmill stress test
c. Obtain Doppler ultrasound of deep veins of lower legs
d. Institute cardioselective beta-blocker therapy
e. Institute respiratory therapy for exercise-induced bronchospasm

Questions 430 and 431 relate to the following scenario.

A 38-year-old man is brought to the emergency department because of obtundation. He has a history of back pain and takes oxycodone. Admission vital signs include BP 90/50 mm Hg, heart rate 50 beats/min, respiratory rate 4 breaths/min, temperature 35.8°C (96°F). Pupils are dilated. Naloxone is administered and within 2 minutes the patient becomes alert and awake. Inquiry into your state Prescription Drug Monitoring Program reveals that he has been receiving prescriptions from multiple providers for large quantities of oxycodone. Four hours later you are preparing to discharge the patient when the nurse reports that he is again unarousable and has a respiratory rate of 6 breaths/min.

430. What is the most likely explanation for the fact that the patient has become unarousable 4 hours after naloxone administration?

a. The half-life of naloxone is shorter than the half-life of oxycodone.
b. The patient has surreptitiously taken opiates in the emergency department.
c. The patient has developed aspiration pneumonia.
d. The patient has developed ketoacidosis.
e. Drowsiness is a side effect of naloxone.

431. Which opiate receptor is primarily responsible for opiate addiction and abuse?

a. Delta (etorphine)
b. Kappa (butorphanol)
c. Mu (morphine)
d. Orphanin
e. Opiate receptors are not associated with addiction and abuse

432. A 42-year-old man sees you because of obesity. He played football in high school and at age 18 weighed 250 lb. He has gradually gained weight since. Many previous attempts at dieting have resulted in transient weight loss of 10 to 15 lb, which he then rapidly regains. He has been attending weight watchers for the past 3 months and has successfully lost 4 lb. Recent attempts at exercise have been limited because of bilateral knee pain and swelling. On examination height is 6 ft 0 in, weight 340 lb, BMI 46. Blood pressure with a large cuff is 150/95. Baseline laboratory studies including CBC, biochemical profile, thyroid-stimulating hormone, and lipids are normal with the exception of fasting serum glucose, which is 145 mg/dL. What is the best next step?

a. Discuss bariatric surgery with the patient
b. Refer to a commercial weight-loss program
c. Recommend a 1000-calorie per day diet
d. Prescribe phentermine
e. Recommend a low-fat diet

433. A 54-year-old man sees you for follow-up of hypertension and a seizure disorder that is well controlled. He established as a new patient 2 months ago and now returns for his second office visit with you. At the time of his initial visit he admitted to a 35-year history of smoking 2 packs of cigarettes per day. At that time he indicated that he was not interested in stopping smoking and seemed irritated when you suggested that he quit. Today his blood pressure is well controlled and there are no new medical issues. With regard to discussing cessation of cigarette smoking during today's visit, what is the best next step?

a. Do not discuss cessation of cigarette smoking because it will likely upset him again.
b. Do not discuss cessation of cigarette smoking, because there is no real benefit to cessation of cigarette smoking after smoking this long.
c. Ask him if he is still smoking, and, if so, advise him to quit and assess his willingness to do so.
d. Recommend bupropion.
e. Recommend that he switch to smokeless tobacco.

434. A 70-year-old man with unresectable carcinoma of the lung metastatic to liver and bone has developed progressive weight loss, anorexia, and shortness of breath. The patient has executed a valid living will that prohibits the use of feeding tube in the setting of terminal illness. The patient becomes lethargic and stops eating altogether. The patient's wife of 30 years now insists on enteral feeding for her husband. Which of the following is the most appropriate course of action?

a. Respect the wife's wishes as a reliable surrogate decision maker.
b. Resist the placement of a feeding tube in accordance with the living will.
c. Ask the daughter to make the decision.
d. Place a feeding tube until such time as the matter can be discussed with the patient.
e. Request a court order to place a feeding tube.

435. A 32-year-old, overweight, diabetic woman is found to have a triglyceride level greater than 1000 mg/dL. Family history is positive for diabetes, pancreatitis, and premature coronary artery disease. TSH is normal. You advise the patient to follow a low-fat diabetic diet, to exercise regularly, and to avoid alcohol. What medication would be most appropriate to start at this time?

a. High-dose rosuvastatin
b. Nicotinic acid
c. Low-dose atorvastatin
d. High-dose fenofibrate
e. Over-the-counter fish oil

436. A 40-year-old obese man presents with intense pain in his left first metatarsophalangeal (MTP) joint for the past few hours. He has no history of trauma, fever, chills, and no previous similar episode. He has no history of renal disease or diabetes though he has been told he is "prediabetic." He does not recall any recent skin infections and no family members have had any reported staphylococcal infection. On examination he has a swollen, red, warm, tender first MTP joint on the left. Uric acid level is 9 mg/dL; serum creatinine is normal. What is the best treatment approach for this patient?

a. Start allopurinol immediately and titrate for a uric acid level below 6. Add colchicine if this is not effective within the first 24 hours.
b. Begin prednisone until symptoms subside.
c. Begin indomethacin. As the patient improves, reduce the dose to minimize gastrointestinal side effects.
d. Prescribe a narcotic until pain is under control.
e. Refer the patient to a rheumatologist.

437. A 42-year-old man with long-standing daily alcohol ingestion comes to the emergency department with visual hallucinations. He stopped drinking alcohol 3 days ago. He has had no vomiting or diarrhea, and takes no medications. His family reports that he has been consuming a normal diet. On examination blood pressure is 140/90 mm Hg, pulse rate is 120 beats/min, respiratory rate is 20 breaths/min, and he is afebrile. He appears anxious and agitated and has a diffuse tremor of the outstretched hands. Laboratory studies include the following: Na = 136, K = 2.9, Cl = 102, bicarb = 25, BUN = 8, creatinine = 0.9. What is the most likely mechanism for the hypokalemia?

a. Laboratory error
b. Renal tubular acidosis
c. Poor oral intake
d. Cellular shift
e. Alcoholic ketoacidosis

438. A 44-year-old woman comes to clinic with concerns about her family history of diabetes and high blood pressure. Her height is 62 in, weight 50 kg (110 lb), BMI is 20 kg/m², waist circumference 33 in (85 cm), and blood pressure 138/88. Laboratory evaluation reveals fasting glucose of 120 mg/dL. Lipid profile shows total cholesterol 240 mg/dL, HDL 38 mg/dL, and triglyceride 420 mg/dL; LDL cannot be calculated. She does not smoke, use alcohol, or take any medications. Which of the following is correct regarding the identification of the metabolic syndrome in this patient?

a. Metabolic syndrome is not present in this case due to the absence of abdominal obesity.
b. Metabolic syndrome is not present because the blood pressure is not sufficiently elevated to be a risk factor.
c. Metabolic syndrome is not present because the glucose is not sufficiently elevated to be a risk factor.
d. Metabolic syndrome is present based on the risk factors given.
e. Metabolic syndrome cannot be identified until the LDL is determined.

Questions 439 to 441

The initial choice of an antihypertensive or the addition of further agent(s) to the regimen may depend on concomitant factors. For each case below, indicate the medication choice that would give the best additional benefit in addition to blood pressure control. Each lettered option may be used once, more than once, or not at all.

a. Alpha-blocker
b. Beta-blocker
c. Calcium-channel blocker
d. Angiotensin-converting enzyme inhibitor
e. Centrally acting alpha agonist
f. Thiazide diuretic
g. Angiotensin receptor blocker (ARB)

439. An obese 54-year-old white woman has a hemoglobin A_{1C} of 9.5 and elevated urine microalbumin.

440. A 62-year-old man has a history of a myocardial infarction and has chronic stable angina.

441. A 49-year-old woman with a history of congestive heart failure and a low ejection fraction (35%) following an episode of viral myocarditis is well controlled with furosemide, low-dose carvedilol, and lisinopril. She develops a persistent dry cough without obvious infectious or allergic etiology.

Questions 442 and 443

Many times the most important step that can be taken to reduce morbidity and mortality from common medical conditions such as diabetes and cardiovascular disease is to focus on lifestyle and/or risk factor modification. For each patient below, choose the most important step to take next. Each lettered option may be used once, more than once, or not at all.

a. Urge the patient to quit smoking and discuss the various available medications to assist in the process.
b. Recommend an exercise program such as brisk walking for at least 30 minutes per day and a low salt, Dietary Approaches to Stop Hypertension (DASH) diet.
c. Prescribe a low-cholesterol diet and statin drug.
d. Recommend aspirin (81 mg) daily.
e. Encourage a diet of smaller portions, lower-fat content, and reduced overall calories.
f. Prescribe chlorthalidone 12.5 mg daily.

442. A 45-year-old, healthy nonsmoking woman with a normal BMI (24) has been found on two occasions to have a blood pressure of 145/95. She has no family history of premature coronary artery disease.

443. A 60-year-old obese man (BMI 32) with coronary artery disease smokes a pack of cigarettes per day. He has recently begun a weight-loss program that includes diet and exercise. He is taking aspirin and a statin. He refuses to take any more prescription medications at this time.

Questions 444 to 447

For each patient below, select the most appropriate screening tests or preventive measures. Each lettered option may be used once, more than once, or not at all.

a. Administer the first dose of one of the available human papillomavirus (HPV) vaccines.
b. Intermediate strength tuberculin skin test followed by a repeat test 1 month later if the first test is negative.
c. Abdominal ultrasonography.
d. Chest x-ray.
e. Rapid plasma reagin (RPR).

444. A 23-year-old asymptomatic unmarried woman who is in a monogamous relationship. She is not pregnant.

445. A 67-year-old male smoker with stable chronic cough.

446. A 32-year-old female smoker who is beginning employment at a hospital as a nurse's aide.

447. A 70-year-old woman admitted to a nursing home with diabetes, hypertension, and Alzheimer disease.

General Medicine and Prevention

Answers

410. The answer is c. Treatment goals for the management of high blood pressure recommended by JCN 8 are 140/90 for all hypertensive persons younger than 60 years. In the past, more stringent blood pressure lowering has been recommended for diabetics and persons with chronic kidney disease, but JCN 8 recommends the same goal (140/90) for these patients as well. Other major recommendations by JNC 8 include (1) a treatment goal for persons aged 60 or older should be 150/90 or below; (2) treatment for adults with chronic kidney disease (including blacks) should include an angiotensin-converting enzyme inhibitor (ACEI) or angiotensin receptor blocker (ARB); (3) initial treatment for nonblack populations (including those with diabetes) should be thiazide-type diuretic, calcium-channel blocker (CCB), ACEI, or ARB; and (4) initial treatment for black populations should include a thiazide-type diuretic or CCB.

411. The answer is b. The controversial 2013 American College of Cardiology/American Heart Association guidelines recommend high intensity statin therapy for (1) patients with a history of a cardiovascular event (myocardial infarction, stroke, stable or unstable angina, peripheral artery disease, transient ischemic attack, or coronary or other arterial revascularization); (2) adults with an LDL-cholesterol of 190 mg/dL or higher; and (3) diabetics age 40 to 75. Either moderate or high-intensity statins are recommended for patients age 40 to 75 years without cardiovascular disease or diabetes who have a 7.5% or higher risk for having a heart attack or stroke within 10 years. Ten-year CVD risk is calculated from the Pooled Cohort data from the Framingham study; patients with a 10-year risk of 5% to 7.5% should be "considered" for statin therapy. Gemfibrozil is used primarily for hypertriglyceridemia; this patient's triglyceride level is normal (<150 mg/dL). ACE inhibitors have no significant effect on lipids. While high-dose fish oil does lower triglyceride levels, it is not effective at lowering LDL cholesterol levels and has not been shown to decrease CVD events. Lowering LDL cholesterol is of prime importance in the prevention of coronary heart disease.

412. The answer is b. In patients who have had a myocardial infarction, beta-blockers are documented to lower the risk of myocardial reinfarction and sudden death, whereas some calcium-channel blockers may increase the risk. Alpha-blockers have been associated with an increased risk of congestive heart failure. ACE inhibitors are beneficial in this setting and should be continued. Despite their decades-long use for the symptomatic treatment of angina, nitrates are not indicated for secondary prevention of infarction. Recently, long-term use of some nonsteroidal anti-inflammatory drugs (including naproxen sodium) has been associated with an increased risk of myocardial infarction.

413 to 415. The answers are 413-b, 414-d, 415-c. Case-control studies (one type of observational study) compare patients with a disease to a group of patients without the disease. Selecting an appropriate control group (patients without the disease) is very important to minimize confounders. Case-control studies are often the only practical way to study rare diseases. Randomized controlled trials are experimental studies in which a group of patients are randomly assigned to a treatment and compared to a group of patients who do not get the treatment. These studies are often expensive but are the best way to determine cause and effect. Another type of observational study is a cohort study, which follows a group of subjects over time (the "cohort") and then determines which patients develop a certain disease, such as a group of miners, some of whom were exposed to uranium. The advantage of cohort studies is that they can determine incidence and often suggest etiology. Another type of observational study is a cross-sectional study, in which a group of patients are studied at one point in time to see if they have a particular disease. These studies are usually easy and inexpensive; they can determine prevalence but not incidence. A meta-analysis combines the results of several studies in order to improve statistical power.

Odds ratio is an estimate of relative risk that case-control studies report. Odds ratios are calculated for each study variable and can be calculated even in studies with relatively few patients. In order for an odds ratio to be considered statistically significant, the entire confidence interval must lie between 0 and 1.0 or be above 1.0 ("not cross 1"). In this instance, the lower limit of the 95% confidence interval for the variable "bicyclist riding against traffic" (0.8) is less than 1, thus the odds ratio would not be considered statistically significant. Statistical significance for odds ratios can also be reported as a p-value; a p-value of 0.05 or less is usually considered statistically significant. Statistical significance may or may not be clinically relevant. If the group of patients treated with a new antihypertensive drug has a statistically significant systolic blood pressure that is 1 mm lower than the control group, we would probably consider this clinically unimportant. Thus, proper interpretation of a study requires more than just looking at p-values and odds ratios.

416. The answer is a. The patient has a valid living will in place that clearly states the wife should make decisions when the patient becomes incapacitated. Ultimately this advance directive must be honored even if the majority of family members wish something different. Consulting an ethics committee may be helpful when documentation of the patient's wishes is unclear, but in this case the advance directive clearly appoints the wife as surrogate decision maker. In general, ethics committees make recommendations and not decisions. When there are differences among family members, a family conference is often more helpful than discussing these issues with family members separately. You should do your best to explain to the children why their mother's decision is not only legally acceptable but ethically acceptable as well. Their father had expressed his wishes, and his current poor quality of life is not something he had wanted to prolong. You could emphasize that no action will be taken to hasten their father's death and that he will be provided compassionate care until the day he dies naturally. Serving as an advocate for the patient, even when the patient has lost decision-making capacity, is an essential role of the physician.

417. The answer is b. This patient has an alcohol use disorder, which is defined as a maladaptive pattern of alcohol use causing clinically significant impairment or distress. Men who consume more than 14 drinks per week or 4 drinks on any one day, and women who consume more than 7 drinks per week or more than 3 drinks on any one day are at risk for this disorder. This patient has had significant marital discord, has been unable to cease alcohol use, and has had an arrest for driving while intoxicated. All of these indicate that the patient has clinically significant impairment from alcohol abuse. Alcohol use disorder may or may not be accompanied by alcohol dependence, which is characterized by symptoms and signs of alcohol withdrawal during periods of abstinence. Patients with alcohol use disorder are usually unable to limit the amount of alcohol that they consume, and therefore complete abstinence from alcohol is recommended. Mutual help groups (such as Alcoholics Anonymous) as well as medications (such as acamprosate and naltrexone) can be helpful in maintaining abstinence. Physician advice alone is usually unsuccessful. Alcohol use disorder is frequently accompanied by other psychiatric disorders such as depression. Alcohol use disorder can aggravate hypertension; blood pressure will improve with abstinence. Current understanding of alcohol use disorder suggests that there is a genetic tendency to this illness.

418. The answer is b. This patient meets criteria for generalized anxiety disorder (GAD). The disorder is more common in woman than men (2:1) and age of onset is usually in the 20s. In general, a combination of pharmacologic and psychotherapeutic interventions is most effective for generalized anxiety disorder. The best agent for a patient with daily symptoms is a serotonin-specific reuptake inhibitor (SSRI). SSRIs are safe and effective. Nausea and sexual impairment (anorgasmia in women, erectile dysfunction in men) are common side effects; patients may be reluctant to volunteer sexual side effects unless specifically questioned. Because worsening of anxiety symptoms may occur shortly after initiating therapy with a SSRI, recommended starting doses are half of those used for treatment of depression. Short-acting benzodiazepines are often used on an "as-needed" basis. Longer-acting benzodiazepines tend to accumulate active metabolites and cause sedation with impairment of cognition and hence are not the first choice. Dependence is a serious problem when any benzodiazepine is used for more than a few weeks or on a scheduled basis. Second-line agents for GAD include buspirone, beta-blockers, and anticonvulsants with GABAergic properties such as pregabalin. Tricyclic antidepressants are rarely used because of side effects and toxicity. Atypical antipsychotic agents would not be used for GAD although they are effective for agitation in patients with bipolar disorder. Clonidine is a centrally acting antihypertensive that has not been shown to be effective for GAD.

419. The answer is c. Patients with symptomatic *Giardia lamblia* infection typically present with several weeks of bloating, loose stools, and weight loss. Most patients respond to metronidazole therapy. This protozoan parasite is contracted by ingesting contaminated food or water from freshwater streams or closed water supplies in developing countries. Giardiasis is rarely associated with fever and person-to-person transmission is responsible for the majority of human cases. Bacterial pathogens such as *Campylobacter jejuni,* enterotoxigenic *Escherichia coli, Salmonella,* and *Shigella* usually cause acute diarrhea, often bloody. These illnesses usually respond to fluoroquinolones or azithromycin. Many bacterial pathogens in developing countries are resistant to trimethoprim-sulfamethoxazole. Oral glucose-electrolyte solution rehydration is the mainstay of *Vibrio cholerae* therapy. Hydration rather than antibiotics is also the key for enterohemorrhagic *E coli.*

420. The answer is b. The Advisory Committee on Immunization Practices (ACIP) is an independent panel of experts and makes evidence-based immunization recommendations for children and adults. Tetanus-diphtheria-acellular pertussis (Tdap) should replace a single dose of tetanus-diphtheria (Td) for all adults who have not previously received this vaccine. Health care workers should be vaccinated with the tetanus-diphtheria-acellular pertussis vaccine (Tdap), especially those health care workers who have direct patient contact with infants. Yearly influenza immunization is recommended for all health care workers. A single dose of trivalent influenza vaccine is recommended each year beginning in October. Booster doses for influenza are not recommended. The ACIP recommends pneumococcal vaccination for all adults aged 65 and older, and for younger adults with certain medical illnesses such as chronic obstructive pulmonary disease, diabetes mellitus, HIV infection, or asplenia. Herpes zoster vaccine is recommended for adults 60 years of age or older. Meningococcal vaccine is recommended for adults with anatomic or functional asplenia, complement deficiencies, and first-year college students who live in dormitories. Up-to-date ACIP recommendations can be found on the website of the Immunization Action Coalition (http://www. immunize.org/).

421. The answer is e. A tetanus-diphtheria booster should be given every 10 years. The tetanus-diphtheria-acellular pertussis (Tdap) vaccination should be used in all adults if they have never received Tdap. A flu shot should be given in this age group, but at the appropriate time in the fall. There is no recommendation to give the *Haemophilus* immunization in adults. This patient is not in one of the high-risk categories for hepatitis B (including health care workers, hemodialysis patients, routine recipients of clotting factors, travelers to endemic areas, persons at elevated risk for sexually transmitted diseases, injection drug users, those in long-term institutional care, and household contacts of hepatitis B carriers) and therefore has no specific indication to receive this series. In persons over age 65 who have previously been vaccinated with the 23-valent pneumococcal polysaccharide vaccine (PPSV23) after age 64, a dose of the 13-valent pneumococcal conjugate vaccine (PCV13) is recommended 1 year later. A booster dose of PPSV23 is recommended 6 months after PCV13 vaccination only for adults who received the PPSV23 before age 65.

422. The answer is b. According to USPSTF recommendations, a woman aged 52 years should have a mammogram every 2 years and a Pap smear at least every 3 years. She should also have had colorectal cancer (CRC) screening (colonoscopy or fecal occult blood testing yearly) starting at age 50 if there is no family history of CRC in a first-degree relative. Chest x-rays are not recommended as a screening tool for lung cancer in smokers. The USPSTF recommends annual screening for lung cancer with low-dose computed tomography in adults aged 55 to 80 years who have a 30-pack-year smoking history and currently smoke or have quit within the past 15 years. Screening should be discontinued once a person has not smoked for 15 years or develops a health problem that substantially limits life expectancy or the ability or willingness to have curative lung surgery. A bone density scan is recommended for women at age 65 unless they have risk factors for fragility fracture (chronic steroid use, low BMI, smoking, alcohol abuse, secondary cause of low bone mass, among others), which this patient does not have. A screening aortic sonogram is recommended for male smokers (or prior smokers) once between the ages of 65 and 75, but is not recommended at all for women. While a CA-125 has been shown to detect ovarian cancer somewhat earlier than without screening, no mortality benefit has been demonstrated; hence it is not recommended.

423. The answer is b. Travel to developing countries is becoming more common and exposes the traveler to uncommon infectious diseases. The physician can obtain up-to-date professional advice for travelers at the CDC Travel Medicine website (http://www.cdc.gov/travel/default.aspx). For travel to most countries outside of North America and Europe, hepatitis A vaccine and typhoid vaccine are recommended. Polio vaccine is recommended for travel to areas where polio is endemic, including a few countries in Africa, Asia, and Southeast Asia. Rabies vaccination is recommended for travelers who will be spending time in rural areas and outdoors where they might encounter rabid animals, especially if it will be several days journey to a major metropolitan area where rabies biologicals would be available. Malaria prophylaxis is recommended for most of Africa, Southeast Asia, the Middle East, and Central and South America. If traveling to an area reporting chloroquine-resistant malaria, mefloquine, atovaquone/proguanil, or doxycycline are usually the drugs of choice. Meningococcal vaccine is recommended before travel to sub-Saharan Africa and for pilgrims to Mecca. There is no vaccine against dengue.

424. The answer is d. This patient has acute low back pain. This is a very common complaint seen by primary care physicians and is the most common cause of occupational disability in young persons. In the absence of certain "red flags," patients with acute low back pain can be treated without imaging studies. Clinical "red flags" that would suggest the need for early imaging include recent trauma, age more than 50 years, fever, weight loss, corticosteroid or illicit drug use, bladder or bowel symptoms, progressive radicular symptoms, and a history of cancer. Evidence-based studies demonstrate that nonsteroidal anti-inflammatory drugs, chiropractic manipulation, massage, and cognitive behavioral therapy shorten the duration of symptoms. Bed rest delays recovery. Lumbosacral spine series can identify fractures, but CT scanning and MRI scanning are much more sensitive for detecting herniated discs, if evaluation becomes indicated. Epidural corticosteroids may help radicular pain that does not respond to initial modalities (evidence of benefit is weak) but would certainly not be indicated for pain localized to the low back and paraspinous muscles.

425. The answer is d. This advertisement reports an impressive relative risk reduction but the relative risk reduction can be misleading, particularly in low-incidence events. Though there were only 5 melanomas in the treatment group versus 55 in the control group, note that melanoma occurs in the baseline population (control group) at a low rate of 55 per 10,000 persons over 5 years. Thus, 10,000 persons had to take the drug for 5 years to prevent 50 melanomas. The absolute risk reduction is 50/10,000 or 0.5%. The number needed to treat is the reciprocal of 0.5% (1/200), that is, 200. The number needed to treat (NNT) is a useful way to think about drug efficacy.

426. The answer is c. This patient's liver enzymes including AST, ALT, and GGT are likely to be at least mildly elevated. On his CBC, the mean corpuscular volume (MCV) may be elevated due to his chronic alcohol intake. Using these laboratory abnormalities, one can explain to the patient that he has a high likelihood of serious physical consequences if he continues drinking. At-risk drinking is considered more than 14 drinks per week or more than 4 drinks at one setting by a man (7 and 3, respectively, for a woman). An ultrasound or CT scan can detect cirrhosis, but cirrhosis does not occur after only 2 years of heavy alcohol use. Surveillance EGD to detect esophageal varices would be recommended if cirrhosis is documented but would be premature at this point. Alpha-fetoprotein is useful in evaluating a liver mass in a patient with cirrhosis as it is usually elevated in the setting of a hepatocellular carcinoma. A CA-19-9 test is used to follow patients with pancreatic cancer.

427. The answer is c. Depression is a common mood disorder which affects up to 30% of the population sometime during their life. It is characterized by a depressed mood lasting longer than 2 weeks and accompanied by other symptoms such as loss of interest and pleasure (anhedonia), difficulty concentrating, feelings of worthlessness or guilt, hopelessness, and fatigue. Patients with depression often have low levels of certain neurotransmitters such as norepinephrine and serotonin. Studies have demonstrated that treatment with a combination of pharmacotherapy and psychotherapy is more effective than treatment with either alone. Psychiatric hospitalization is usually reserved for people who have a major depressive disorder with accompanying suicidal ideation or psychosis. Electroconvulsive therapy may be helpful, but is generally reserved for refractory cases.

428. The answer is c. Medications which inhibit hepatic cytochrome activity (including fluoroquinolones and many other broad-spectrum antibiotics) can potentiate the effect of warfarin (Coumadin). Patients taking warfarin should be advised to review any medication change with their health care provider. ACE inhibitors, benzodiazepines, and famotidine have no effect on the metabolism of warfarin. Nonsteroidal anti-inflammatory drugs may occasionally enhance warfarin's effect, so discontinuing naproxen, if anything, should lower the INR. If the H_2 blocker cimetidine or the proton pump inhibitor omeprazole had been used for gastric acid reduction in this case, either of these can potentiate warfarin and increase the INR. Of interest, the over-the-counter herbal product ginkgo biloba can also potentiate the anticoagulant effect of warfarin.

429. The answer is a. The question of cocaine and/or amphetamine use must be raised in virtually all young adults with cardiovascular symptoms, despite a professed negative history. Therefore, a urine drug screen should be obtained early on. In the absence of dyspnea, recent immobilization, or physical examination evidence of venous thrombosis, workup for asthma or DVT would not be warranted. Beta-blockers can be used for symptomatic treatment of PVCs but not until the more serious issue of substance abuse has been addressed. Cardiovascular complications from cocaine and methamphetamine use include hypertension (which may be severe), arrhythmias, myocardial infarction, stroke, and sudden death.

430. The answer is a. Opiate overdose is characterized by drowsiness or obtundation, hypotension, bradycardia, slow respiratory rate, hypothermia, and dilated pupils. Treatment of opiate overdose includes supportive therapy and administration of naloxone, an opiate antagonist. Naloxone has a relatively short half-life (just a few hours) and repeated doses may be required when the patient has overdosed on a longer acting opiate such as oxycodone or methadone. Patients with opiate addiction may surreptitiously take drugs in the hospital, but this is a less likely explanation in this case. Patients with opiate overdose are at risk for aspiration pneumonia, but this would be associated with tachypnea and not a low respiratory rate. Ketoacidosis can be associated with drowsiness but the normal compensatory response is a respiratory alkalosis which requires tachypnea. Drowsiness is not a side effect of naloxone. Oxycodone is now the most commonly abused opiate, ahead of heroin and morphine.

431. The answer is c. The abuse potential of opiates is primarily related to the Mu (morphine) receptor. This receptor is responsible for sedation analgesia, euphoria, decreased respiratory drive, and suppressed appetite. The Delta receptor is responsible for hormone changes and results in dopamine release. The Kappa receptor also results in analgesia and decreases respirations and appetite, but it is associated with dysphoria and can result in psychosis. The orphanin receptor also results in analgesia, but it is not affected by opiate medications.

432. The answer is a. This patient has morbid obesity (BMI over 40) and has comorbidities of hypertension, diabetes, and osteoarthritis of the knees. At least two large meta-analyses have established that bariatric surgery is more effective than nonsurgical therapy for achieving sustained weight loss and controlling comorbid conditions for patients with morbid obesity. Surgical mortality is low (<1%) and surgery is associated with long-term sustained weight loss of 45 to 65 lb. Several professional organizations, including the American College of Physicians, now recommend bariatric surgery as the treatment of choice for patients with morbid obesity, especially if they have comorbid conditions and have failed dietary therapy. Controlled trials have established that caloric restriction and physical activity can achieve modest weight reduction, usually on the order of 2% to 8%. A review of commercial weight-loss programs demonstrated that Weight Watchers was the most effective but only produced sustained weight reduction of 3% at 2 years. Medications such as orlistat and phentermine are FDA approved for weight reduction but have demonstrated only modest effectiveness. Sibutramine has been removed from the U.S. market due to increased risk of cardiovascular events. This patient has morbid obesity with comorbid conditions and has failed dietary therapy and exercise program. Therefore his physician should discuss the possibility of bariatric surgery for treatment of his obesity.

433. The answer is c. Despite overwhelming evidence of the adverse health effects of cigarette smoking that has accumulated over the past 50 years, 20% of Americans still smoke cigarettes. Cigarette smoking is the most common health behavior associated with preventable death in the United States. Physicians can play a major role in encouraging patients to stop smoking. Evidence shows that even very brief counseling (as little as 3 minutes) in the physician's office can improve smoking cessation rates. Even in long-term smokers, smoking cessation has major health benefits. After cessation of smoking, the risk of myocardial infarction declines by over 50% in 1 year and the risk of lung cancer declines by 3% to 5% per year even in long-term cigarette smokers. Many professional organizations (including the American Medical Association) recommend that physicians should ask their patients whether they are smoking at each visit, advise them to quit, and assess their willingness to do so. If the patient is willing to consider smoking cessation, the physician should assist them in their attempt to quit and arrange follow-up to assess compliance. Behavioral counseling and drug therapy improve the likelihood of smoking cessation. Nicotine replacement therapy, bupropion, and varenicline are FDA-approved for smoking cessation. Nicotine replacement therapy is contraindicated in patients with recent myocardial infarction, angina, and severe arrhythmias. Bupropion is contraindicated in patients who have preexisting seizures. Varenicline has been associated with depression and behavioral abnormalities. Smokeless tobacco carries the risk of oral cancer and is not recommended as treatment for cessation of cigarette smoking.

434. The answer is b. The patient's autonomy as directed by the living will must be respected. This autonomy is not transferred to a surrogate decision maker, even one who is very credible, when a valid living will is in effect. Living wills and other advance directives are completed when patients are competent, and give instructions for their treatment if they become incompetent or unable to express their wishes. A medical power of attorney (POA) assigns decision-making capacity to another person (surrogate) when the patient lacks decisional capacity and when no documentation of the patient's previous wishes is available. A court order is not necessary given clear written evidence of the patient's wishes.

435. The answer is d. A normal triglyceride (TG) level is below 150 mg/dL. A moderate to high triglyceride level is between 150 and 499 mg/dL, and over 500 is considered very high. Obesity increases TG levels by causing increased hepatic very-low-density lipoprotein (VLDL) production. In diabetes, insulin insufficiency leads to decreased lipoprotein lipase activity and impairment of VLDL catabolism. In addition, this patient may have familial hypertriglyceridemia or familial combined hyperlipidemia. All such patients should be advised to follow a low-fat diet. Because of the risk of acute pancreatitis with such high levels of TG, medication should be instituted as well. Patients with levels over 500 should be started on a fibrate such as fenofibrate or gemfibrozil.

While potent statins such as rosuvastatin and atorvastatin decrease TG modestly, they are second-line agents in this situation. Nicotinic acid also reduces TG levels but often elevates the blood glucose level in diabetics. Fish oil in high doses can lower the TG level but not as effectively as fenofibrate or gemfibrozil.

436. The answer is c. This patient is experiencing his first episode of acute gout. The first MTP joint is the most commonly affected, and 80% of acute gout attacks will be monoarticular. Predisposing conditions include trauma, surgery, starvation, high intake of beer and hard liquor (not wine), or diets high in meat and seafood. Certain medications also increase the chances of acute gout including thiazide and loop diuretics and even the initiation of uric acid lowering drugs such as allopurinol and uricosuric agents. Appropriate initial treatment must be tailored to the patient and their comorbidities. The patient in this question has no contraindication, so a potent NSAID (indomethacin) can be used and is likely to be highly effective. Other acceptable alternatives would have been to start colchicine immediately or oral prednisone in relatively high doses. Since this patient is "prediabetic," steroids may result in overt hyperglycemia and hence would not be the first choice. Allopurinol should not be started until the acute attack has been controlled by anti-inflammatory regimens. All agents that lower uric acid levels (either allopurinol or uricosuric agents) can cause worsening of joint pain, probably by mobilizing uric acid microcrystals previously deposited in the synovial membrane. While narcotics may lessen the pain, they are less effective than anti-inflammatories. Referring the patient to a rheumatologist is unnecessary and would leave the patient in pain and suffering in the meantime.

437. The answer is d. Hypokalemia can occur when potassium shifts into cells. This occurs with alkalosis, hyperthyroidism, in the periodic paralysis syndromes, and by the influence of certain substances such as insulin and beta-agonists. Alcohol withdrawal is characterized by high intrinsic catecholamine levels, often resulting in hypokalemia. Hypomagnesemia is often an additional contributing factor. Lysis of red blood cells due to difficult phlebotomy can sometimes result in erroneous hyperkalemia ("pseudohyperkalemia"), but not hypokalemia. Hypokalemia may also occur due to renal potassium losses, when patients are taking diuretics and in congenital renal tubular acidosis. This patient does not have acidosis as evidenced by normal serum bicarbonate. Hypokalemia on rare occasions may be due to poor oral intake, but this patient's history does not suggest dietary insufficiency. Since potassium is the major intracellular cation, dietary potassium deficiency requires a diet free of either plant or animal cells; distilled liquor (as well as the so-called "tea-and-toast" diet) provides such a diet. Acute alcohol ingestion may occasionally result in the accumulation of beta-hydroxybutyrate and other ketoacids ("alcoholic ketoacidosis"), but this would again cause acidosis and a tendency to hyperkalemia (not hypokalemia).

438. The answer is d. The metabolic syndrome represents a cluster of metabolic risk factors for coronary heart disease that are closely linked to insulin resistance. The syndrome can be identified when any three of the following five items are present: abdominal obesity (waist circumference in women >88 cm [>35 in] or in men >102 cm [40 in]), hypertriglyceridemia (>150 mg/dL), low HDL (<50 mg/dL in women or <40 in men), blood pressure greater than or equal to 130/85, and fasting glucose >110 mg/dL. In this case, four risk factors are present, all except abdominal obesity. In addition, hyperinsulinemia decreases the renal excretion of uric acid, resulting in hyperuricemia, although this finding is not part of the metabolic syndrome definition. Persons with metabolic syndrome are at risk for developing diabetes as well as coronary artery disease. The initial management of metabolic syndrome focuses on intensive lifestyle modification including diet, exercise, and weight loss, all of which will improve insulin sensitivity.

439 to 441. The answers are 439-d, 440-b, 441-g. ACE inhibitors give renal protective effect in diabetics with proteinuria, are helpful in CHF, and are protective after ST-elevation MI. Beta-blockers are indicated post-STEMI, in CHF with reduced systolic function, and in various tachyarrhythmia settings; they may help prevent migraines and treat essential tremor. Beta-blocker use in other hypertensive patients has now been relegated to fourth-line status. A dry cough is a common side effect of angiotensin-converting enzyme inhibitors such as lisinopril. The cough occurs in approximately 10% to 20% of patients on this class of medication. ACE inhibitors have been shown by extensive evidence to play an important role in the control of heart failure as well as in reducing mortality in patients with reduced ejection fractions (<40%). An ARB should be substituted in this case, as ARBs have similar cardiac- and renal-protective benefits to ACE inhibitors and rarely cause cough.

Calcium-channel blockers and thiazide diuretics are very useful antihypertensives but have no particular advantage in the above cases. Both are excellent choices in American-American patients, who tend to have volume- rather than RAAS-mediated hypertension. Thiazides significantly decrease the incidence of stroke and are the drug of choice in isolated systolic hypertension of the elderly. Alpha-blockers can improve symptoms in men with BPH but are no longer considered first-line agents for hypertension. Central alpha-agonists (such as clonidine) can rapidly lower blood pressure in a matter of hours; their long-term use is limited by side effects such as drowsiness, constipation, and erectile dysfunction.

442 and 443. The answers are 444-b, 447-a. The first patient can now be diagnosed with hypertension. Given the fact that she is still stage 1, lifestyle modification can safely be attempted before beginning a medication. She should be instructed in a 2.4-g sodium diet, daily aerobic exercise, and a restriction in alcohol intake to no more than one serving per day. If the patient does not respond to lifestyle interventions, then starting with monotherapy such as chlorthalidone at low dose would be a good option.

Chlorthalidone is a thiazide diuretic that has a longer half-life (24-72 hours vs 7-12 hours for HCTZ).

Helping the second patient to quit smoking is the best therapeutic maneuver at this time. A brief discussion regarding the use of nicotine gum, nicotine patches, bupropion, or varenicline should follow. Exploring the living situation (ie, other smokers in the home) and attempting to enlist other family member help in the quitting process can also be helpful. The patient has already instituted many of the other measures, though none of these are as important as quitting smoking.

Statins are important medications in patients with diabetes or established cardiovascular disease and those with a greater than 7.5% chance of developing CVD over the next 10 years. Prophylactic aspirin is modestly helpful in men at increased risk of heart attack and in women at increased risk of stroke; population-wide use is not recommended because of increased risk of hemorrhagic stroke and gastrointestinal bleeding in long-term ASA-treated patients. A portion-limited, low-calorie diet will help promote weight loss in overweight or obese patients.

444 to 447.   The answers are 444-a, 445-c, 446-b, 447-b. The human papillomavirus (HPV) vaccine is approved and recommended by the Advisory Committee on Immunization Practices (ACIP) for young women ages 11 to 26 for the prevention of HPV infection with the goal of reducing the risk of cervical cancer. It is best if the full regimen of the vaccine is given prior to first sexual experience, but it should be given to women in this age group even if they have previous known HPV infection. Two different vaccines are available (Gardasil, a quadrivalent vaccine and Cervarix, a bivalent vaccine); both have been shown to be effective at reducing the incidence of cervical intraepithelial neoplasia and cervical cancer. While checking an RPR would be routine if this patient were pregnant, there is no recommendation for the test at this point and there is no reason to order the other listed tests.

The U.S. Preventive Services Task Force (USPSTF) recommends a single screening aortic ultrasound in men who have ever smoked and who are between the ages of 65 and 75 to identify abdominal aortic aneurysm. There is no such recommendation for women at any age or for men who are older or younger than the listed ages. The USPSTF also recommends annual screening for lung cancer with low-dose computed tomography in adults aged 55 to 80 years who have a 30-pack-year smoking history and currently smoke or have quit within the past 15 years. Anyone entering one of the health care professions or who will have contact with patients should be tested for tuberculosis. People with active tuberculosis or latent tuberculosis should be identified and treated for the protection of the patients and the public. A booster effect can be seen if a person with a negative TB skin test is retested 1 to 4 weeks after the initial test. While this practice reduces the specificity of the test somewhat (since the positive skin test may be related to a previous BCG vaccination, atypical mycobacterium exposure, or remote TB infection), it does increase the sensitivity of the test. If the TB skin test returns positive, the patient will need a chest x-ray to assess for active disease. If the x-ray shows no pulmonary disease suggestive of tuberculosis, the patient with a positive TB skin test is said to have latent TB infection (LTBI). To reduce the risk of reactivation of their tuberculosis, patients should be offered either 6 to 9 months of isoniazid, 4 months of rifampin or isoniazid plus rifapentine once weekly for 12 weeks. Chest x-rays have not proven beneficial in screening programs, even in high-risk groups such as current cigarette smokers.

The USPSTF and the Centers for Disease Control and Prevention (CDC) recommend targeted screening for the detection of latent tuberculosis infection in persons who are at risk for being infected or developing active tuberculosis. This includes persons who live in congregant settings (such as prisons, homeless shelters, and nursing homes), persons who are severely immunocompromised (such as those with HIV infection), persons recently exposed to an active case of tuberculosis, and health care workers. Health care workers and persons entering congregant settings are tested initially and, if negative, then yearly thereafter to detect the acquisition of infection.

Suggested Readings

1. Kasper DL, Fauci AS, Hauser SL, Longo DL, Jameson JL, Loscalzo J. *Harrison's Principles of Internal Medicine.* 19th ed. New York: McGraw-Hill; 2015. Chapters 4, 17e, 29, 97, 148, 416, 421.
2. Immunization Action Coalition, available at: http://www.immunize.org/
3. U.S. Preventative Services Task Force, available at: http://www.uspreventiveservicestaskforce.org/
4. CDC. Traveler's Health Website, available at: http://www.cdc.gov/travel/default.aspx
5. James PA, Oparil S, Carter BL, et al. 2014 evidence-based guideline for the management of high blood pressure in adults: Report from the panel

members appointed to the Eighth Joint National Committee (JNC 8). *JAMA*. 2014;31:507-520. doi:10.1001/jama.2013.284427. Available at: http://jama.jamanetwork.com/article.aspx?articleid=1791497

6. Stone NJ, Robinson J, Lichtenstein AH, et al.;   American College of Cardiology/American Heart Association Task Force on Practice Guidelines. 2013 ACC/AHA guideline on the treatment of blood cholesterol to reduce atherosclerotic cardiovascular risk in adults: A report of the American College of Cardiology/American Heart Association Task Force on Practice Guidelines. *J Am Coll Cardiol*. 2014 Jul 1;63(25 Pt B): 2889-2934. doi: 10.1016/j.jacc.2013.11.002. Available at: http://circ. ahajournals.org/content/early/2013/11/11/01.cir.0000437738.63853.7a. full.pdf

Allergy and Immunology

Questions

448. A 20-year-old woman develops urticaria that lasts for 6 weeks and then resolves spontaneously. She gives no history of weight loss, fever, rash, or tremulousness. She denies any use of medication or drugs; the hives are not related in time to the ingestion of fresh fruits, shellfish, peanuts, or dairy products. Physical examination shows no abnormalities except for a few residual hives in the antecubital fossae. Which of the following is the most likely cause of the urticaria?

a. Connective tissue disease
b. Hyperthyroidism
c. Chronic infection
d. Food allergy
e. Not likely to be determined

449. A 22-year-old man is evaluated because of recurrent pneumonias. He had two sinus infections in childhood, but over the past 18 months he has been treated with antibiotics on seven occasions for sinus infection and/or pneumonia. Review of previous chest x-rays shows that infiltrates were located in several different lobes and segments, and that all have responded to antibiotics, only to recur a few months later. The patient denies weight loss, gastrointestinal (GI) symptoms, or infertility. He does not have chronic fever or other systemic symptoms between episodes. CBC, comprehensive metabolic panel, and urinalysis are normal. What are the best next tests to help understand his recurrent infections?

a. Skin testing with common antigens such as candida or mumps
b. Measurement of antibody response to a protein vaccine such as tetanus-diphtheria
c. HIV testing and measurement of quantitative serum immunoglobulin levels
d. Serum and urine protein electrophoresis
e. Bronchoscopy to exclude endobronchial lesion

450. A 25-year-old woman complains of watery rhinorrhea and pruritus of the eyes and nose. She had mild asthma as an adolescent, but her lower respiratory symptoms have resolved. The nasal symptoms occur throughout the year but are worse in spring and fall. She has no pets in the home and avoids exposure to pollens and grass as much as possible. She has had inadequate symptom relief with month-long trials of daily oral loratadine and cetirizine. She does not use over-the-counter (OTC) decongestants. On physical examination, vital signs are normal. Nasal mucosa is pale and boggy, and she has an "allergic crease" on her nose. There is no sinus tenderness or lymphadenopathy. What is the best next step in the management of her symptoms?

a. Referral to allergist for immunotherapy.
b. Addition of montelukast 10 mg daily to the oral antihistamine.
c. Addition of prednisone 10 mg daily until symptoms are controlled, then taper to lowest dose that controls her symptoms.
d. Addition of daily intranasal glucocorticoid.
e. Addition of daily intranasal cromolyn.

451. A 20-year-old nursing student complains of asthma while on her surgical rotation. She has developed dermatitis of her hands. Symptoms are worse when she is in the operating room. Which of the following statements is correct?

a. This is a benign contact reaction.
b. The patient should be evaluated for latex allergy by skin testing.
c. This syndrome is less common now than 10 years ago.
d. Oral corticosteroid is indicated.
e. She will have to change her career since there is no substitute for latex gloves.

452. A 59-year-old man develops skin rash, pruritus, and mild wheezing 20 minutes after a coronary arteriogram. The symptoms respond to a single dose of epinephrine and diphenhydramine. The angiogram, however, reveals 95% stenosis of the right coronary artery. The cardiologist recommends repeat study with percutaneous angioplasty. What is the best recommendation for this patient's management?

a. The patient cannot receive intravenous contrast agents. Medical management of his coronary stenosis should be pursued.
b. Premedicate the patient with oral N-acetylcysteine and intravenous normal saline and proceed with contrast study.
c. Make sure that a nonionic contrast agent is used, premedicate the patient with corticosteroids, and proceed with the angioplasty.
d. Premedicate the patient with subcutaneous epinephrine and inhaled albuterol and proceed with the angioplasty.
e. Proceed with the angioplasty, with epinephrine and endotracheal tube readily available in the heart catheterization suite.

453. A 16-year-old adolescent girl develops weakness, wheezing, and shortness of breath 5 minutes after receiving intramuscular ceftriaxone for gonorrhea. She is on no other medications. On examination, she is anxious and in respiratory distress. BP is 80/50, HR is 142, and RR is 40. She has large hives on her chest, and her tongue is edematous. She has both wheezing and stridor. Which of the following is most important immediate treatment?

a. Intramuscular or intravenous epinephrine 0.3 mg STAT
b. Intravenous epinephrine 1 mg IV push
c. Intravenous methylprednisolone 100 mg and diphenhydramine 50 mg
d. Intravenous normal saline 1 L over 20 minutes
e. Intravenous dopamine titrated to a mean arterial pressure of 60 mm

454. A 32-year-old woman complains of severe seasonal allergies. Every year from April through July she is miserable with sneezing, nasal congestion, and watery itchy eyes. Antihistamines, nasal corticosteroids, nasal saline washes, oral montelukast, and attempts to avoid potential antigens have proven unsuccessful. She requests referral to an allergist for "allergy shots." What advice should you give her about immunotherapy (hyposensitization) for her allergic symptoms?

a. Immunotherapy is useful in asthma but not in allergic rhinitis.
b. Immunotherapy is used in allergic rhinitis because there is no risk.
c. The beneficial effect of immunotherapy goes away as soon as the shots are discontinued.
d. Immunotherapy against respiratory organisms can decrease the incidence of bacterial sinusitis.
e. Immunotherapy requires the identification of specific antigen by dermal or serum testing.

455. A 55-year-old farmer develops recurrent cough, dyspnea, fever, and myalgia several hours after entering his barn. He has had similar reactions several times previously, especially when he feeds hay to his cattle. Which of the following statements is true?

a. The presence of fever and myalgia indicates that this is an infectious process.
b. Immediate-type IgE hypersensitivity is involved in the pathogenesis of his illness.
c. The causative agents are often thermophilic actinomycete antigens.
d. Demonstrating precipitable antibodies to the offending antigen confirms the diagnosis of hypersensitivity pneumonitis.
e. Chronic lung disease does not occur in this setting.

456. A 35-year-old woman is concerned that she may be allergic to certain foods. She gets a rash several hours after eating small amounts of peanuts. In evaluating the possibility of food allergies, which of the following is correct?

a. At least 30% of the adult population is allergic to some food substance.
b. Symptoms usually occur hours after ingestion of the food substance.
c. The foods most likely to cause allergic reactions include egg, milk, seafood, nuts, and soybeans.
d. The organ systems most frequently involved in allergic reactions to foods in adults are the respiratory and cardiovascular systems.
e. Immunotherapy is of proven benefit for food allergies.

457. A 32-year-old woman with a history of migraine headaches on prophylactic propranolol experiences a severe anaphylactic reaction following a sting from a yellow jacket (wasp). She is treated successfully with parenteral epinephrine and is dismissed from the hospital. What is the best recommendation for prevention of recurrent hospitalizations?

a. Pursue desensitization injections against *Hymenoptera* species.
b. Discontinue beta-blockers.
c. Avoid exposure to bees as well as wasps.
d. Carry an epinephrine self-injector (Epi-pen) with her during outdoor activities.
e. Take loratadine 10 mg daily.

458. A 62-year-old man is diagnosed with neurosyphilis. Seven years ago he had an anaphylactic reaction to a penicillin shot which was administered for streptococcal pharyngitis. He required treatment with epinephrine and reports that he "almost died." What is the best approach to the management of his neurosyphilis?

a. Oral doxycycline
b. Intravenous ceftriaxone
c. Oral erythromycin
d. No treatment available
e. Penicillin desensitization followed by parenteral penicillin G

459. A 31-year-old homeless man is admitted with a diffuse pneumonia. He has a history of alcohol and IV drug abuse and has not been in the health care system since leaving high school at age 16. He is found to be HIV positive with a CD4 count of 11/mm^3. His pneumonia responds to trimethoprim-sulfamethoxazole. His nutritional status improves, and a long-term care bed is secured to make sure he gets his medications and nutritional support. You want to make sure that all appropriate vaccines have been given. Which vaccine is contraindicated in this patient?

a. Pneumococcal conjugate vaccine
b. Hepatitis B vaccine
c. Influenza vaccine
d. Herpes zoster vaccine
e. Hepatitis A vaccine

Questions 460 and 461

For each clinical description, select the one most likely immunologic deficiency. Each lettered option may be used once, more than once, or not at all.

a. Wiskott-Aldrich syndrome
b. Ataxia telangiectasia
c. DiGeorge syndrome
d. Immunoglobulin A deficiency
e. C1 inhibitor deficiency
f. Severe combined immunodeficiency (SCID)

460. A 16-year-old adolescent boy has recurrent episodes of nonpruritic, nonerythematous, angioedema. There is a family history of angioedema. The patient has also complained of recurring abdominal pain.

461. A 42-year-old man requires transfusion for blood loss resulting from an automobile accident. During the infusion, he develops urticaria, stridor, and hypotension requiring IV epinephrine. Further history reveals frequent episodes of sinusitis and bronchitis.

Questions 462 and 463

For each patient, select the most likely immunologic deficiency. Each lettered option may be used once, more than once, or not at all.

a. Complement deficiency C5-C9
b. Postsplenectomy
c. Drug-induced agranulocytosis
d. Interleukin-12 receptor deficit
e. Hyper-IgE (Job) syndrome
f. Adenosine deaminase deficiency

462. A 30-year-old man has developed fever, chills, and neck stiffness. Cerebrospinal fluid shows gram-negative diplococci. He has had a past episode of sepsis with meningococcemia.

463. A 22-year-old man has been healthy except for abdominal surgery after an auto accident. He is admitted with clinical signs of pneumonia and meningitis. Cultures of blood, sputum, and cerebrospinal fluid grow gram-positive diplococci.

Allergy and Immunology

Answers

448. The answer is e. Urticaria (hives) presents as well-circumscribed wheals with raised serpiginous borders. Individual lesions usually persist less than 24 hours, only to be replaced by other hives at other locations. The process may be triggered by a specific antigen such as food, drugs, or pollen. It may also be bradykinin-mediated, such as in hereditary angioedema, or complement-mediated, as in hypocomplementemic vasculitis. Some chemical agents cause urticaria by direct (ie, non-IgE mediated) effect on mast cells, either by mast cell degranulation (narcotics, radiocontrast agents) or by affecting arachidonic acid metabolism (aspirin, NSAIDs). These causes should be sought in the history; however, in the great majority of patients with urticaria, a cause is never found. Very rarely, urticaria accompanies illnesses such as chronic infection, myeloproliferative disease, collagen vascular disease, or hyperthyroidism. Usually, however, the patient with one of these illnesses displays clinical evidence of the underlying process.

449. The answer is c. Evaluation of patients with recurrent infections starts with history, physical examination, and review of microbiological records. A history of infertility would raise the issue of immotile-cilia syndrome or cystic fibrosis. Lymphadenopathy might indicate an underlying lymphoma. Patients with T-cell disorders tend to have infections like those seen in acquired immunodeficiency syndrome, mucocutaneous candidiasis, *Pneumocystis* pneumonia, cryptococcal meningitis, and disseminated fungal or mycobacterial infections. Patients with neutrophil disorders have serious infections with gram-positive cocci (especially *Staphylococci*), gram-negative rods, and invasive fungal infections such as *Aspergillus* or *Mucor*. Patients with terminal complement deficiencies have disseminated infections with gonococci or meningococci. Patients with asplenia have sepsis with encapsulated organisms (pneumococcus, *Haemophilus influenzae*, *Salmonella*). In this patient with recurrent common bacterial infections, evaluation for an immunoglobulin production problem should start with assessment of quantitative immunoglobulins (including IgG subclass quantification). As patients with HIV infection have disordered immunoglobulin production early in their illness (eg, 100-fold increased incidence of pneumococcal pneumonia), HIV status should be assessed as well. If this patient is found to have common variable immunodeficiency, he would benefit from monthly IgG infusions.

Skin testing for common antigens to assess delayed hypersensitivity (T-cell function) is no longer felt to be reliable enough for clinical use. Measurement of antibody response to Td vaccination is used in some research laboratories but is not the first study ordered. This young patient without bone pain is unlikely to have multiple myeloma as a cause of his B-cell dysfunction. If the patient had recurrent pneumonias in the same lobe or segment, bronchoscopy would be considered; an endobronchial lesion, however, would not account for the sinus infections.

450. The answer is d. Allergic rhinitis is caused by allergens that trigger a local hypersensitivity reaction. Specific IgE antibodies attach to mast cells or basophils. Mast cell degranulation leads to a cascade of inflammatory mediators. This woman's other atopic symptoms, seasonal exacerbations, and negative medication history suggest that other causes of rhinitis (vasomotor rhinitis, rhinitis medicamentosa) are unlikely. Itching and sneezing are more common in allergic rhinitis than in vasomotor rhinitis, where nasal discharge and congestion are the dominant complaints. In allergic rhinitis, nasal turbinates appear pale and boggy (rather than red and inflamed as in viral rhinosinusitis).

Avoidance measures alone are often ineffective. Oral nonsedating antihistamines are useful in mild cases (although they are ineffective at relieving nasal congestion). The most effective treatment is daily use of a potent nasal corticosteroid, which provides symptom relief in 70% of patients. Side effects are uncommon, although with prolonged use the risks of osteopenia and hypothalamic-pituitary-adrenal (HPA) axis suppression are increased. The leukotriene antagonist montelukast and immunotherapy are reserved for patients who fail to respond to nasal steroids. Long-term use of systemic steroids should be avoided because of the high risk of serious side effects. Intranasal cromolyn can be tried in mild cases but is less effective than a potent intranasal corticosteroid.

451. The answer is b. Latex allergy has become an increasingly recognized problem. This is an IgE-mediated hypersensitivity to latex products, particularly surgical gloves. Patients present with localized urticaria at the site of contact, but can also have serious manifestations such as generalized urticaria, wheezing, laryngeal edema, and hypotension. A scratch test with latex extract is the most sensitive approach to diagnosis. The test must be done with caution since anaphylaxis can occur. Education with avoidance of latex products is the best approach to management. Vinyl gloves can be substituted for latex, although she will still need to be cautious because latex is present in so many medical devices (including mundane objects such as enema tubes). Corticosteroids might be used in severe asthma or anaphylaxis but, because of long-term side effects, would not be part of routine management.

452. The answer is c. Signs and symptoms of radiocontrast media sensitivity include tachycardia, wheezing, urticaria, facial edema, and hypotension, occurring within 20 minutes of the injection of a radiocontrast agent. The risk is greater if ionic contrast agents are used, if the patient has a history of dye reaction, and if the patient has a history of asthma. Use of a beta-blocker increases the risk slightly and also blunts response to adrenergic agents used in treatment of dye reactions. The most important preventive measure is making sure that a nonionic agent is used (most procedures in the United States already use these more expensive agents). Although some controversy exists, the standard of care in the United States is to premedicate the patient with corticosteroids, often starting with oral agents the day before the procedure if possible.

Intravenous saline and (occasionally) oral *N*-acetylcysteine are used to prevent dye-mediated acute kidney injury but have no effect on direct mast-cell degranulation. Epinephrine might precipitate myocardial ischemia in this patient and should be used only if anaphylactic shock occurs; pre-procedure albuterol has not been studied. Resuscitative drugs and equipment are available in every catheterization laboratory but should be supplemented in this case by preventive measures.

453. The answer is a. This patient has severe anaphylaxis (anaphylactic shock) and immediate treatment may be lifesaving. Epinephrine is the cornerstone of treatment. For mild to moderate cases, subcutaneous epinephrine is recommended. If the patient is in shock, cutaneous perfusion may be compromised and IM or IV epinephrine is preferable. The proper dose is 0.3 mg (0.3 mL of the 1:1000 solution, diluted if given intravenously), repeated if necessary at 5- to 10-minute intervals. The 1-mg container of epinephrine, available on the "crash cart," is reserved for cardiac arrest. Antihistamines such as diphenhydramine can be used for mild urticaria but are ineffective in anaphylaxis. Corticosteroids are not helpful acutely; they are given to prevent the "second wave" of mediator release that can occur 8 to 12 hours after the initial event. Intravenous saline is important in the management of shock, but will not relieve the laryngospasm and bronchospasm. Epinephrine will elevate the blood pressure more promptly than saline. Dopamine is less effective than epinephrine in anaphylactic shock; in addition it takes longer to uptitrate the infusion rate than it does to give every-5-minute boluses of epinephrine.

454. The answer is e. Antigen immunotherapy has been proven to be more effective than placebo in the management of severe allergic rhinitis, but the specific antigen(s) must be identified before allergy shots are begun. Ideally, the test result should correlate with the patient's symptoms (time of year of attacks, exposure history, etc). Immunotherapy requires a long-term commitment; treatment duration of less than a year is ineffective. Once a 3- to 5-year course is completed, however, the beneficial effect can persist for years. Evidence for benefit in asthma is LESS compelling than in allergic rhinitis. The chief drawbacks to allergy shots are the time-commitment, expense, and the risk of severe allergic reaction to the injected immunogen. Thirty to fifty deaths are reported each year from anaphylaxis to allergy shots. There is no evidence that specific immunotherapy to bacterial pathogens decreases the incidence of sinusitis or respiratory infections.

455. The answer is c. Hypersensitivity pneumonitis is characterized by an immunologic inflammatory reaction in response to inhaled organic dusts, the most common of which are thermophilic actinomycetes, fungi, and avian proteins. In the acute form of the illness, exposure to the offending antigen is intense. Cough, dyspnea, fever, chills, and myalgia typically occur 4 to 8 hours after exposure. Patients are often suspected of having an infection, especially pneumonia, but the history of previous similar symptoms on antigen exposure should suggest hypersensitivity pneumonitis. In the subacute form, antigen exposure is moderate, chills and fever are usually absent, and cough, anorexia, weight loss, and dyspnea dominate the presentation. In the chronic form of hypersensitivity pneumonitis, progressive dyspnea, weight loss, and anorexia are seen; pulmonary fibrosis is a permanent and sometimes fatal complication.

Almost all patients have IgG antibody to the offending antigen, although positive serology is common in asymptomatic patients and is therefore not diagnostic. While peripheral T-cell, B-cell, and monocyte counts are normal, a suppressor T-cell functional defect can be demonstrated in these patients. IgE does not play a role, so the symptoms begin hours (not minutes) after antigen exposure. Inhalation challenge with the suspected antigen and concomitant testing of pulmonary function can confirm the diagnosis but are seldom used. Therapy involves avoidance; steroids are administered in severe cases. Bronchodilators and antihistamines are not effective.

456. The answer is c. Food allergy is an IgE-mediated reaction to antigens in food. It is caused by glycoproteins found in shellfish, peanuts, eggs, milk, nuts, and soybeans. Symptoms occur within minutes (not hours) of ingestion in most patients. The incidence of true food allergy in the general population is uncertain but is likely to be about 1% of patients—less than might be generally perceived. Studies have demonstrated that breastfeeding can decrease the incidence of allergies to food in infants genetically predisposed to developing them. Food allergy symptoms most commonly affect the gastrointestinal tract (cramping, diarrhea) and the skin (urticaria). Respiratory and cardiovascular symptoms are rare. Food allergic reactions are diagnosed by the medical history, skin or radioallergosorbent tests (RASTs), and elimination diets. The best test, however, remains the double-blind, placebo-controlled food challenge. If the diagnosis of a food allergy is confirmed, the only proven therapy is avoidance of the offending food. At present, there is no proven role for immunotherapy in the treatment of food allergy.

457. The answer is d. Approximately 40 deaths per year occur as a result of *Hymenoptera* stings. Additional fatalities undoubtedly occur and are unknowingly attributed to other causes. Both atopic and nonatopic persons experience reactions to insect stings. The responses range from large local reactions with erythema and swelling at the sting site to acute anaphylaxis.

Although each of the first four recommendations might be beneficial, the most important measure is for this patient to keep an epinephrine self-injector with her during activities where *Hymenoptera* species might be encountered. These devices are very effective when used properly. Desensitization injections are probably effective, although they carry some risk of anaphylaxis (albeit in a controlled setting). Beta-blockers increase the risk of anaphylaxis and impair response to epinephrine if an allergic reaction should occur. The venom of honeybees (apids) cross-reacts moderately with that of wasps (vespids), although the latter are the most dangerous species. Antihistamines have not been shown to block anaphylaxis.

Numerous mediators other than histamine are present in mast cell granules. The majority of fatal reactions occur in adults, with most persons having had no previous reaction to a stinging insect. Reactions can occur with the first sting and usually begin within 15 minutes. Enzymes, biogenic amines, and peptides present in the insects' venom are the sensitizing allergens. Venoms are commercially available for testing and treatment. Venom immunotherapy is indicated for patients with a history of sting anaphylaxis and positive skin tests. Although epinephrine self-injectors can be lifesaving; they are contraindicated in the presence of ischemic heart disease.

458. The answer is e. As a general rule, a history of respiratory distress or anaphylactic shock associated with an antibiotic use precludes the use of that or similar agents. However, in circumstances where penicillin is the clearly superior therapy and the consequences of treatment failure are dire (as in this case), desensitization is recommended. First, skin testing with several penicillin-related antigens is performed to confirm the diagnosis. Then, gradually increasing doses of penicillin are administered, starting with low oral doses and finally progressing to parenteral doses. IV access and epinephrine must be available, as even in the most meticulous hands, anaphylaxis can occur. Remember that there is 20% cross-reactivity between penicillins and cephalosporins (ie, ceftriaxone). A history of severe reaction to one class generally contraindicates use of other beta-lactams. Oral antibiotics are of no use in the treatment of neurosyphilis; only high-dose IV penicillin is effective. Syphilis in the pregnant, penicillin-allergic patient also requires desensitization rather than alternative antibiotics.

459. The answer is d. Live virus vaccines are contraindicated in severely immunocompromised patients. Live virus vaccines include varicella or zoster vaccines, measles-mumps-rubella vaccine, oral polio vaccine, and certain vaccines used in international travelers. If this patient responds to antiretroviral treatment with immune reconstitution (CD4 count above 200), he may receive live virus vaccines, if indicated, at that time. Other patients who should not receive live virus vaccines include pregnant women, patients with severe congenital immunological problems (eg, SCID), and patients who have received solid organ or stem cell transplants. Live virus vaccines are generally well-tolerated in patients with milder degree of immunosuppression, such as patients on low dose steroids (<10 mg daily prednisone or equivalent). Patients with HIV have increased risk of pneumococcal pneumonia, hepatitis B, and several other vaccine-preventable diseases and can safely receive the other listed vaccines.

460 to 461. The answers are 460-e, 461-d. C1 inhibitor deficiency prevents the proper regulation of activated C1. As a consequence, levels of C2 and C4—substrates of C1—are also low. Recurrent angioedema is the result of uncontrolled action of other serum proteins normally controlled by C1 inhibitor. The disease may be acquired but is usually inherited in an autosomal dominant pattern as a result of a deficiency of C1 inhibitor. There is no pruritus or urticarial lesions. Recurrent gastrointestinal attacks of colic commonly occur, probably due to angioedema of the bowel wall.

Immunoglobulin A deficiency is the commonest immunodeficiency syndrome, occurring in 1 in 600 patients. It is especially common in Caucasians. The most well-defined aspect of the syndrome is the development of severe allergic reactions to the IgA contained in transfused blood. Patients probably have an increased incidence of sinopulmonary infections and chronic diarrheal illness, although the increased susceptibility may be attributed to concomitant IgG subclass (especially IgG2 and IgG4) deficiency. There is no effective treatment for the IgA deficiency although those with IgG subclass deficiency and recurrent bacterial infections may benefit from immunoglobulin infusions.

Ataxia-telangiectasia is an uncommon genetic syndrome of immunodeficiency, cerebellar ataxia, and facial and ocular telangiectasias. The patients have abnormal DNA repair and suffer from an increased incidence of cancer, especially lymphomas. The abnormal gene is called the *ATM* gene; approximately 1% of the population is deficient in one allele. Interestingly, heterozygotes, although otherwise normal, are susceptible to increased radiation damage because of the abnormal DNA repair mechanism. Wiskott-Aldrich syndrome causes immunodeficiency (T cells more severely affected than B cells), thrombocytopenia, and eczema. A mutation in the *WASP* gene, whose protein product is involved in organizing the cytoskeleton, gives rise to severe bleeding, recurrent viral infections, and lymphomas. DiGeorge syndrome causes the classic isolated T-cell dysfunction; immunoglobulin levels are normal. In DiGeorge syndrome, thymic cells do not migrate normally from their origin in the pharyngeal pouches. Severe combined immunodeficiency (SCID) is associated with severe dysfunction in both B-cell and T-cell lineages. Genetics can be either X-linked or autosomal recessive; without stem cell transplantation, death occurs in infancy.

462 and 463. The answers are 462-a, 463-b. Patients who have a deficiency of one of the terminal components of complement have a remarkable susceptibility to disseminated *Neisseria* infection, particularly meningococcal disease. This association with meningococcal disease is related to the host inability to assemble the membrane attack complex—a single molecule of complement components that creates a discontinuity in the bacteria's membrane lipid bilayer. The complement deficiency results in inability to express complement-dependent bactericidal activity.

The pneumococcus is the most important cause of postsplenectomy sepsis, making up about 67% of all cases. (*Haemophilus influenzae* is the second most common organism.) The spleen serves a variety of immunologic functions, but, as the main production site for opsonizing antibody, it is especially important for the clearance of encapsulated bacteria from the bloodstream. A polysaccharide capsule surrounds all invasive pneumococci, and a deficiency in opsonizing antibody post-splenectomy can result in overwhelming sepsis with pneumonia, bacteremia, meningitis, and death.

Drug-induced agranulocytosis causes acute pharyngitis ("agranulocytic angina"), fever, and sepsis. Absolute neutrophil count is close to 0; recovery occurs 7 to10 days after withdrawal of the offending drug. Antibiotics, antithyroid, or antiepileptic drugs are the common offenders. Interleukin-12 receptor deficiency impairs production of interferon-gamma, leading to disseminated mycobacterial infection, often with nontuberculous species. The hyper-IgE syndrome causes recurrent staphylococcal abscesses, sometimes leading to pneumatoceles in the lung. The genetics of this syndrome is not well understood. Adenine deaminase deficiency accounts for 50% of cases of autosomal recessive SCID. Accumulation of purine metabolites leads to rapid apoptosis of both T and B cells.

Suggested Readings

1. Kasper DL, Fauci AS, Hauser SL, Longo DL, Jameson JL, Loscalzo J. *Harrison's Principles of Internal Medicine*. 19th ed. New York: Mc-Graw Hill; 2015. Chapters 74, 374, 376.
2. Allergy Clinical Practice Guidelines, available at: www.aaaai.org/practice-parameters-and-other-guidelines-page.aspx.
3. Primary Immunodeficiency Clinical Practice guidelines, available at: https://primaryimmune.org.
4. Bershed SV. In the clinic. Atopic dermatitis (eczema). *Ann Intern Med*. 2011;155:ITC5 1-15.
5. Casale TB. Clinical practice. Hymenoptera-sting hypersensitivity. *JAMA*. 2014;370:1432-1439.

Geriatrics

Questions

464. A 75-year-old woman is accompanied by her daughter to your clinic. The daughter reports that her mother fell in her yard last week while watering flowers. Her mother suffered scratches and bruises but no serious injury. The daughter is concerned that her mother might fall again with serious injury. The patient has hypertension and osteoarthritis of the knees. She takes hydrochlorothiazide (HCTZ), lisinopril, naproxen, and occasional diphenhydramine for sleep. The daughter reports some mild forgetfulness over the past 2 years. The patient gets up frequently at night to urinate.

Blood pressure is 142/78 lying and 136/74 standing. Pulse is 64 lying and standing. Except for some patellofemoral crepitance of the knees, her physical examination is normal. A Folstein Mini-Mental Status Examination (MMSE) is normal except that she only remembers two of three objects after 3 minutes (29/30). She takes 14 seconds to rise from sitting in a hard backed chair, walk 10 ft, turn, return to the chair, and sit down (timed up-and-go test, normal less than 10 seconds). CBC, chemistry profile, and thyroid tests are normal. What is the best next step?

a. CT scan of the brain
b. Holter monitor
c. Discontinue hydrochlorothiazide and prescribe donepezil
d. Discontinue diphenhydramine, assess her home for fall risks, and prescribe physical therapy
e. Electroencephalogram (EEG)

465. A 78-year-old woman with mild renal insufficiency complains of pain in the right knee on walking. The pain interferes with her day-to-day activities and is relieved by rest. There is no redness or swelling. There is minimal joint effusion. An x-ray of the knee shows osteophytes and asymmetric loss of joint space. Erythrocyte sedimentation rate (ESR) and white blood cell count are normal. Which of the following is the best initial management of this patient?

a. Naproxen
b. Indomethacin
c. Intra-articular corticosteroids
d. Acetaminophen
e. Total knee arthroplasty

466. An 82-year-old man is admitted to a long-term care facility after a right hemiplegic stroke. He is unable to walk and has limited ability to move himself in bed. He is frequently incontinent of urine. He has a history of type 2 diabetes mellitus. On examination you note a 3-cm area of persistent erythema on the right buttock. Which of the following treatments would you recommend at this time?

a. Sharp surgical debridement to remove the area of erythema.
b. Application of a hydrocolloid dressing (such as DuoDerm) to be left in place for 5 days.
c. Placement of a Foley catheter.
d. Use of a foam mattress, repositioning at least every 2 hours, and scheduled voidings.
e. Admission to the hospital for IV antibiotics.

467. A 65-year-old man has had symptoms of progressive cognitive dysfunction over a 1-year period. Memory and calculation ability are worsening. The patient has also had episodes of paranoia and delusions. Antipsychotic medication resulted in extrapyramidal signs and was stopped. The patient has recently complained of several months of visual hallucinations. There is no history of alcohol abuse. Which of the following is the most likely diagnosis?

a. Lewy body dementia
b. Alzheimer disease (AD)
c. Early parkinsonism
d. Delirium
e. Vascular dementia

468. An 80-year-old nursing home patient has become increasingly confused and unstable on her feet. On one occasion she has wandered outside the nursing home. In considering the issue of restraints for this individual, which of the following is correct?

a. A Geri chair would provide the best approach to safety and restraint.
b. Physical restraints are the best method to prevent falls.
c. Restraints cause many complications and increase the risk of falls.
d. Sedative medication should be used instead of restraints.
e. Wrist restraints are more effective than ankle restraints.

469. An 86-year-old woman lives alone. Her husband died 2 years ago; since then her self-care has deteriorated. She has lost weight and has become increasingly frail. She has fallen on several occasions and appears bewildered when faced with simple household decisions. Physical examination shows no focal neurological deficits and a Folstein Mini-Mental Status Examination (MMSE) score is 19 (out of possible 30). A workup for reversible causes of dementia is negative, and treatment in a balance disorder clinic is not helpful because the patient cannot remember her instructions. The patient appears in your office, accompanied by her daughter, who is concerned about her mother's safety. She inquires about nursing home placement but is worried about the financial implications of this decision. Which of the following statements is true?

a. Medicare will pay 80% of the costs associated with nursing home care.
b. The patient will need to be hospitalized for 3 days before Medicare will pay for her care.
c. Medicaid will pay for nursing home care if her income falls below the national poverty level.
d. Medicaid will pay for her nursing home care if she falls below her state's eligibility levels.
e. The patient should not be placed in a nursing home since the daughter can take her into her own home.

470. A frail 80-year-old nursing home resident has had several episodes of syncope, all of which have occurred while she was returning to her room after breakfast. Before each episode she has complaints of light-headedness and states she feels cold and weak. She takes nitroglycerin in the morning for a history of chest pain, but denies recent chest pain or shortness of breath. Which of the following is the best initial test?

a. Carotid Doppler ultrasound
b. Postprandial blood pressure monitoring
c. Holter monitoring
d. CT scan of the head
e. EEG

471. A 68-year-old woman was recently diagnosed with major depression. She has a history of hypertension and a seizure disorder. She is currently treated with lisinopril and levetiracetam (Keppra). On examination blood pressure is 165/90, temperature 37°C (98.6°F), pulse 68/min, and BMI 34. Other than obesity, physical examination is normal. Along with behavioral therapy, which of the following medications is most appropriate for treatment of her depression?

a. Venlafaxine
b. Sertraline
c. Mirtazapine
d. Bupropion
e. A tricyclic antidepressant

472. A 78-year-old man complains of slowly progressive hearing loss. He finds it particularly difficult to hear his grandchildren and to appreciate conversation in a crowded restaurant. On examination, ear canal and tympanic membranes are normal. Audiology testing finds bilateral upper-frequency hearing loss with difficulty in speech discrimination. Which of the following is the most likely diagnosis?

a. Presbycusis
b. Cerumen impaction
c. Ménière disease
d. Chronic otitis media
e. Acoustic neuroma

473. A 75-year-old woman is seen because of memory loss. Her only medical condition is hypertension. Her son states that he has noticed increasing memory difficulty in his mother for over 2 years. In the past several months she has had difficulty maintaining her household because she will forget to pay bills and has missed important appointments. There is no history of stroke, head injury, or hospitalization. She takes lisinopril and aspirin. On examination her vital signs are normal. A neurological examination is normal, except for a score of 20/30 on a Mini Mental Status Examination (MMSE). On laboratory testing, serum electrolytes, glucose, creatinine, calcium, and vitamin B_{12} are normal. Rapid plasma reagin (RPR) is negative. What is the most likely diagnosis?

a. Alzheimer disease
b. Pseudo-dementia of depression
c. Mild cognitive impairment (MCI)
d. Vascular dementia
e. Delirium

474. A 79-year-old man who has not had routine medical care presents for a physical examination and is found to have blood pressure of 165/80. He has no other risk factors for heart disease. He is not obese and walks 1 mile a day. Physical examination shows no retinopathy, normal cardiac examination including point of maximal impulse, and normal pulses. There is no abdominal bruit, and neurological examination is normal. ECG, electrolytes, blood glucose, and urinalysis are normal. A low-sodium DASH diet is recommended. The patient returns 6 weeks later, having strictly followed the diet; blood pressure is 168/76. Which of the following is the best next step in management?

a. Obtain renal artery Doppler
b. Begin therapy with low-dose thiazide diuretic
c. Follow patient; avoid toxicity of antihypertensive agents
d. Begin therapy with a beta-blocker
e. Begin therapy with a short-acting calcium channel blocker

475. A 75-year-old man comes for routine follow-up of his hypertension. He receives the influenza vaccine yearly but has never received a pneumococcal vaccine. When you consult the Advisory Committee on Immunization Practices (ACIP) guidelines, you learn that both the 23-valent polysaccharide vaccine (PPSV23, Pneumovax®) and the 13-valent pneumococcal conjugate vaccine (PCV13, Prevnar 13®) are recommended for all persons age 65 and older. What is the most important reason that the ACIP recommends two different pneumococcal vaccines?

a. The pneumococcal serotypes covered by the two vaccines are completely different.
b. The PPSV23 also contains antigens against *Haemophilus influenzae*.
c. PPSV23 boosts the antibody response of the PCV13.
d. PCV13 results in a better antibody response than PPSV23 but does not cover as many pathogens.
e. Some people respond to one vaccine but not the other.

476. An 82-year-old patient presents with nausea and weakness. She has a 3-year history of type 2 diabetes mellitus, as well as essential hypertension and congestive heart failure. Her medications include insulin glargine, hydrochlorothiazide, lisinopril, metoprolol, and digoxin. Medication doses have not recently been changed. Physical examination reveals clear lung fields, regular heart rhythm at 56 beats/minute, a soft systolic murmur that radiates to the axilla, and normal liver size. There is no peripheral edema or jugular venous distension. Chest x-ray shows cardiomegaly without pulmonary vascular congestion. Her CBC is normal. Multichannel chemistry profile shows potassium of 4.0 mEq/L and serum creatinine of 1.2 mg/dL (normal range 0.5-1.3). Digoxin level is 2.2 (therapeutic 0.8-1.5). What condition is most likely to account for her symptoms?

a. Decreased glomerular filtration rate
b. Polypharmacy
c. Progressive decline in cardiac output
d. Diabetic gastroparesis
e. "Senile" emphysema

477. A 67-year-old man is brought by his wife for evaluation of memory loss. Over the past 2 years he has had difficulty recalling the names of friends. On two occasions he has become lost in his own neighborhood. Recently, he has become suspicious that his wife is trying to put him in a nursing home.

He has hypertension. He has never used alcohol. He does not have urinary incontinence. His only medication is hydrochlorothiazide 25 mg daily. His mother was diagnosed with Alzheimer disease at age 60.

Blood pressure is 130/76. There are no focal neurologic findings and gait is normal. He is not oriented to date and cannot recall any of three objects at 3 minutes. He cannot speak the name of common objects such as a pen or watch. His clock-drawing test is abnormal. Complete blood count, blood chemistries, liver function tests, serologic test for syphilis, thyroid-stimulating hormone, and vitamin B_{12} levels are all normal. CT scan of the brain reveals age-related atrophic changes but is otherwise normal. Of the following choices, which is the best next step?

a. Begin treatment with donepezil 5 mg daily
b. Order *APOE* gene testing
c. Refer the patient for neurocognitive testing
d. Begin treatment with ginkgo biloba
e. Begin treatment with olanzapine 25 mg at bedtime

478. A 65-year-old female is recently diagnosed with a compression fracture of the second lumber vertebra. She was diagnosed with osteoporosis 3 years ago with T-score of −2.6 on bone densitometry. Her mother and sister were both treated for breast cancer. Her medical history includes hypertension and a deep venous thrombosis. Current medications include lisinopril, omeprazole, calcium, and vitamin D. Physical examination is normal except for midline tenderness over the lower back. In addition to continuing calcium and vitamin D and advising weight bearing exercise, which of the following is the most appropriate management for this patient's osteoporosis?

a. Alendronate
b. Calcitonin
c. Raloxifene
d. Estradiol
e. No additional treatment

Questions 479 and 480

Match the patient with the most likely type of urinary incontinence. Each lettered option may be used once, more than once, or not at all.

a. Stress incontinence
b. Urge incontinence
c. Overflow incontinence
d. Functional incontinence
e. Mixed incontinence

479. A 70-year-old woman complains of leakage of urine in small amounts. This occurs when laughing or coughing. It has also occurred while bending or exercising. The patient has five children who are concerned about her urinary problems.

480. An 85-year-old man has a history of long-standing diabetes mellitus and prostatic hypertrophy. He complains of dribbling urine. There is a sense of incomplete voiding and of a decrease in urinary stream. Postvoiding residual is 300 mL.

Geriatrics

Answers

464. The answer is d. Falls in the elderly are common. Nearly one-third of community dwelling adults over 65 years of age fall at least once yearly. Minor imbalances are common in everyday life. Falling in the elderly is usually associated with decreased ability of the elderly to compensate for these imbalances. Age-related declines in vestibular function, autonomic function, hearing and eyesight, and muscular strength all contribute to the inability of the elderly to correct for minor imbalances. Medical illnesses and medications may also contribute to this difficulty. The evaluation of falling in the elderly includes a careful history to exclude syncope, a careful medication history, and a review of medical conditions that may aggravate falling. Persons who have fallen more than once in the past 6 months are at high risk of falling again. The timed up-and-go (TUG) test also predicts who is likely to fall again in the next year. In an elderly person who presents with falling, evidence-based literature supports three measures to prevent future falls: elimination of medications with sedating and anticholinergic properties, elimination of environmental and structural hazards in the home, and physical therapy. Diphenhydramine has both sedating and anticholinergic effects.

In the absence of syncope and focal neurologic findings, CNS imaging, EEG, and Holter monitoring are unnecessary. Since the patient does not have orthostatic hypotension, discontinuing HCTZ is not indicated. Donepezil is indicated for dementia but not just forgetfulness.

465. The answer is d. This patient has osteoarthritis. In addition to physical therapy, the best symptomatic treatment would be acetaminophen because it is frequently effective in providing pain relief and has an excellent safety profile in the elderly. Nonsteroidal anti-inflammatory drugs should be avoided, at least initially, because they tend to cause gastrointestinal upset and impairment of renal function. Indomethacin is relatively contraindicated in the elderly because of its long half-life and central nervous system side effects. Intra-articular steroids are indicated for large effusions in joints unresponsive to first-line therapy. Arthroplasty is highly effective in treating osteoarthritis of a single joint and is not contraindicated in the elderly. Such surgery is usually considered if attempts at physical therapy, education, and pain control with pharmacotherapy do not provide adequate symptom relief.

466. The answer is d. Pressure ulcers are a serious problem in the elderly. They result when skin is damaged by compression between a bony prominence and hard surface for prolonged periods. Pressure ulcers are classified using a standard staging system. A stage I ulcer consists of persistent erythema. A stage II ulcer is characterized by partial-thickness skin loss involving the epidermis or dermis or both. These ulcers are superficial. A stage III ulcer is characterized by full-thickness skin loss involving subcutaneous tissue but not extending through underlying fascia. A stage IV ulcer is a stage III ulcer that extends through fascia and results in damage to underlying structures such as muscle or bone. The treatment of all pressure ulcers includes frequent monitoring of the ulcer, modifying the support surface (such as prescribing a foam mattress), frequent repositioning, and keeping the skin dry and clean from urine and stool. Scheduled urinary voidings are preferable to Foley catheters, which increase risk for urinary tract infection. In order to remove devitalized tissue, debridement is recommended for stages II, III, and IV ulcers. Hydrocolloid gels are recommended for stages II and III ulcers. Neither of these interventions would be indicated for this patient's stage I ulcer. All pressure ulcers eventually become colonized with bacteria. Local wound care is the first management of these infections. Topical antibiotics are reasonable if the ulcer is unimproved after 2 weeks of local wound care. Intravenous antibiotics are reserved for patients with cellulitis, sepsis, or underlying osteomyelitis.

467. The answer is a. Lewy body dementia has been recently recognized as a specific type of dementia different from Alzheimer disease or Parkinson disease. On autopsy Lewy bodies are present throughout the brain, including the cortex. Mild extrapyramidal signs and/or symptoms may or may not be present. Paranoia and delusions are more common than in Alzheimer disease, and treatment with antipsychotic drugs characteristically worsens the underlying condition. Visual hallucinations are characteristic of Lewy body dementia and uncommon in Alzheimer disease. Parkinson disease causes dementia late in its course, when the characteristic tremor, bradykinesia, and balance disturbance are easily recognized. Delirium is an acute confusional state that would not present with progressive cognitive deterioration or repeated hallucinations over time. Vascular dementia is characterized by stepwise progression (due to numerous lacunar strokes) and upper motor neuron signs.

468. The answer is c. Restraints are being used less and less in nursing homes as their complications and alternatives become more appreciated. The four Ds—*d*econditioning, *d*epression, *d*isorientation, and *d*ecubiti— are all complications of restraints. A Geri chair is just another form of physical restraint and promotes the same difficulties. Effective alternatives to restraints usually require an individual care plan. In this case, alarm bells for the institution's exits and evaluation of the patient's gait would be important. All physical restraints, either wrist or ankle restraints, should be avoided if possible. Sedation leads to complications such as pneumonia and may, in fact, also promote falls.

469. The answer is d. Medicare is a federally sponsored health insurance program for the elderly (age 65 and older). Medicare part A provides for acute hospitalization. Medicare part B, which requires a monthly premium, pays the fees of doctors and certain other health providers. Part B also covers some transitional services such as short-term Skilled Nursing Facilities. Medicare part D covers some prescription drug costs. Although Medicare covers some groups of nonelderly patients (eg, chronic dialysis patients, disabled patients) it does not pay for long-term custodial care even in the elderly. Medicare will provide payment for hospice care if the patient is near the end of life; these services are usually provided in the patient's home.

Medicaid is a program to provide health care to the poor. Whereas Medicare is administered by the federal government, Medicaid is administered by the states (often supplemented by funds from the federal government). The eligibility threshold for Medicaid, therefore, varies from state to state. Generally, adults who qualify for Medicaid must be poor. Coverage was expanded in many states under the Affordable Care Act to include most poor adult citizens. Unlike Medicare, Medicaid pays for chronic nursing home care.

The decision to place a frail parent in assisted living, nursing home, or Alzheimer unit is a difficult one for many families. Still, 30% of frail elderly are in chronic nursing facilities, often at a monthly cost of $3500 to $7000. Over 50% of patients above age 90 are unable to care for themselves at home.

470. The answer is b. Postprandial hypotension has been increasingly recognized in the frail elderly. In one study, a quarter of all patients had a reduction in systolic blood pressure of greater than 20 mm Hg occurring after meals. Much of the decrease is attributed to splanchnic blood pooling. Those on nitrates and other drugs that cause postural hypotension are at greatest risk. Older patients with this condition should avoid large meals. Diagnosis is confirmed by monitoring blood pressure after eating. Carotid studies are indicated in those with focal weakness/numbness or amaurosis fugax suggestive of focal carotid disease; this woman's symptoms instead suggest global brain underperfusion. Cardiac arrhythmia is unlikely to cause the symptoms described. Arrhythmic symptoms are usually of sudden onset and are typically *not* preceded by warning symptoms such as coldness and light-headedness. If initial evaluation is negative a Holter monitor may be of value. CT scan is rarely helpful in the evaluation of syncope in a patient without focal neurologic findings. In the absence of clinical features to suggest seizure, EEG is not recommended in the diagnostic workup of syncope.

471. The answer is b. Depression can be more difficult to diagnose in older adults, who often attribute lack of interest and other depressive symptoms to aging and other health problems. A number of standard screening tools are available to assist with the diagnosis of depression, such as the Patient Health Questionnaire-9 (PHQ-9). Pharmacologic therapy is often combined with nonpharmacologic therapy in the treatment of major depression in the elderly. All FDA-approved antidepressants have comparable response rates. Medication should be chosen based on patient tolerability and preferences and side effect profile. Sertraline, an SSRI, is well tolerated in the elderly. Venlafaxine acts as an SSRI at lower doses but at higher dose it acts as SNRI. Major side effects include hypertension and sexual dysfunction. Given this patient's high blood pressure, venlafaxine would not be the best choice. Mirtazapine works as a norepinephrine, $5\text{-}HT_2$ and $5\text{-}HT_3$ antagonist. Mirtazapine is often associated with increased appetite and weight gain. Given this patient's obesity, mirtazapine would also not be the best choice. Bupropion, a norepinephrine and dopamine reuptake inhibitor, is generally well tolerated but it can lower seizure threshold and is contraindicated in patients with a seizure disorder. Tricyclic antidepressants are generally avoided in the elderly because of their strong anticholinergic effects.

472. The answer is a. Presbycusis is the most common cause of sensorineural hearing loss in the elderly. Probably the result of cochlear damage over time, it is characterized by bilateral high-frequency hearing loss above 2000 Hz. Diminished speech discrimination is more apparent compared to other causes of hearing loss. Both Ménière disease and chronic otitis media are causes of hearing loss in the elderly; they usually present as unilateral hearing loss. Acoustic neuroma is uncommon and also causes unilateral neurosensory hearing loss. Otoscopy should always be used to rule out hearing loss associated with cerumen impaction in the elderly patient.

473. The answer is a. Dementia is a common problem in the elderly, and is characterized by chronic and progressive decline in cognition. Alzheimer disease (AD) makes up about 2/3 of cases dementia in the elderly. Risk factors for AD include advanced age, female gender, and a family history of dementia. AD is a diagnosis of exclusion, but is suggested by the clinical features and by a slowly progressive course that is insidious in onset. The most common cognitive defects present in early AD are recent memory loss and difficulty with executive function. Other cognitive defects which typically occur later in the illness include disorientation, difficulty with language (such as anomia), and apraxia (difficulty performing skilled motor activity). Depression can sometimes mimic dementia but usually has more decreased motivation on testing; the depressed patient is usually quite concerned about the memory loss. Mild Cognitive Impairment (MCI) is characterized by mild memory loss but preservation of functional abilities. In general the MMSE scores in patients with MCI are between 25 and 30. Vascular dementia is characterized by a more abrupt onset and focal neurologic deficits on physical examination. Delirium is distinguished from dementia by its more recent onset, a fluctuating course, and prominent inattention on examination. Very often symptoms of delirium can be seen in AD patients especially in advanced cases.

474. The answer is b. There is now general agreement that systolic hypertension in the elderly should be treated and that low-dose thiazide diuretic is the initial regimen of choice. Treatment, recommended when systolic blood pressure exceeds 160, reduces the risk of stroke and cardiovascular events. Side effects appear to be minimal. Long-acting calcium channel blockers or ACE inhibitors are generally recommended as second-step therapy. Short-acting calcium channel blockers should be avoided. Workup for secondary causes is not indicated, as they are less common in the elderly; such a workup may be appropriate if hypertension is refractory to medication. Renal artery stenosis due to atherosclerosis (detected by renal artery Doppler) is a common cause of refractory hypertension in the elderly; unfortunately, revascularization is less often curative than in young patients with fibromuscular dysplasia.

475. The answer is d. In 2014, the ACIP revised its recommendations regarding the use of pneumococcal vaccines in adults, recommending that all adults aged 65 and older receive both the 23-valent and 13-valent vaccine. The 23-valent vaccine contains 12 of the 13 serotypes in the PCV13, but the PCV13 is much more immunogenic, provides a better antibody response, and randomized controlled trials have established the efficacy of the PCV13 vaccine in preventing community-acquired pneumonia in adults aged 65 and older. PPSV23 is still recommended since it covers 11 serotypes that are not in the conjugate vaccine. Thus the ACIP recommends that the vaccines be given in series. Neither vaccine contains antigens against bacteria other than the pneumococcus, and a boosting response is not seen. Adults develop an antibody response to both vaccines.

476. The answer is a. In the usual patient, glomerular filtration rate (GFR) drops by about 1 mL/min every year after the age of 60. However, muscle mass and therefore creatinine production and excretion decline proportionately. Therefore, the serum creatinine can remain within the normal range despite considerable renal dysfunction. Age-related decline in GFR can lead to the accumulation of drugs that are cleared by renal mechanisms. This problem can be avoided if an "estimation formula" (ie, the Cockcroft-Gault or the MDRD equation) is used; they provide an accurate estimation of GFR, similar to a 24-hour urine collection for creatinine clearance.

Although polypharmacy is a common cause of gastrointestinal side effects in the elderly, this patient has been on a stable regimen; of her medications, only digoxin is likely to cause nausea or vomiting. Congestive heart failure can cause nausea by causing passive congestion of the liver, but this patient's heart failure appears clinically well compensated. In particular, she does not have tender hepatomegaly or hepatojugular reflux. The combination of an ACE inhibitor and beta-blocker is often very effective in preserving myocardial function. Diabetic gastroparesis can cause nausea and vomiting but rarely occurs after such a short history of diabetes. Lung capacity (including forced vital capacity and lung elastic recoil) often deteriorates with the aging process and can cause dyspnea and fatigue even in the nonsmoker, but would not cause her gastrointestinal symptoms.

477. The answer is a. This patient meets the diagnostic criteria for Alzheimer disease: the gradual development of multiple cognitive defects (which must include memory impairment) resulting in significant social impairment, not explained by another physical or psychiatric disease.

The primary treatment is a cholinesterase inhibitor. Many clinicians initiate therapy with donepezil. Neurocognitive testing may confirm the diagnosis but is not necessary. The *APOE* gene on chromosome 19 influences the risk for late-onset Alzheimer disease, but it is not a clinically useful test for influencing diagnosis or treatment. In prospective trials, ginkgo biloba has been demonstrated to be ineffective in the treatment of Alzheimer dementia. Antipsychotics do not affect the course of Alzheimer disease and are reserved for severe behavioral disturbances, which have not responded to nonpharmacological therapy. Long-term use of antipsychotics in patients with dementia increases the risk of sudden death.

478. The answer is a. Calcium, vitamin D, smoking cessation, and weight-bearing exercise are recommended for all women with established osteoporosis. Additional pharmacologic therapy is generally recommended for women with a hip or vertebral compression fracture. Because of their established efficacy and relatively low cost, oral bisphosphonates such as alendronate are usually recommended as first-line therapy. Intravenous bisphosphonates are a more expensive but reasonable alternative for patients who are intolerant of oral bisphosphonates. The most common side effect of oral bisphosphonates is reflux esophagitis, therefore oral bisphosphonates should be taken on an empty stomach with patient being in upright position. Raloxifene is a selective estrogen-receptor modulator and has estrogenic effect on bone. Raloxifene increases the risk of thromboembolic events and is unsuitable for this patient with a history of deep vein thrombosis. Calcitonin is available in subcutaneous injections and as a nasal spray. Calcitonin is less effective than other antiresorptive drugs, though there is some evidence that it may have some analgesic effect in painful vertebral fractures.

479 and 480. The answers are 479-a, 480-c. The 70-year-old woman with episodes of leaking small amounts of urine while laughing or coughing has stress incontinence. Stress incontinence occurs when the internal urethral sphincter fails to remain closed in response to increasing intra-abdominal pressure caused by laughing, coughing, or lifting. The problem is usually seen in postmenopausal women who have weakening of their pubococcygeus muscle after multiple childbirths.

Diabetes and prostatic hypertrophy may be contributing to this 85-year-old man's overflow incontinence. Overflow incontinence occurs when there is a mechanical or functional obstruction at the bladder outlet.

This leads to overfill of the bladder and leakage with detrusor contraction. A similar picture can occur in a diabetic with an atonic bladder.

Urge incontinence occurs due to hyperactivity of the detrusor muscle. Urge incontinence is frequently preceded by a sudden urge to urinate that cannot be voluntarily suppressed. Patients with mixed incontinence have clinical features of both stress and urge incontinence. Functional incontinence is incontinence due to conditions that are not urologic (such as high urine flow rates with diabetes insipidus or inability to ambulate to the toilet).

Suggested Readings

1. Kasper DL, Fauci AS, Hauser SL, Longo DL, Jameson JL, Loscalzo J. *Harrison's Principles of Internal Medicine.* 19th ed. New York: McGraw-Hill; 2015. Chapters 10, 11, 27, 34, 35, 94e.
2. Durso SC, Sullivan GM. *Geriatric Review Syllabus.* 8th ed. New York: American Geriatric Society; 2013. Chapters 10, 32-39.
3. American Geriatrics Society. Clinical Practice Webpage available at http://www.americangeriatrics.org/health_care_professionals/clinical_practice/clinical_guidelines_recommendations/
4. Clinical Practice Guidelines for Treatment of Major Depressive Disorder, available at http://psychiatryonline.org/pb/assets/raw/sitewide/practice_guidelines/mdd.pdf
5. McKhann GM, Knopman DS, Chertkow H, et al. The diagnosis of dementia due to Alzheimer disease: Recommendations from the National Institute on Aging-Alzheimer Association workgroups on diagnostic guidelines for Alzheimer disease. *Alzheimer's Dement.* 2011;7:263-269.
6. Sessums LL, Zembrzuska H, Jackson JL. Does this patient have medical decision-making capacity? *JAMA.* 2011;306:420-427. doi: 10.1001/jama.2011.1023.
7. Saxena S, Lawley D. Delirium in the elderly: A clinical review. *Postgrad Med J.* 2009;85:405-413. doi: 10.1136/pgmj.2008.072025.
8. Reuben DB. Medical care for the final years of life: "When you're 83, it's not going to be 20 years". *JAMA.* 2009;302:2686-2694. doi: 10.1001/jama.2009.1871.

Women's Health

Questions

481. A 23-year-old woman with a 5-pack-year history of cigarette use wonders if she is a candidate for human papillomavirus (HPV) vaccination. She has been sexually active for 5 years with three partners. Her Pap smear is normal, but her examination reveals two small wart-like nontender vaginal lesions. You first educate her that quitting smoking will help her immune system fight the strain of HPV that she already has acquired. What advice should you give her?

a. She is already infected with one strain, but the vaccine will still be effective against acquiring other strains.
b. The vaccine will protect her from every HPV strain.
c. If she receives the vaccine, she will never have to have another Pap smear.
d. She is already infected with one strain, and there is no benefit in vaccination against the others.
e. The vaccine will help cure her genital warts.

482. A 45-year-old woman presents to your office to establish care. She has been watching television programs hosted by doctors recommending various screening tests, and she wishes to have "everything done." She has a history of gastroesophageal reflux and seasonal allergies, and no family history of diabetes or cancer. Her best friend was recently diagnosed with ovarian cancer, so she would like to be tested for that. Which of the following recommendations (based on the United States Preventive Services Task Force) would be appropriate?

a. Dual-x-ray absorptiometry (DXA) bone density scan
b. Annual Pap smear
c. CA-125 and pelvic sonogram every 5 years
d. Annual mammogram
e. Alcohol counseling

483. A 60-year-old white woman presents for an office visit. Her mother recently broke her hip, and the patient is concerned about her own risk for osteoporosis. She weighs 165 lb and is 5 ft 6 in tall. She has a 50-pack-year history of tobacco use. Medications include a multivitamin and levothyroxine 50 µg/d. Her exercise regimen includes mowing the lawn and taking care of the garden. She took hormone replacement therapy for 6 years after menopause, which occurred at age 49. Which recommendation for osteoporosis screening is most appropriate for this patient?

a. Nuclear medicine bone scan
b. Dual-x-ray absorptiometry (DXA) scan
c. Quantitative CT bone densitometry
d. Peripheral bone densitometry
e. No testing is recommended at this time

484. An orthopedic surgeon asks you to help him manage an 82-year-old woman who just received a hip replacement as a result of a hip fracture. The patient was watering her flowers when she tripped on the water hose and heard her hip crack as she fell to the ground. She has a history of hypothyroidism, mild cerebrovascular accident (CVA), and hypertension. Her mother had lost about 5 in of height in her older years. She believes that she has lost "a few inches" in comparison to her husband. On review of systems, she admits to chronic diarrhea. Her only home medication is metoprolol. On physical examination, her blood pressure is 158/90; pulse 88 and regular; the hip is tender to palpation. Laboratory tests show normal calcium, renal function, and alkaline phosphatase. TSH, celiac panel, and 25-OH vitamin D level are also normal. Which of the following medications would be the best choice in preventing another fracture?

a. Raloxifene
b. Calcitonin-salmon nasal spray
c. Estradiol
d. Hydrochlorothiazide
e. A bisphosphonate

485. A 50-year-old woman presents with chest discomfort for 2 days. It lasted for 3 hours on the first day and 6 hours on the second. She describes it as indigestion. She walks 2 miles a day, and has never smoked. She has a family history of atherosclerosis in her father. Her BMI is 25, blood pressure is 124/74, and heart rate is 72. HDL is 55, LDL is 78, TG 120, and total cholesterol is 188. She is in mild discomfort as you examine her. Her ECG during the discomfort shows 3-mm ST elevation in inferior leads. Troponin I is 4.2 µg/L (normal <0.04). Cardiac catheterization shows no luminal defects. How does her clinical course differ from that of a man with a similar disorder?

a. She is more likely to have high degree coronary obstruction than a male.
b. She is more likely to have atypical symptoms and to be diagnosed later than a male.
c. Her mortality rate with the acute event is less than that of a male.
d. Fibrates will be more important than statins in secondary prevention.
e. She is more likely to undergo coronary stenting than a male.

486. A 25-year-old woman presents to your office with complaints of pain during intercourse for 2 months. The pain occurs with initial penetration and continues throughout the entire episode. She relates that she and her husband have been married for a year and previously had a pleasurable, pain-free relationship. She tells you that she has been to several area doctors, and had a "full work-up" without a diagnosis, including a pelvic examination, Pap smear with cultures, and pelvic sonogram. On examination, she has a normal pelvic examination with no pain. You are unsure of the differential diagnosis, so you continue taking more history. She admits to vaginal dryness and low libido during this same timeframe. You ask if anything in her life changed 2 months ago. She suddenly begins to cry and states she found evidence of her husband's infidelity 2 months ago. What is the most appropriate recommendation for your patient?

a. Marriage counseling
b. Estrogen vaginal cream for vaginal dryness
c. Vaginal dilators for treatment of vaginismus
d. Antidepressant therapy
e. Low dose testosterone for hypoactive sexual desire disorder

487. A 46-year-old diabetic woman complains of vaginal discharge which has been present for several days. She denies fever or dysuria, but has noticed vulvar itching and discomfort. She has never had similar symptoms before. She has a monogamous relationship with her husband of 24 years. She takes metformin for her diabetes; a recent hemoglobin A1C level was 8.6% (goal <7.0%). She has not recently used antibiotics. She has tried over-the-counter miconazole cream without benefit. General examination is unremarkable; she is afebrile. Pelvic examination shows vulvar erythema and thick, non-malorodous, whitish vaginal discharge. The walls of the vagina are mildly erythematous; the cervix is normal and nontender to manipulation. Vaginal pH is 4.0. A wet prep shows no motile organisms or clue cells. KOH slide shows budding yeasts and hyphae. What is the best treatment for her symptoms?

a. Fluconazole 150 mg po X1
b. Fluconazole 150 mg po, repeated once after at least 72 hours
c. Metronidazole 2 grams po X1
d. Metronidazole 500 mg po BID for 7 days
e. Azithromycin 1 gram po and ceftriaxone 250 mg IM X1

488. A 33-year-old woman presents to your office because of abnormal hair growth. She has noticed gradually increasing coarse hair on her upper lip, chin, and lower abdomen for the past 3 years. She notices mild facial acne but denies frontal balding or deepening of voice. Her menses are irregular, occurring every 28 to 60 days. She and her husband use condoms for contraception. They have no children. She uses over-the-counter benzoyl peroxide for the acne but otherwise takes no medications or supplements. On examination, her BMI is 29.0 and her waist circumference is 36 in. Her voice is normal; she has mild facial acne. There is mild acanthosis nigricans of the axillae. Pelvic examination is normal without ovarian mass or clitoromegaly. Evaluation of her hirsutism should include which of the following?

a. Glucose tolerance test
b. Serum testosterone and dehydroepiandrosterone-sulfate (DHEA-S) level
c. Overnight dexamethasone suppression test with 8 am cortisol level
d. CT scan of adrenals
e. Therapeutic trial of spironolactone

489. A 42-year-old nurse sees you in the office to establish care. She is asymptomatic, does not use tobacco, and exercises regularly. She practices monthly breast self-examination and has had Pap smears according to USPSTF recommendations in the past. On social history she tells you that she is a lesbian and is in a committed relationship with a single partner. Her blood pressure and vital signs are normal, as is the general physical examination. How should the information about her sexual self-identification affect your subsequent care?

a. She will not need further pelvic examinations or Pap smears.
b. Her breast cancer risk is less; so she will need less frequent mammography.
c. You will need to discuss and document durable power for health care.
d. Her risk of developing a sexually transmitted disease is nil.
e. Her risk of alcohol-use disorder is less than a heterosexual woman.

490. A 51-year-old woman presents to your office with questions about whether postmenopausal hormone therapy (HT) is "dangerous." She heard this on the news and read about it in a women's magazine. She denies hot flushes, irregular menses, emotional lability, or vaginal dryness. She has hypertension, but is otherwise healthy. Her family history is negative for breast cancer and cardiovascular disease. According to data from the Women's Health Initiative study, what advice should you give her?

a. She should start HT for cardiovascular protection.
b. HT is not indicated for this patient.
c. She should start vaginal estrogen cream.
d. She should start HT for breast cancer risk reduction.
e. Hormone therapy is too risky to give to any woman.

491. A 21-year-old woman complains of fatigue and difficulty swallowing. She describes the difficulty swallowing as a choking sensation that occurs randomly and not with eating. She denies fever, chills, nausea, or vomiting. She notes intermittent abdominal cramping, decreased sexual desire, and difficulty sleeping at night. Physical examination reveals normal vital signs and normal thyroid gland. Abdomen shows mild diffuse tenderness without organomegaly. After you notice bruising of the thigh and a vaginal laceration, you ask about her home safety, and she admits that her husband has coerced her into sexual intercourse against her will and that he has "hurt" her when she doesn't comply. What should you recommend?

a. You should advise her to leave her spouse immediately.
b. You should contact the police and file a report against her husband.
c. You should recommend paroxetine to decrease her somatic symptoms.
d. You should refer her to a therapist who specializes in hypoactive sexual desire disorder.
e. You should inquire about suicidal ideation and provide her with the contact information for a domestic violence center.

492. A 28-year-old nonsmoking woman presents to discuss birth control methods. She requests a contraceptive option that is not associated with weight gain. She and her husband agree that they desire no children for the next few years. Her periods are regular, but heavy and painful. She frequently stays home from work on the first day due to severe lower abdominal cramping and back pain. She changes her pad every 4 hours. This pattern of bleeding has been present since she was 15 years old. For a week before her period begins, she is uncharacteristically tearful, irritable, and depressed. These behavioral changes are beginning to affect her personal relationships. Her physical examination reveals blood pressure 110/75, BMI 22, and moderate acne on her face and neck. What recommendation would best address her mood, skin, and contraceptive needs?

a. Tubal ligation
b. Drospirenone/ethinyl estradiol combination pill
c. Progesterone-infused intrauterine device
d. Depo-progesterone shots every 3 months
e. Regular condom use

493. You are asked to evaluate a 24-year-old pregnant woman for abnormal liver enzymes. She is in the 34th week of her first pregnancy, which has been complicated by mild preeclampsia. She was doing well until 1 week ago, when she developed nausea, which has become progressively severe. Over the past 3 days, she has developed mild jaundice and headache. On examination, she has moderate scleral icterus; her blood pressure is 164/86 and she is afebrile. Abdominal examination reveals a gravid uterus at the anticipated size. She has mild right upper quadrant tenderness and 1+ pretibial edema. Neurological examination is nonfocal but she is mildly somnolent. Flapping tremor is present bilaterally. Laboratory studies include CBC with WBC of 17,500, hemoglobin 11.3 g/dL, and platelet count 142,000. No fragmented red blood cells are seen on the peripheral blood smear. Liver enzymes show bilirubin 7.2 mg/dL, alkaline phosphatase 233 U/L (normal <120), AST 332 U/L (normal <40), ALT 267 U/L (normal <40), and prothrombin time 17.5 seconds (normal 12 seconds). Blood glucose is 51 mg/dL. What is the most likely diagnosis?

a. Acute alcoholic hepatitis
b. Intrahepatic cholestasis of pregnancy
c. Hemolysis, elevated liver enzymes, low platelet count (HELLP) syndrome
d. Acute fatty liver of pregnancy
e. Acute hepatitis A virus infection

494. A 40-year-old woman presents to discuss breast cancer prevention. Her mother was diagnosed with breast cancer at the age of 45, and the patient carries the *BRCA1* gene. The patient is menstruating regularly. In addition to recommending daily exercise and minimal alcohol use, what is your best advice to this patient?

a. Raloxifene use for 5 years is indicated for high-risk premenopausal women.
b. Bioidentical hormone replacement carries less breast cancer risk than estradiol/progestin combinations.
c. Oophorectomy does not affect breast cancer risk.
d. Screening her daughters, but not her sons, for *BRCA* mutation is appropriate.
e. Screening with MRI and mammogram improves sensitivity of screening.

495. A 40-year-old woman presents to your office regarding a breast lump she found on self-examination 2 weeks ago. The patient does not regularly examine her breasts. Her last clinical breast examination was 2 years ago; she had a normal mammogram 9 months ago. She has no family history of breast cancer. Her father had colon cancer diagnosed at age 50. She takes no medications regularly. On examination, she has a well-localized nontender nodule in the left breast at 2 o' clock. It is 1.5 cm in diameter with irregular borders. Diagnostic breast imaging includes a negative mammogram and a sonogram showing solid nodule in the left breast at the site of the palpable abnormality. What is the most appropriate next step in the management of this woman's breast abnormality?

a. Reassure her that she has a fibroadenoma and reassess in 6 months.
b. Refer the patient for needle biopsy.
c. Tell the patient to discontinue caffeine and wear a supportive bra.
d. Schedule breast MRI.
e. Start the patient on NSAIDs and vitamin E.

496. A 57-year-old white woman with history of breast cancer stage II, ER+, PR+, presents to the emergency room complaining of the sudden onset of chest pain and shortness of breath. The pain is sharp and stabbing in the left posterior lung area. The pain does not increase on exertion but increases with deep breathing. The patient denies any history of cardiovascular or pulmonary disease. Her only medications are tamoxifen for 2 years and OTC vitamins. Pulse is 110, RR 26, and BP 150/94; lungs are clear bilaterally. Cardiovascular examination shows regular rate and rhythm with fixed splitting of S_2. ECG shows S wave in lead I, Q wave in lead III, and inverted T in lead III. Pulse oximetry is 90% on room air. Chest x-ray is unremarkable. Which factor is most likely to be contributing to this patient's respiratory distress?

a. Myocardial infarction
b. Asthma
c. Tamoxifen use
d. Anxiety
e. Pneumonia

497. A 46-year-old woman presents for her annual examination. Her main complaint is frequent sweating episodes with a sensation of intense heat starting at her upper chest and spreading up to her head. These have been intermittent for the past 6 to 9 months but are gradually worsening. She has three to four flushing/sweating episodes during the day and two to three at night. She occasionally feels her heart race for about a second, but when she checks her pulse it is normal. She reports feeling more tired and has difficulty with sleep due to sweating. She denies major life stressors. She also denies weight loss, weight gain, or change in bowel habit. Her last menstrual cycle was 3 months ago. Physical examination is normal. Which treatment is most appropriate in alleviating this woman's symptoms?

a. Levothyroxine
b. Estrogen
c. Estrogen plus progesterone
d. Citalopram
e. Gabapentin

498. A 60-year-old woman presents with complaints of pain during intercourse. She describes the pain as sharp and constant during sexual activity, and there is a lack of lubrication. This discomfort is very bothersome to her because she wishes to continue an active sex life. She underwent surgical menopause at age 44 due to uterine fibroids and heavy bleeding. She used oral estrogen until age 50; she has used no hormonal therapy since then. On physical examination you note significant urethral and vaginal atrophy. Which of the following is the best treatment option for this patient?

a. Commercial lubricant (such as K-Y lubricating jelly)
b. Oral estrogen
c. Vaginal estrogen preparation
d. Sildenafil
e. Topical testosterone

499. A 43-year-old woman presents to your office because of musculo-skeletal pain and weight gain. Over the past 6 months, she has noted gener-alized aches and pains of muscles and joints, fatigue, and poor sleep quality. She admits to wanting to stay in bed rather than socialize with her friends and family. She does not enjoy usual daily activities as she did before. She denies fever, night sweats, morning stiffness, joint redness, blood loss, easy bruising, or daytime somnolence. Physical examination reveals normal BMI, normal thyroid, normal cardiovascular examination, normal joints, and no tenderness to palpation. CBC, TSH, ESR, ANA, rheumatoid factor, electrolytes, liver enzymes, and kidney function tests are normal. She wants pain control. Which treatment is most likely to relieve her symptoms?

a. Long-acting opiates
b. Oral acetaminophen/hydrocodone combination
c. Prednisone
d. Methotrexate
e. Antidepressant

500. You are reviewing your office records as part of a performance review mandated by an insurance company. One criterion is appropriate to use of low-dose aspirin for prevention of heart attack or stroke. According to the United States Preventive Services Task Force recommendations, which of the following patients should be treated with low-dose (81 or 162 mg daily) aspirin?

a. A 46-year-old healthy woman to prevent heart attack.
b. A 42-year-old healthy man to prevent heart attack.
c. A 66-year-old healthy woman to prevent stroke.
d. A 66-year-old healthy man to prevent stroke.
e. A 95-year-old healthy woman to prevent heart attack and stroke.

Women's Health

Answers

481. The answer is a. Human papillomavirus (especially subtypes 16, 18, 33, and 45) has an established relationship to genital warts and cervical cancer. Both current multivalent vaccines are highly effective in establishing immunity to the subtypes included in the vaccine, even if one or more of the subtypes is already acquired. Both vaccines cover strains 16 and 18. Gardasil is a quadrivalent vaccine which also covers strains 6 and 11, common causes of genital warts. Cervarix is a bivalent vaccine but may provide cross-protection against strain 45. One or the other vaccine should be chosen. The vaccines are not effective in treatment of any disease (ie, vaginal warts) caused from prior infection. Because over 40 sexually transmitted HPV subtypes exist and the vaccine includes the types responsible for about 70% of cervical cancer, there is still a risk of cervical dysplasia caused from other subtypes not covered in the vaccine. Therefore, continued Pap screening is needed. This patient's likelihood of clearing her current HPV infection increases with tobacco cessation.

482. The answer is e. The USPSTF recommends screening for alcohol use disorder in all adults. Maximum recommended consumption is one or less standard drink per day for adult women, and two or fewer standard drinks per day for adult men. On average, women have higher blood alcohol levels than men after ingestion of the same amount of alcohol. Evidence also supports that women have accelerated development of fatty liver, hypertension, malnutrition, and GI hemorrhage with excessive alcohol use. A meta-analysis of studies examining the association between all-cause mortality and average alcohol consumption found that men averaging at least four drinks per day and women averaging two or more drinks per day experienced increased mortality relative to nondrinkers.

Bone density screening by DXA is recommended for all women over 65 years of age or for women whose fracture risk is equivalent to that of a 65-year-old woman. Risks for low bone mass include personal history of fracture, secondary cause of low bone mass (eg, celiac disease, hyperparathyroidism, liver disease, long-term use of systemic steroids or anti-epileptic drugs), cigarette smoking, alcohol abuse, low body mass index, and first-degree family member with hip fracture. The newest recommendations for screening frequency for cervical cancer for a woman age 30 and older are every 3 years (or every 5 years when combined with HPV testing). CA-125 and pelvic sonogram are not recommended for screening of ovarian cancer because of their low sensitivity. Mammogram screening is recommended every-other-year for a normal-risk woman beginning at age 50; screening between ages 40 and 49 should be individualized.

483. The answer is b. This woman has an increased risk of fragility fracture; so screening before age 65 is recommended. Her risk factors include estrogen deficiency, positive family history of hip fracture, and tobacco use; therefore peripheral bone densitometry, such as a heel quantitative ultrasound, would not be sufficient. The heel ultrasound, which does predict fracture risk in women over 65, is less accurate than DXA and is useful for population-wide screening programs, not individual treatment recommendations. A nuclear medicine bone scan has no role in the diagnosis of osteoporosis. Quantitative CT allows for adequate prediction of vertebral fractures, but is not considered standard of care at this time, and exposes the patient to greater radiation than DXA.

484. The answer is e. This patient has a diagnosis of osteoporosis based on the occurrence of her fragility fracture (fall from normal walking height), regardless of her T-score. Bisphosphonate therapy is proven to reduce the high risk of subsequent hip and vertebral fractures. Raloxifene is less appropriate for this patient with her history of a CVA, as it has been associated with increased incidence of thromboembolic events and stroke. The effect of nasal calcitonin on fracture risk is unproven. Estrogen therapy is approved by the FDA for the prevention of osteoporosis, but not for treatment. Estrogens and raloxifene are equally thrombogenic. Hydrochlorothiazide decreases urine calcium loss and helps maintain bone density. Epidemiologic data suggest decreased first fracture risk with long-term use, but it is not proven to decrease risk of subsequent fractures.

485. The answer is b. This patient's laboratory and testing prove she has suffered a myocardial infarction. Ischemic heart disease is an area where gender differences between men and women carry important implications. Women with coronary disease develop symptoms 10 years later in life than men and often present with atypical symptoms, such as shortness of breath, nausea, vomiting, indigestion, fatigue, or upper back pain. Hence, women go to the hospital later in the course of a myocardial infarction and actually have an increased mortality rate. Women with an MI are more likely to present with cardiac arrest, hypotension, or cardiogenic shock.

Conversely, women with myocardial infarction have lesser degrees of coronary obstruction than men; as many as 20% have no coronary obstruction at all. This has led to the hypothesis that vasospasm and endothelial dysfunction are more important than plaque instability and obstruction in women. This may partly account for the fact that women receive coronary stenting less often than men. Other factors include more advanced age, smaller coronaries, and perhaps disparities in how seriously women's symptoms are addressed. Statins are as important in secondary prevention of coronary artery disease (CAD) in women as in men. Fibrates have shown very modest if any benefit in long-term prevention of coronary events in either sex.

486. The answer is a. An organic cause of this patient's sexual dysfunction is unlikely. Her pain during intercourse, poor desire, and lack of sufficient lubrication probably stem from the psychological stress from her husband's infidelity. Marital counseling may aid in resolving the issues that resulted in the infidelity, and the aftermath. Female sexual dysfunction consists of four broad categories: dyspareunia, orgasmic disorder, arousal disorder, and impaired sexual drive. Sexual dysfunction may result from physical conditions, such as neuropathy or sleep deprivation, or from psychological conditions, such as depression or a history of abuse. A thorough evaluation should include medical conditions as well as psychosocial questions pertaining to the health of her relationship with her partner and personal issues that contribute to her sexual well-being. Topical intravaginal estrogens are useful for perimenopausal vaginal dryness, and vaginal dilators are often tried for vaginismus, but neither would help her obvious psychological distress. Antidepressants would not address the cause of her symptoms. Low-dose testosterone has not been approved for the management of hypoactive sexual desire disorder and would not address the cause of this woman's distress.

487. The answer is b. Vaginal discharge can be the result of vaginitis or cervicitis. Vaginitis due to *Trichomonas vaginalis* or cervicitis due to *Chlamydia trachomatis* or *Neisseria gonorrhoeae* indicate important sexually transmitted diseases and require partner contact, but vulvovaginal candidiasis (VVC) and bacterial vaginosis (BV) are not sexually transmitted (although the incidence of BV is higher in sexually active women). This patient's diabetes, her prominent vulvar symptoms, and the thick cottage-cheese discharge all suggest VVC; the findings on examination of the vaginal discharge confirm the diagnosis. VVC is classified as uncomplicated (which usually responds to topical imidazoles or one dose of oral fluconazole) or complicated (which requires a prolonged course of topical antifungals or at least two doses of oral fluconazole for cure). Criteria for complicated VVC include diabetes, pregnancy, immunosuppression, and severe or recurrent disease. Because of her diabetes (especially with marginal control), this patient will require the more intense regimen to achieve cure.

Single dose metronidazole is recommended treatment for trichomoniasis. The sexual partner(s) should be treated as well. *Trichomonas* usually causes a profuse malodorous yellow-green discharge with vaginal pH >4.5 and motile organisms on wet-prep. One week of metronidazole is recommended for bacterial vaginosis. BV is associated with a vaginal pH >4.5 and thin whitish-grey discharge, which has a "fishy" odor (especially after KOH has been dropped onto a sample of the exudate). "Clue" cells (squamous vaginal epithelial cells plastered with coccobacilli) are characteristic of BV. Single dose azithromycin plus ceftriaxone is the treatment of choice for gonococcal or chlamydial cervicitis; this patient has no cervical erythema or exudate. Remember that the history of a monogamous relationship does NOT rule out an STD, since we don't know the sexual history of her partner.

488. The answer is b. Abnormal growth of terminal hair in androgen-dependent areas in a woman is termed hirsutism. It is a common problem, affecting 5% to 10% of premenopausal women. Hirsutism should be distinguished from virilization, which includes frontal balding, deepening of the voice, and clitoromegaly in addition to hirsutism. Virilization (especially of recent onset) is worrisome for an androgen producing tumor of the adrenal gland or ovary. Women with moderate hirsutism (as in this case) or any evidence of virilization should undergo endocrine testing with DHEA-S (to rule out adrenal androgen overproduction), testosterone (to rule out ovarian androgen overproduction), TSH, prolactin, and follicular phase 17-hydroxy progesterone (to rule out late-manifesting congenital adrenal hyperplasia).

This woman likely has polycystic ovarian syndrome (PCOS). PCOS and idiopathic hirsutism are the two most common causes of hirsutism in women. PCOS is classically diagnosed with any 2 of these 3 criteria:

oligomenorrhea (with anovulatory bleeding), clinical or biochemical evidence of hyperandrogenism (excluding other causes of hyperandrogenemia), and polycystic ovaries by ultrasound. Most women with PCOS will have elevated serum DHEA-S and testosterone concentrations; facial acne is common but full virilization is rare. Hyperinsulinemia and insulin resistance, seen clinically as acanthosis nigricans, are also common findings. Women with PCOS are at increased risk of metabolic syndrome, diabetes, and cardiovascular disease. Exercise and weight loss are first-line recommendations, and may restore normal ovulation without medications. Treatment for women not pursuing pregnancy includes oral contraceptives (which improve the hirsutism) or metformin (which improves insulin resistance and often restores ovulatory periods).

Although checking fasting blood glucose is reasonable, glucose tolerance test is not part of the first-line workup for hirsutism. The overnight dexamethasone suppression test is sometimes used for the diagnosis of Cushing syndrome, but in the absence of other features of hypercortisolism (ecchymoses, purplish abdominal striae) it would not be recommended. In addition, 24-hour urine free cortisol should be the first test for suspected Cushing syndrome. Women with testosterone levels of >200 ng/dL or DHEA-S levels of >700 µg/dL should have imaging of the ovaries and adrenal glands, but ordering a CT scan of the adrenals would be premature until the hormone levels are available. Spironolactone (which has antiandrogenic as well as antimineralocorticoid properties) is often used to treat idiopathic hirsutism, but by definition patients with this condition have normal menses and normal androgen levels. Starting spironolactone before ruling out other, more serious conditions would be premature.

489. The answer is c. From 1% to 3% of American women self-identify as lesbians; so a women's health practitioner will need to become familiar with the special characteristics and needs of this population. Although an increasing number of states recognize the legal status of same-sex unions or marriages, this is not universally the case. This woman with a committed partner may wish to designate that partner as her surrogate decision-maker for health care. If so, you should keep documentation for durable power of attorney in her chart. Without such documentation, most states will designate her next of kin as the decision maker if she is incapacitated.

Although women who have never had sexual intercourse are at low risk for cervical cancer, between 50% and 80% of lesbians have a history of sexual intercourse with a man. Recommendations for Pap smears for lesbians do not differ from those for heterosexual women. Nulliparity increases a woman's breast cancer risk; although it has not been definitively proven that the risk of breast cancer is higher in the lesbian population, standard recommendations for mammography also apply in this population. Certain sexual practices such as genital-genital contact and sharing of sex toys are considered high-risk practices for STDs including HIV infection; the incidence of bacterial vaginosis is increased in the lesbian population compared with those who abstain from sexual contact. Frequent use of alcohol (>7 drinks per week) is actually increased in the lesbian population, although serious consequences (such as cirrhosis and alcohol dependency) have not been shown to be increased.

490. The answer is b. Data from the Women's Health Initiative randomized trial of estrogen and progesterone in healthy postmenopausal women found a 26% increase in the risk of breast cancer over a mean follow-up of 5.2 years. This trial confirmed the benefit of HT in prevention of osteoporotic fractures, but did not show a benefit in prevention of coronary heart disease. Routine use of postmenopausal HT for prevention of coronary heart disease is no longer recommended. Vaginal estrogen cream is safe and effective treatment for postmenopausal vaginal atrophy but would not be indicated in this asymptomatic woman. Short-term use of HT (<5 years) for relief of menopausal symptoms in a healthy perimenopausal woman remains a reasonable and highly effective option. In this woman without perimenopausal symptoms, however, treatment would be premature.

491. The answer is e. Women who have suffered intimate partner violence (IPV) often present with somatic symptoms (especially abdominal and pelvic pain) and depression. The provider should maintain a high index of suspicion; many organizations recommend screening with open-ended, nonthreatening questions such as "Do you feel safe at home?" A positive response should elicit further questions to determine the pattern of violence (ie, a recent increase in frequency, situational triggers), the severity (is a weapon involved?), the type of violence (emotional, physical, or sexual abuse), and whether the patient has suicidal ideation or plan. The patient should be given contact information for a domestic violence center or hotline, and a follow-up visit should be scheduled.

A victim's greatest risk of harm or even death at the hands of the partner occurs when she attempts to leave the relationship. Assessment of risk of leaving and provision of a safe haven are best accomplished by the experts at the domestic violence center. It is the patient's responsibility to contact law enforcement. Your contacting the authorities without her consent would be a violation of her autonomy and privacy and could backfire. Antidepressants are minimally effective for situational depression and, even if effective, would only be covering up the true cause of her symptoms. Even if hypoactive sexual desire disorder had preceded the violent behavior, a spouse's disagreement about the frequency of intercourse in a relationship would never justify sexual coercion or violence.

492. The answer is b. While each of the options will provide contraception, only the combination pill fulfills all of her requests. Tubal ligation represents permanent sterilization and will not help her mood swings or dysmenorrhea. Progesterone-infused IUDs provide convenient and effective reversible contraception; they usually decrease menstrual flow and do not cause significant weight gain. IUDs, however, are not effective in treating acne or premenstrual dysphoric disorder (PMDD). Progesterone intramuscular injections are associated with weight gain. Condoms do not provide benefits beyond contraception and protection against sexually transmitted infections. The only FDA-approved contraceptive pill for PMDD is a drospirenone/ethinyl estradiol combination.

493. The answer is d. This woman has acute fatty liver of pregnancy, a medical and obstetrical emergency. She needs IV glucose and immediate induction of labor and delivery. Acute fatty liver of pregnancy occurs in the third trimester and is often associated with preeclampsia. Initial symptoms are usually nausea and RUQ pain, but evidence of liver failure occurs rapidly. In this case, somnolence and asterixis indicate failure of the detoxification of ammonia. The prolonged prothrombin time indicates synthetic failure of clotting factor production, and the hypoglycemia indicates failure of gluconeogenesis. Liver pathology shows microvesicular fat deposition, similar to another life-threatening condition, Reye syndrome (this is in distinction to the macrovesicular fat seen with alcohol consumption and nonalcoholic steatohepatitis). Immediate delivery is lifesaving for both mother and baby.

Elevated liver enzymes are not uncommon in pregnancy. An elevation of alkaline phosphatase is expected due to placental production of alkaline phosphatase. Acute alcoholic hepatitis causes modest transaminase elevation (rarely above 300) and typically elevates the AST higher than the ALT. It would be uncommon for a patient with alcoholic hepatitis to present with acute liver failure. Intrahepatic cholestasis of pregnancy causes alkaline phosphatase and occasionally bilirubin elevation but not liver synthetic failure. The main problem in benign cholestasis is pruritus, which is uncommon in acute fatty liver of pregnancy. In the HELLP syndrome, thrombocytopenia and hemolysis due to RBC fragmentation are the most prominent features. Schistocytes would be seen on peripheral blood smear. The HELLP syndrome is also managed with induction of labor. Acute viral hepatitis can occur during pregnancy as at any other time. However, hepatitis severe enough to cause jaundice usually causes transaminase elevation above 1000. It would be unusual for hepatitis A to present with hepatic encephalopathy.

494. The answer is e. The addition of annual MRI to mammogram in women with *BRCA* mutations improves the sensitivity, but also the false-positive rate, of screening programs. MRI should not replace a screening mammogram. This combination should begin at age 30.

Raloxifene is indicated for breast cancer prevention only in high-risk postmenopausal women. Tamoxifen can be used for prevention in high-risk premenopausal women, but has been associated with the development of uterine cancer in women ages 50 and older. Both of these medications are associated with a twofold increased risk of thromboembolic events. The most effective method to prevent breast cancer occurrence in *BRCA*-positive women is prophylactic bilateral subcutaneous mastectomy. Bioidentical hormones have no proven advantage over FDA-approved hormones. Premenopausal women with *BRCA* gene mutations who undergo prophylactic oophorectomy reduce their risk of breast cancer by 75%, and their risk of ovarian cancer by 85% to 95%. Carrying the *BRCA* gene increases the likelihood that this patient has passed the gene to her children. *BRCA* mutations in men convey increased risk for breast and prostate cancer, and possibly an increased risk of pancreatic cancer.

495. The answer is b. Evaluation of a breast nodule should determine whether the patient has a true mass or prominent physiologic glandular tissue. The next step is to determine whether the dominant mass represents a cyst, a benign solid mass, or cancer. Worrisome characteristics of this patient's mass include irregular borders, size larger than 1 cm, and location in the upper outer quadrant of the breast. Her age (>35) also places her at slightly higher risk. Even with a negative mammogram, a noncystic mass on ultrasound should be examined and biopsied by a breast surgeon or a comprehensive breast radiologist. Six months is too long to wait for reevaluation. In a younger woman (<35 years), repeat examination after the next menstrual cycle might be warranted (ie, <1-month reevaluation). To assume breast changes are benign without further investigation is not appropriate. MRI of the breast is a useful screening tool in complicated cases, such as a woman with dense breasts on mammography or *BRCA* positivity. Negative breast MRI, however, does not rule out breast cancer nor obviate biopsy of a clinically palpable nodule. To treat the patient for fibrocystic disease of the breast (answers c and e) without further evaluation would be risky.

496. The answer is c. This patient's history and physical examination are consistent with a diagnosis of pulmonary embolus (PE). The combination of respiratory distress, mild hypoxia, sinus tachycardia, clear chest x-ray, and typical ECG changes warrants emergent treatment and testing to confirm the diagnosis. Tamoxifen, a selective estrogen-receptor modulator, is associated with an increased risk of thromboembolic events. Myocardial infarction is less likely with this ECG pattern, which is classic for PE. Asthma rarely presents with pleuritic chest pain. An anxiety attack would not cause hypoxia or these ECG changes. There is no infiltrate on chest x-ray to suggest pneumonia.

497. The answer is c. The differential diagnosis for palpitations and sweating is broad, but major consideration should be given to hyperthyroidism, panic attacks, cardiac arrhythmias, malignancy, and vasomotor instability. This patient denies symptoms of malignancy such as weight loss. She does not have symptoms of clinical depression such as decreased concentration, apathy, weight changes, sleep changes, sadness, irritability, or suicidal thoughts. She reports no change in bowel habits or weight, which would indicate a thyroid disorder. The most likely diagnosis for this patient is vasomotor symptoms associated with the menopause transition. The best treatment option would be a combination estrogen and progesterone low-dose oral contraceptive. Her symptoms are more suggestive of hyperthyroidism than hypothyroidism; so levothyroxine would be of no benefit. Estrogen alone would increase the risk of endometrial hyperplasia and cancer. Fluoxetine and gabapentin have been used to treat hot flushes but are much less effective than hormone replacement.

498. The answer is c. This patient has dyspareunia or pain during intercourse. She has been postmenopausal for many years without hormone (estrogen) replacement. A commercial lubricant would be helpful for vaginal dryness but will not treat the underlying cause of her urogenital atrophy, which is hypoestrogenemia. She has no other symptoms of menopause (such as vasomotor symptoms or sleep disturbance) that impair quality of life. Therefore oral estrogen with its increased risk of thromboembolic event would not be justified. She denies depressive symptoms. The best treatment option for this patient is to treat the underlying disorder of urogenital atrophy with topical estrogen applied to the vagina. A commercial lubricant could be used as needed, but would be in addition to the vaginal hormone cream. Though sildenafil has been shown to be efficacious in the treatment of antidepressant-associated sexual dysfunction, it is not FDA-approved for use in women. Topical testosterone is used to treat lichen sclerosus, which manifests as a characteristic well-demarcated atrophic white plaque, often affecting the vulva and perianal skin in a figure-of-eight pattern. This patient's physical examination does not suggest lichen sclerosus.

499. The answer is e. This patient is suffering from the emotional and physical symptoms of depression. Initiation of an antidepressant is the most appropriate pharmacologic management, either with a selective serotonin reuptake inhibitor (SSRI), or with a serotonin-norepinephrine reuptake inhibitor (SNRI). An SNRI may provide more relief from her physical symptoms than SSRI therapy. Opiate therapy for the pain of depression is inappropriate and exposes the patient unnecessarily to potential addiction. Steroids are not clinically indicated. Methotrexate is reserved for specific rheumatologic diseases, not nonspecific musculoskeletal symptoms.

500. The answer is c. Prevention of cardiovascular diseases is another area where gender differences between cohorts of women and men are important. In general, low-dose aspirin has been found to be more useful in stroke prevention in woman and more useful in heart attack prevention in men. In each group, preventive treatment should be targeted to those most likely to benefit. The United States Preventive Services Task Force (USPSTF) currently strongly recommends the use of low-dose aspirin for women between ages 55 and 79 for ischemic stroke reduction when the potential benefit outweighs the potential harm. It also strongly recommends the use of low-dose aspirin in men between ages 45 and 79 to reduce the risk of myocardial infarction when the potential benefit outweighs the potential harm. The USPSTF recommends against the use of aspirin for stroke prevention in women younger than 55 years or aspirin for myocardial infarction prevention in men younger than 45 years. There is insufficient evidence that the use of aspirin for primary prevention of cardiovascular events in men and women over the age of 80 exceeds the potential harm of GI hemorrhage from aspirin use.

Suggested Readings

1. Kasper DL, Fauci AS, Hauser SL, Longo DL, Jameson JL, Loscalzo J. *Harrison's Principles of Internal Medicine*. 19th ed. New York: McGraw-Hill; 2015. Chapters 6e, 8, 67, 68, 69, 413, 425.

2. Legato M. *Principles of Gender Specific Medicine*. 2nd ed. Philadelphia: Elsevier; 2011.

3. Osteoporosis Screening and Treatment guidelines, available at: www.guidelines.gov/content.aspx?id=47543

4. Faubion SS, Litin SC, Bundrick JB. Clinical pearls in women's health. *Dis Mon*. 2014;60:363-372.

5. McNamara M, Walsh JM. Update in women's health: Evidence published in 2012. *Ann Intern Med*. 2013;159:203-209.

6. Mosca L, Benjamin EJ, Berra K, et al. Effectiveness-based guidelines for the prevention of cardiovascular disease in women—2011 update: A guideline from the American Heart Association. *Circulation*. 2011;123:1243-1262.

7. Hsia J, Langer RD, Manson JE, et al. Conjugated equine estrogens and coronary heart disease: The Women's Health Initiative. *Arch Intern Med*. 2006;166:357.

Index